Management of Speech and Swallowing Disorders
in Degenerative Diseases

MANAGEMENT OF SPEECH AND SWALLOWING DISORDERS IN DEGENERATIVE DISEASES

(Second Edition)

Kathryn M. Yorkston

Robert M. Miller

Edythe A. Strand

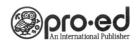

pro·ed
An International Publisher

8700 Shoal Creek Boulevard
Austin, Texas 78757-6897
800/897-3202   Fax 800/397-7633
www.proedinc.com

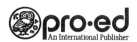

© 1995, 2004 by PRO-ED, Inc.
8700 Shoal Creek Boulevard
Austin, Texas 78757-6897
800/897-3202   Fax 800/397-7633
www.proedinc.com

Library of Congress Cataloging-in-Publication Data

Yorkston, Kathryn M., 1948–
    Management of speech and swallowing in degenerative diseases / by Kathryn M.
Yorkston, Robert M. Miller, Edythe A. Strand.—2nd ed.
      p. cm.
    Includes bibliographical references and index.
    ISBN 0-89079-966-0
    1. Speech disorders.   2. Deglutition disorders.   3. Nervous
system—Degeneration—Complications.   I.   Miller, Robert M. (Robert Michael), 1946–
II.   Strand, Edythe A.   III.   Title.

RC423.Y57   2003
616.8'3—dc21

2002036820

This book is designed in Janson Text and Officina Sans ITC.

Printed in the United States of America

1 2 3 4 5 6 7 8 9 10   07 06 05 04 03

Contents

Preface

Management of Speech and Swallowing Disorders in Degenerative Diseases was written for clinicians who serve individuals with amyotrophic lateral sclerosis, Parkinson disease, Huntington disease, or multiple sclerosis. In most service-delivery settings, clinicians see a relatively small number of adults with degenerative neurologic disease each year. Management of these populations is a challenge, however, because of their diversity and the urgency of their needs. Table P. 1 provides a comparison of important features of each of the neurologic diseases described in this text. A review of the table suggests that each disease is unique in its neuropathology, symptoms, and medical management. In some diseases, such as amyotrophic lateral sclerosis, the rate of progression may be rapid. In others, such as Parkinson disease, progression is slow. In multiple sclerosis, rate of progression is highly variable from individual to individual and from one point in time to another for one individual. Typical age of onset ranges from young adulthood in multiple sclerosis to the 60s and 70s in Parkinson disease. Degree of cognitive impairment also varies from one disease to another. Although dysarthria and dysphagia are common in all these diseases, the characteristics of the speech and swallowing disorders vary. These differences in disease features dictate differing approaches to management of speech and swallowing disorders.

We were spurred to prepare this text by our work in an outpatient setting. In 1988 we established the Neuromuscular Clinic for Speech and Swallowing Disorders through the Department of Otolaryngology, University of Washington. The goal of this clinic is to evaluate degenerative speech and swallowing disorders in their mild stages and to follow patients as progression occurs, providing intervention when it is appropriate. The clinic is staffed by a neurologic nurse specialist, a nutritionist, speech–language pathologists, and an otolaryngologist. We frequently consult with professionals in other specialties, including neurology, rehabilitation medicine, radiology, gastroenterology, and pulmonary medicine. In the 14 years since the clinic was established, we have seen hundreds of individuals with degenerative neurologic disease and their families. We have followed many people through a number of stages of their diseases and have been impressed by a number of aspects of this clinical work:

1. The inability to communicate (or the potential of it) and the inability to eat normally are the most distressing aspects of neurologic diseases such as amyotrophic lateral sclerosis.

2. The role of the medical team in patient education is critical. Although there is no cure for any of the diseases described in this text, patients and their families need information in order to make appropriate decisions about their care.

3. There is an urgent need for appropriate staging of intervention, that is, sequencing of management so that current problems are addressed and future problems anticipated. This staging should be

based on knowledge of disease progression and provision of that information to patients and their families in a timely fashion. A balance must be struck between providing intervention too early—before the individual is ready—and providing intervention too late—when there is an atmosphere of crisis or when secondary complications have arisen.

4. Finally, we have learned to appreciate that diagnosis of a degenerative disease is not synonymous with a loss of hope. It is the task of the medical team to be honest, realistic, and hopeful as our patients and their families cope with the day-to-day challenges they face.

Management of Speech and Swallowing Disorders in Degenerative Diseases was first published in 1995. This second edition provides an update on the many advances that have been made in our understanding and treatment of degenerative diseases. This text is organized into four chapters, each devoted to one medical diagnosis: amyotrophic lateral sclerosis, Parkinson disease, Huntington disease, and multiple

TABLE P.1

Comparison of Features of Four Degenerative Diseases

	Amyotrophic Lateral Sclerosis	Parkinson Disease	Huntington Disease	Multiple Sclerosis
Changes in Neural Tissues	Upper and lower motor neuron degeneration	Deficiency of dopamine affects basal ganglia function	Deficiency of neuro-transmitter GABA in the basal ganglia	Scattered multiple lesions in the CNS
Typical Symptoms	Include weakness and spasticity	Include tremor, rigidity, and bradykinesia	Include chorea, hypo-tonia, and rigidity	May include ataxia, tremor, weakness, and spasticity
Pharmacologic Intervention	No significant pharma-cologic intervention	Drugs are important in symptom management	Medical treatment is symptomatic	Medical treatment is generally symptomatic, but antiviral agents may affect the frequency and severity of attacks
Natural Course	May be rapidly progressive	Slowly progress	Death typically occurs 15–20 years postonset	Highly variable; most frequent pattern is remission–relapsing
Age of Onset	Mean age in 50s	Usually in 60s or 70s	In midlife, usually 35–40 years	Usually in young to middle-aged adults, 18–40 years
Onset of Dysarthria and Dysphagia	Dysarthria, dysphagia may be initial symptoms	Dysarthria, dysphagia usually appear later in the disease	Onset of dysarthria, dys-phagia vary considerably	Not universal, depends on site of lesions
Type of Dysarthria	Mixed spastic flaccid	Hypokinetic	Hyperkinetic	Mixed spastic ataxic
Cognition	Cognition usually intact	May exhibit cognitive problems	Cognitive changes may occur early and worsen as disease progresses	May exhibit cognitive problems
Awareness of Dysphagia	Good awareness of dysphagia	May be unaware of dysphagia	Dysphagia is not univer-sal; patient's subjective reports are not reliable	Varies depending on sites of lesion

sclerosis. Each chapter is organized around a series of questions, which were chosen to reflect information that speech–language pathologists need to know in order to manage people with degenerative disorders appropriately. Some of the questions relate to the nature of the underlying problem: "What changes in neural systems are associated with the disease?" "What symptoms are associated with the disease?" or "How is the diagnosis made?" Other questions relate to speech and swallowing symptoms: "How rapidly do speech changes occur in the disease?" "What information is obtained in a clinical examination of speech and swallowing disorders in adults with degenerative disease?" For each of the diseases, we have organized the intervention into stages such as mild dysarthria, moderate dysarthria, and severe dysarthria. Scales rating speech and swallowing function are provided for each disease, along with clinical examination forms and checklists. References and Web sites are provided so that interested readers can explore each topic in more depth. Finally, a glossary of operational definitions will serve to familiarize readers with some of the medical and technical terms used in the text.

Management of Speech and Swallowing Disorders in Degenerative Diseases also contains patient information. Our clinical experience indicates that such material is critical. Patients and their families often meet four or five professionals during the course of one clinic visit, and they are provided with a considerable amount of information in a very short time. Much of this information is not retained unless patients are provided with written information that they can review repeatedly and without time pressure. The handouts are organized into brief descriptions of normal speech and swallowing, information on each of the diseases, and how speech and swallowing are typically affected by each of the diseases. Suggestions for improving speech and swallowing are also provided, along with diagrams of the speech and swallowing mechanisms. These drawings may be helpful in patient education. These handouts are found in the Appendix: Handouts for Patients and Families at the back of the book. A resource list containing addresses of pertinent national organizations is also provided.

The planning and preparation of this text have spanned a number of years. During that time, many people have been generous in their assistance and support. We wish to acknowledge Judy Brown, a special nutritionist, who helps our patients to prepare a rich menu of calorie-dense foods; Al Hillel, MD, otolaryngologist, who had the idea for the Speech and Swallowing Clinic in the first place; Nancy Schuman, neurologic nurse specialist, who keeps the clinic organized and running; Katie Hauser, who ably assists our patients with their assistive technology needs; and Patricia Waugh, who advises and assists us in laryngeal examinations. We also are grateful for the assistance of Estelle Klasner, a doctoral candidate who offered her considerable clinical experience in Huntington disease to the revision of that chapter. Finally, we wish to acknowledge the contributions of our patients and their families. They have supported our efforts, educated us, and asked some of the difficult questions that led us to write this text.

1

AMYOTROPHIC LATERAL SCLEROSIS

Nature of the Problem

This section covers the symptomatology of amyotrophic lateral sclerosis (ALS) and what is known about its etiology and course. The information about medical treatment forms the foundation for discussions of speech and swallowing that follow. A brief summary of information is found in the handout "Amyotrophic Lateral Sclerosis" in the Appendix of Handouts for Patients and Families at the back of the book.

What Is Amyotrophic Lateral Sclerosis (ALS)?

Amyotrophic lateral sclerosis is a rapidly progressive degenerative disease of unknown etiology involving the motor neurons of both the brain and spinal cord. It is also known as Lou Gehrig's disease in the United States, motor neuron disease in Great Britain, and Charot's disease in France. The most common presenting symptom is weakness, with approximately one third of people with the disease reporting upper extremity weakness, one third leg weakness, and one quarter bulbar weakness manifested in dysarthria and dysphagia. As the disorder progresses, both upper and lower motor neurons typically become involved. The signs and symptoms are generally divided into two areas: bulbar features and spinal features. The bulbar symptoms are those associated with speech function and swallowing function, whereas the spinal symptoms are those associated with upper extremity function and lower extremity function. Respiratory symptoms, also significant in ALS, are usually considered to be a function of both bulbar and spinal involvement. Respiratory failure is the usual cause of death in ALS. Please see Chapter Appendix 1.1 for a "Clinical Examination for ALS" form.

The term ALS is often used synonymously with motor neuron disease, even though it is only one of a group of motor neuron diseases. See Table 1.1 for a comparison of neuropathologies, signs, and symptoms of the various motor neuron diseases. ALS is by far the most common of these and is often distinguished from other motor neuron diseases with restricted presentation, including progressive bulbar palsy (pure bulbar), progressive muscular atrophy (pure lower motor neuron), and primary lateral sclerosis (pure upper motor neuron), because of the varying disease course. Although the rate of progression of motor neuron disease with restricted presentation is slower than ALS, many of these diseases may evolve into ALS if the patient is followed for a long enough time (Belsh, 1999).

What Changes in Neural Systems Are Associated with ALS?

ALS is characterized by pathology in both the central and peripheral nervous systems. In the central nervous system, one finds degeneration and loss of large motor neurons in the

TABLE 1.1

Comparison of Motor Neuron Diseases

Disease	Neuropathology	Signs and Symptoms	Percentage of MND Population[a]	Gender Ratio (M/F)[a]	Survival Data[a]
Amyotrophic Lateral Sclerosis (ALS)	Degeneration of lateral, corticospinal tracts, anterior horn cells, anterior roots and peripheral nerves, nuclei of cranial nerves V, VII, IX, and XII, and corticobulbar tracts	Combination of weakness and spasticity in bulbar and spinal systems	81.6	1.7:1	Median survival 4.08 years
Progressive Bulbar Palsy (PBP)	Degeneration of bulbar nuclei	Flaccid weakness of bulbar musculature	9.3	.76:1	Equal to that of ALS
Primary Progressive Muscular (Spinal) Atrophy (PMA)	Degeneration of ventral horn cells of the spinal cord	Weakness and wasting of extremities	7.3	1.4:1	Longer than ALS or PBP
Primary Lateral Sclerosis (PLS)	Degeneration of motor cells-cortex and corticospinal tracts	Spastic weakness of trunk and extremities	1.8	1.33:1	Longer than ALS or PBP
Kennedy Syndrome (Spinobulbar Muscular Atrophy)[b]	Loss of primary motor neurons in the anterior horn of the spinal cord and brainstem motor nuclei and sensory neurons in the dorsal root ganglia	Weakness and wasting of extremities and bulbar musculature	Rare: prevalence 1 in 40,000	All male (X-linked inherited disease)	Lifespan unaffected

[a]Based on a series of 397 cases (Caroscio, Mulvihill, Sterling, & Abrams, 1987). [b]See Orrell and Figlewicz (2001) and Fischbeck (1997).

cerebral cortex, brain stem, and cervical and lumbar spinal cord. There is degeneration of the large pyramidal neurons (Betz cells) of layer 5 of the motor cortex. These pyramidal cells constitute the origin of the descending corticospinal motor pathway, which is responsible for voluntary movement.

In the periphery, nerves show reduced numbers of large myelinated fibers, acute axonal degeneration at all levels, and distal axonal atrophy. Cranial nerves V, VII, IX, X, and XI are frequently involved and are responsible for some of the features of dysarthria and dysphagia. The extraocular muscles, served by cranial nerves III, IV, and VI, are usually functionally spared, although there is subclinical evidence of pathology. There is also subclinical evidence for changes in sensory nerves (Theys, Peeters, & Robberecht, 1999). Loss of upper and lower extremity function is associated with the loss of large myelinated nerve axons from ventral roots and peripheral nerves in the anterior horn cells in the cervical, thoracic, and lumbar regions. The sacral segment of the cord is typically spared, thus explaining the absence of bowel and bladder symptoms.

What Symptoms Are Associated with ALS?

The symptoms characteristic of ALS are generally classified by site of involvement (i.e., upper motor neuron vs. lower motor neuron) and by whether spinal nerves (those innervating the arms and legs) or bulbar nerves (those innervating the muscles of speech and swallowing) are involved. See Table 1.2 for a summary of symptoms. Initially, either upper motor neuron or lower motor neuron involvement may predominate. As ALS progresses, both usually become involved. Hence, initial symptoms may involve weakness in one or more extremities or weakness in the speech musculature. As the disease progresses, both spinal and bulbar symptoms usually appear.

Upper motor neuron involvement affects neurons from the cortex to the anterior horn cells of the spinal cord. This involvement results in weakness, increased tone, spasticity without muscle wasting, hyperreflexia, plantar extensor response, or clonus. Muscle cramping may also occur. Lower motor neuron involvement, on the other hand, affects neurons from the anterior horn cells to the muscles and is responsible for a different pattern of symptoms. These include weakness, flaccid muscle tone with muscle wasting or atrophy, hyporeflexia, plantar flexor response, fasciculations, and fibrillations.

What Is Known About the Cause of ALS?

Although the cause of ALS is currently unknown, researchers from a variety of disciplines are actively pursuing many lines of evidence. The field of epidemiology contributes population-based studies of risk factors for the disease. Several epidemiology observations in individuals with ALS are commonly accepted (Armon, 2001). One is that ALS shares three features with Alzheimer's disease and Parkinson disease: (a) specific incidence increases with age, (b) all take either a sporadic or a familial form, and (c) all appear in the Western Pacific foci with increased incidence. Taken together, these features suggest that these three major neurodegenerative diseases have common risk factors. The observation that sporadic ALS occurs more frequently in men than women is also robust. Because of mixed findings, it appears that environmental factors such as metal toxicity are not causally related to the development of ALS (Armon, 2001).

TABLE 1.2   Summary of Symptoms Associated with ALS

	Site of Neural Involvement	
	Upper Motor Neuron	**Lower Motor Neuron**
Bulbar Nerves	Weakness, slow movement, increased tone of lips, tongue, soft palate, and jaw; voice may be strained/strangled	Weakness, muscle atrophy, and fasciculation of lips, tongue, and soft palate; voice may be breathy
Spinal Nerves	Weakness, slow movement, increased tone of arms and legs	Weakness, muscle atrophy, and fasciculations in arms and legs

The pathophysiologic mechanisms underlying ALS have been described as complex, multifactorial, and interrelated (Eisen, Schulzer, MacNeil, Pant, & Mak, 1993). Several theories exist including glutamate excitotoxicity, free radical oxidative stress, neurofilament accumulation, and autoimmunity (Jackson & Bryan, 1998). The excitotoxicity theory suggests that glutamate, the primary excitatory neurotransmitter in the central nervous system, accumulates to toxic concentrations at synapses and causes neurons to die (Bensimon, Lacomblez, & Meininger, 1994). Further, defective glutamate transport activity has been found in the motor areas of the spinal cords of individuals with ALS (Rothstein, Martin, & Kuncl, 1992).

From 5% to 10% of ALS cases are inherited as an autosomal dominant trait. The underlying cause of hereditary ALS has also come under close attention. In 1993 Rosen et al. identified the gene responsible for this form of the disorder. This gene encodes an enzyme that in a healthy cell will deactivate free radicals (molecular byproducts of normal metabolism that can destroy cells if left untamed). Thus, freeradical toxicity may be implicated in at least one type of ALS.

What Is the Typical Course of ALS?

ALS is generally considered a relentlessly and rapidly progressive disease. Although many individuals with ALS survive for more than 5 years, most do not. The rate of deterioration is strikingly linear (Caroscio, Mulvihill, Sterling, & Abrams, 1987; Pradas et al., 1993). However, despite the fact that weakness increases at the same rate over time for an individual, there is considerable variability in rate of progression from one individual to another. Appel, Stewart, Smith, and Appel (1987) followed 74 individuals with ALS for at least 1 year and found that while 34% exhibited rapid change (predicting progression to a terminal stage in less than 2 years), 19% showed slow change (predicting progression to a terminal stage over at least 5 years). In a study of 28 individuals, Caroscio and colleagues (1987) found that 25% achieved a plateau lasting at least 9 months.

Associated symptoms within an individual also appear to progress at similar rates. High correlations were found between deterioration rates in arm strength and leg strength (Pradas et al., 1993) and between speech function and swallowing function (Yorkston, Strand, Miller, Hillel, & Smith, 1993). As noted earlier, symptoms typically start in one location—for example, the arms or legs—then spread to other locations. The spread of symptoms of ALS appears to be a function of the distance between the original site of pathology and sites of subsequent impairment. For example, the spread to various areas within the spinal cord is faster than the spread from the spinal cord to the bulbar region. Furthermore, the time for spread from the arms to the brain stem is shorter than from the legs to the brain stem. Although the mechanism that underlies this spread is uncertain, evidence suggests that it relates to distance between the neural segments (Brooks, 1991; Eisen & Krieger, 1993).

Progression of ALS is commonly studied using mean survival durations. When data from 138 patients were examined, men tended to survive longer than women, and those with early onsets (before 40 years of age) survived longer than those with onsets later in life (Eisen & Krieger, 1993). Evidence also suggests that the trend toward later age at onset and shorter survival holds for familial as well as sporadic ALS (Strong, Hudson, & Alvord, 1991).

Survival durations can be predicted on the basis of a number of related factors, including age at onset, type of initial symptoms, pulmonary status, and psychological factors. As noted earlier, studies suggest that the older the person at onset of symptoms, the shorter the survival time. Furthermore, the 5-year survival rate of people with initial spinal symptoms is 3 times better than that of people with initial bulbar symptoms (Rosen, 1978). Because decline in pulmonary function is closely correlated with death (Ringel et al., 1993), respiratory status is also an important indicator of survival duration. Psychological factors have also been implicated. McDonald, Wiedenfeld, Hillel, Carpenter, and Walter (1994) followed 144 individuals with ALS for 3½ years. Subjects were grouped according to a number of measures of psychologic well-being. During the study period, death rates for those with "high psychological well-being" were 32% compared with 82% for those with psychological distress. Even when confounding factors such as length of illness, disease severity, and age were controlled, individuals with psychological distress had a greater risk of mortality during the study period than those with psychological well-being. Finally, survival rates may be changing as a result of new drugs and better management of nutritional and respiratory symptoms.

The functional status of individuals with ALS has been described with rating systems developed for clinical drug trials. One such system, called the ALS Functional Rating Scale–R, rates extremity, bulbar, and respiratory function (Cedarbaum et al., 1999). Another called the ALS Health State Scale (Riviere, Meininger, Zeisser, & Munsat, 1998) categorized individuals with ALS in the following health states:

- *State 1 (Mild):* Recently diagnosed with mild deficits in only one of three regions (i.e., speech, arms, and legs). These individuals are functionally independent in speech, upper extremity activities of daily living, and ambulation.
- *State 2 (Moderate):* Individuals at this state exhibit mild deficits in all three regions or moderate to severe deficits in one region, while the other two regions are normal to mildly affected.
- *State 3 (Severe):* These individuals need assistance in two or three regions. Speech is dysarthric or individuals need assistance to walk or need assistance with upper extremity activities of daily living.
- *State 4 (Terminal):* These individuals have no functional use of at least two regions and at least moderate limitations in the use of the third region.

The major outcome measure for the drug studies was the number of days after initial observation that passed before the individual entered the next more severe health state.

How Is the Diagnosis of ALS Made?

There are no laboratory tests or neuroimaging studies that directly confirm the diagnosis of ALS. Diagnosis is typically based on a clinical history of progressive motor involvement in the absence of sensory findings, together with results of electromyography, measures of nerve conduction velocity that show widespread denervation patterns with fibrillations and fasciculations, neuroimaging techniques including magnetic resonance imaging (MRI) and computerized tomography (CT) of the spine and brain to exclude other neurologic disease, genetic testing, and occasionally muscle biopsy that shows a characteristic pattern of denervation atrophy. Because of the seriousness of an ALS diagnosis, a variety of treatable conditions of the central or peripheral nervous system—such as tumors or pressure lesions of the spinal cord— must be ruled out before it is made.

In 1994 the World Federation of Neurology Research Group on Neuromuscular Disease published what is called the El Escorial criteria for diagnosis of ALS. The diagnosis of ALS requires the presence of (a) signs of lower motor neuron degeneration, (b) signs of upper motor neuron degeneration, and (c) progression of signs within a region or to other regions over at least 6 to 12 months after disease onset. The diagnosis requires the absence of electrophyisological or neuroimaging evidence of other disease processes. The El Escorial criteria also list findings that are inconsistent with a diagnosis of ALS, if they are not explained by aging or another disease process, including

1. sensory dysfunction,
2. sphincter abnormalities,
3. autonomic nervous system dysfunction,
4. anterior visual pathway abnormalities,
5. movement abnormalities associated with Parkinson disease, and
6. cognitive abnormalities associated with Alzheimer's disease.

These criteria are now being used by researchers to accurately include individuals with ALS in clinical trials.

The diagnosis of ALS usually involves three persons—the family practitioner, a community neurologist, and an ALS specialist (Eisen, 1999). The need for early diagnosis is increasing with the advent of drugs that maintain individuals for longer periods in the early phases of the disease. See Table 1.3 for a listing of the benefits of early diagnosis. Despite the trend toward early diagnosis, the period between the initial onset of symptoms and diagnosis may be lengthy, ranging from 10 to 19 months (Belsh & Schiffman, 1996; Chio, 1999; Househam & Swash, 2000). The diagnostic delay tends to be shorter for individuals with bulbar symptoms or fasciculations and longer for those who are initially misdiagnosed or those with coexistent diseases.

What Drugs Are Used To Manage ALS?

Until recently the only drug management in ALS has focused on controlling the symptoms. For example, physicians prescribed medications to help reduce fatigue, ease muscle cramps, or control spasticity, pain, depression, and sleep disturbances. Many drugs have been tried and have not been effective. This lack of success is in part due to our incomplete understanding of the causes of ALS. Over the last century,

TABLE 1.3	Benefits of Early Diagnosis of ALS	
• The right of the patient to know the truth	• Appropriate and individualized treatment
• Psychological benefits for the patient	• Admission to clinical trials before ALS is advanced
• The chance for earlier decision making for patient and family	• A chance to retard the disease using new drugs
• Prevention of mismanagement	

Note. Adapted from "The Amyotrophic Lateral Sclerosis Patient Perspective on Misdiagnosis and Its Repercussions," by J. M. Belsh and P. L. Schiffman, 1996, *Journal of Neurologic Science, 139*(Suppl.), pp. 110–116.

over 60 medications or treatments have been reported anecdotally or tested in clinical trials (Cwik, 2000). Until recently none has been shown to alter the progression of the disease.

Many individuals with ALS also take vitamin E, an antioxidant and probably the most commonly used treatment for ALS over the last century. The rationale for its use is based on two facts: (a) the gene associated for familial ALS is responsible for an endogenous antioxidant, and (b) vitamin E appears to delay the onset and slow the progression of symptoms in a mouse model of ALS (Gurney et al., 1996). Unfortunately, clinical trials with individuals with ALS have not shown benefits.

Creatine, a dietary supplement, is used by muscle-building athletes to increase lean body mass and strength. Some nonblinded studies on humans and animals have been encouraging (Klivenyi et al., 1999; Tarnopolsky & Martin, 1999). Controlled clinical trials are now under way.

A number of drugs are in development. They typically fall into three categories: antiglutamate agents, neurotrophic factors, and antiapoptotic agents (including antioxidants). To date only one drug has been shown to alter the course of ALS. In 1995 the Food and Drug Administration approved Riluzole for the management of ALS. Riluzole is thought to decrease the release of glutamate into the extracellular space, thus decreasing the damage to the motor neurons by ridding the synaptic cleft of extra glutamate that is toxic to the cell. Riluzole has been studied in double-blind, placebo-controlled clinical trials (Bensimon et al., 1994). Although Riluzole does not cure ALS or reverse the damage already done to motor neurons, the results are encouraging. In the bulbar-onset group, 35% of patients on placebo were alive after 1 year, whereas 73% of patients on Riluzole were alive at the same period. Riluzole may increase liver enzymes that usually peak within 3 months and then stabilize (Neatherlin, 1998). Liver enzyme monitoring is suggested every 3 months. Other common adverse effects include asthenia (increased weakness), nausea, dizziness, diarrhea, vomiting, vertigo, circumoral paresthesia, anorexia, and somnolence.

As is obvious from this brief review, the study of drugs to alter the course of ALS is an extremely active area of research. A number of clinical trials are under way. Current information about drug development and clinical trials can be found on the Web site managed by the ALS Association (http://www.alsa.org/research/drugdev.cfm).

What Is the Role of Rehabilitation Medicine in the Management of ALS?

Because there is no cure for ALS, rehabilitation medicine focuses on management of the many symptoms associated with the condition.

GOALS OF REHABILITATION

The multiple consequences of ALS necessitate that rehabilitation needs are met using a coordinated multidisciplinary team approach employing the skills of physiatrists; neurologists; rehabilitation nurses; speech–language pathologists; pulmonologists; respiratory, physical, and occupational therapists; psychologists; and social service providers (Francis, Bach, & DeLisa, 1999). Goals are frequently established using a problem-based approach such as the one presented in Table 1.4. A review of this table reveals that participation in activities of daily living (ADLs) for as long as

TABLE 1.4

Management of Selected Problems in Patients with ALS

Problem	Expected Outcome	Management
Increasing weakness	Maintain patient mobility and participation in activities of daily living for as long as possible	Let patients plan activities important for them. Offer assistance in other areas to prevent fatigue.
		Give the patient time to participate in care to reduce frustration.
		Provide rest breaks between activities.
		Provide braces and other devices to permit patients to use stronger muscle groups and compensate for loss of other weaker groups in the extremities, for example, hand splints and ankle–foot orthoses.
		Move bedroom to the first floor.
		Add hand rails and ramp to the home to maintain accessibility.
		Instruct in use of safety precautions (avoid slippery floors and loose rugs).
		Encourage use of a wheelchair when weakness becomes too great.
Muscle cramping and spasms	Patient comfort and decreased hazards of immobility	Change the position of the patient every 2 hours or more often.
		Instruct about use of satin sheets and polyester pajamas at home to make turning easier and not disrupt the patient's sleep.
		Massage muscles.
		Use supportive pillows, collar, and pads.
		Teach passive range of motion for extremities to prevent adhesions and other joint pain.
Grief and depression	Patient and family gradually work through grief process and perhaps find a purpose in life	Encourage the patient and family to talk about their losses.
		Give the family an opportunity to express feelings, concerns, and anger in separate sessions.
		Encourage the family to take time for rest and activities away from the patient.
		Put patient and family in touch with ALS support groups.
		Encourage patients to continue in job or other activities for as long as possible.

Note. Adapted from "Amyotrophic Lateral Sclerosis: A Challenge for Constant Adaptation," by N. Stone, 1987, *Journal of Neuroscience Nursing*, *19*(3), pp. 166–173. Copyright 1987 by the American Association of Neuroscience Nursing. Adapted with permission.

possible is encouraged by modifying environment or activities and by providing assistive devices to prevent fatigue. Intervention for individuals with ALS generally occurs in episodes that coincide with critical periods or crisis points (Baumann, 1991), that is, when there is a sudden decline in ability to function. Critical periods commonly occur when individuals with ALS can no longer work, walk safely, communicate using natural speech, eat safely, and, finally, breathe without assistance. The management team needs to anticipate these periods and prepare the patient and family for the decisions that must be made during each critical period. Management of critical periods for communication and swallowing will be reviewed in detail later. Table 1.5 illustrates the staging of critical periods for ambulation and some activities of daily living.

USE OF EXERCISE

The role of exercise in the management of ALS is a topic of considerable interest and controversy. Because of the variable rates of progression of ALS, the efficacy of exercise is difficult to document. The possibility that weakness and muscle fiber degeneration may be accelerated by overwork or heavy exercise has been suggested in both animal and human studies (Francis et al., 1999). Sanjak, Reddan, and Brooks (1987) provide an excellent review of this topic. They conclude that the question of whether or not to exercise does not have a simple answer. First, exercise is not a single entity. Rather, there are a number of different types of exercise that place different demands on the muscles. Second, muscles differ in terms of fiber types and motor unit properties. Different muscle types respond to each type of exercise differently.

TABLE 1.5 Clinical Stages of Ambulatory Function in ALS

Stage	Description	
Free ambulatory	The patient is able to perform normal life activities, although mild discomfort or limitation of performance and endurance may be apparent.	Simplification and energy conservation method training.
		Mild, aerobic exercises for unaffected muscles, to compensate for weakness in other muscles and to improve or maintain joint mobility.
		Swimming and bicycling to benefit general conditioning.
		Evaluation of baseline muscle strength, joint range-of-motion, respiratory capacity, posture and gait analysis and ADLs.
		Simple adaptive devices such as splints, soft cervical collars, and properly fitting shoes.
Ambulatory with mild-to-moderate limitation of function	The patient demonstrates muscle imbalance, increased muscle fatigue caused by excessive energy expenditure, decreased mobility and function.	Bracing to support weak muscles, decrease energy expenditure, and ensure the patient's safety.
		An elastic lumbosacral binder to alleviate back pain and improve breathing.
		Assistive walking devices such as canes, tripod, quad canes, and rolling walkers.
		Several brief exercise periods a day but no excessive exercise because of possible falls, injuries, and overfatigue.
		Stretching of tightened muscles to prevent or decrease contractures.
		In cases where spasticity is present, baclofen (Lioresal) may be helpful.
Wheelchair-bound and ADL-dependent	This stage is characterized by progressive weakness of axial muscles, and deterioration of mobility and endurance. The patient requires a wheelchair to go long distances, and later is wheelchair-bound.	Wheelchairs capable of reclining, with a head support, leg elevators, padded armrests, a safety belt, and a lapboard.
		Range-of-motion exercises.
		Encourage the family to take time for rest and activities away from the patient.

Note. ADLs = activities of daily living. Adapted from "Amyotrophic Lateral Sclerosis: A Comprehensive Rehabilitation Approach," by D. W. Janiszewski, J. T. Caroscio, and L. H. Wisham, 1983, *Archives of Physical Medicine and Rehabilitation, 64*, pp. 304–307.

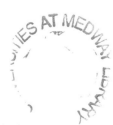

Although clinical opinions vary, there appears to be some agreement that exercise to the point of fatigue is not beneficial. Decreased strength may result from overwork in individuals with polio and in others with partially denervated muscles (Bennett & Knowlton, 1958). In a recent review, Francis and colleagues (1999) suggested that exercise programs requiring submaximal levels of intensity are probably appropriate and helpful for those with a slowly progressive course in those muscles without marked weakness. DeLisa, Mikulic, Miller, and Melnick (1979) suggest that exercise may be helpful in averting fatigue, preventing disuse weakness, and strengthening unaffected muscles so that they can compensate for impaired ones. Recent reports suggest that regular moderate exercise has a short-lived positive effect on disability in ALS (Drory, Goltsman, Goldman Reznik, Mosek, & Korczyn, 2001). Later in the course of the disease, energy conservation and work-simplification methods should be taught. Range of motion exercises and stretching exercises are also helpful in this stage of the disease. A more complete discussion of the types of exercise appropriate at each stage of ALS can be found elsewhere (Dal Bello-Haas, Kloos, & Mitsumoto, 1998). The role of exercise in speech intervention will be discussed later.

PATIENT AUTONOMY

In discussions of physician–patient relationships, there is a growing appreciation of the principle of patient autonomy (Pasetti & Zanini, 2000). This principle suggests that a well-informed patient should actively participate in the decision-making process. In any discussion of medical management, it is appropriate to ask the question, "What do patients want from the medical team?" Beisecker, Cobb, and Ziegler (1988) interviewed 41 individuals with ALS in an attempt to understand their perspective. Patients expected physicians to evaluate the progress of the disease, help with immediate problems, and continue research to find a cure. In addition, patients expected the medical team to provide emotional support, information, and access to assistive devices. When asked how they should be told of the diagnosis of ALS, patients indicated that there is no good way to tell a person "you have ALS." Patients appreciated physicians who were straightforward and honest but not premature, sensitive to patients' readiness for information, and able to convey some degree of hope.

PALLIATIVE CARE

Palliative care is active total care of patients whose disease is not responsive to curative treatment (World Health Organization, 1990). It includes control of pain and management of psychological, social, and spiritual problems. The goal of palliative care is achievement of the best possible quality of life for patients and their families. Studies of individuals with ALS suggest that quality of life is independent of physical function and may depend instead on spiritual and psychological factors (Robbins, Simmons, Bremer, Walsh, & Fischer, 2001). Palliative care starts at the time of diagnosis and may coexist with other care such as course-altering drugs (Oliver, 1996; Oliver, Borasio, & Walsh, 2001). In the terminal stages of ALS, palliative care may be provided through hospice organizations. Because most hospice patients are dying of malignancies, some special issues related to ALS have been outlined for hospice caregivers (Carter, Bednar-Butler, Abresch, & Ugalde, 1999; Francis et al., 1999). Hospice services are available for individuals with a terminal illness (a life expectancy of 6 months or less) and who are not undergoing treatment. Generally, tracheostomy and mechanical ventilation disqualifies the patient, but noninvasive ventilation may be acceptable if it is viewed as comfort care rather than active treatment. Table 1.6 outlines the criteria for hospice admission for individuals with ALS. Speech and swallowing problems occur very frequently in individuals in the terminal stages of

ALS. Results of a retrospective review of patients served by a hospice organization suggested that 90% experienced symptoms of dysphagia and 71% experienced dysarthria.

Do Individuals with ALS Experience Cognitive Changes?

12

The topic of cognition and ALS has received considerable research attention in the past decade. Classically, ALS has been viewed as a disease involving only the upper and lower motor neurons, with clinical features restricted to motor function. This traditional view suggests that ALS does not include involvement of extramotor systems or loss of cognitive function or memory problems. The traditional view has recently come under critical review (Bak & Hodges, 1999, 2001; Strong, Grace, Orange, & Leeper, 1996). Speech–language pathologists need to be aware that cognitive changes in ALS, although not universal, are possible. Because these changes may involve executive function, verbal skills, memory, and new learning, they have ramifications for learning to use augmentative communication systems. At least four categories of cognitive status are possible. Each is described in the following section in order of its frequency of occurrence.

NORMAL COGNITION

The first and probably the largest category is normal cognitive function. This has been referred to as classic ALS. Although precise estimates of the proportion of indi-

TABLE 1.6	Criteria for Hospice Admission in ALS

Increased Respiratory Distress

- Vital capacity less than 30% of predicted
- Significant dyspnea at rest
- Supplemental oxygen required at rest
- Patient has refused intubation, tracheostomy, and mechanism ventilation

Severely Impaired Nutrition

- Tube feeding not elected or discontinued
- Oral intake insufficient due to dysphagia
- Continued weight loss in spite of tube feeding
- Dehydration or hypovolemia

Life-Threatening Complications

- Recurrent aspiration pneumonia
- Decubitus ulcers, multiple, stage 3–4, particularly if infected
- Upper urinary tract infection
- Sepsis
- Fever recurrent after antibiotics

Note. Adapted from "Expanding the Role of Hospice Care in Amyotrophic Lateral Sclerosis," by G. T. Carter, L. M. Bednar-Butler, R. T. Abresch, and V. O. Ugalde, 1999, *American Journal of Hospice & Palliative Care, 16*(6), pp. 707–710. Copyright 1999 by Prime National Publishing Corporation. Adapted with permission.

viduals with ALS in this category are not available, an estimate of over 60% seems reasonable in light of the occurrence of the other categories discussed.

ALS WITH MILD COGNITIVE IMPAIRMENTS ASSOCIATED WITH FRONTAL LOBE SYNDROME

The second category includes individuals with ALS without overt dementia who exhibit often subtle changes in cognitive function. The literature contains a growing number of studies documenting these changes using various neuropsychological tests (see Table 1.7). A review of this table suggests a trend toward slight but definite differences between individuals with ALS and matched controls in a variety of cognitive functions, particularly impairments in executive function, reasoning, response generation, initiation, abstraction, planning and organization, new learning, verbal fluency, and picture recall. These measures of cognitive functioning, along with some evidence from brain imaging, suggest a mild frontal dysfunction. These deficits tend to be more pronounced in individuals with dysarthria (bulbar involvement) and pseudobulbar palsy. Estimates of the prevalence of these cognitive changes range from 25% to 35%. Evidence for the association cognitive changes and changes in neuroimaging are also available (Abrahams et al., 1996; Kiernan & Hudson, 1994; Lloyd, Richardson, Brooks, Al-Chalabi, & Leigh, 2000). These studies suggest the presence on extramotor areas of involvement in a subgroup of individuals with ALS.

FRONTOTEMPORAL DEMENTIA/ALS (FTD/ALS)

Montgomery and Erickson (1987) suggested that overt dementia occurs in 1% to 2% of sporadic cases of ALS. The prevalence of dementia in familial ALS may be somewhat higher. Hudson (1981) estimated that approximately 15% of individuals with familial ALS have presented with dementia. Although dementia in ALS is rare, its occurrence may be underestimated because referrals to specialty centers typically exclude patients with very advanced or rapidly progressing disease (Montgomery & Erickson, 1987). Other factors leading to underestimation may include lack of testing with sufficiently sensitive neuropsychological instruments and misinterpretation of compromised cognition as depression or withdrawal due to motor dysfunction.

A syndrome of frontotemporal dementia and motor neuron disease has been described (Neary, Snowden, & Mann, 2000). FTD/ALS is characterized by profound personality change and breakdown in social conduct. Although not a primary aphasic disturbance, speech output is reduced. Most patients fail on tests of executive function and exhibit poor abstraction, planning, set shifting, and organizational skills.

Neurological signs are usually absent in the early stages. FTD/MND is relatively rare. Frequently, the onset of dementia precedes other physical symptoms (Rakowicz & Hodges, 1998). It is unclear whether this FTD/ALS constitutes the extreme end of range of disease or alternatively whether it represents a separate disease entity.

MOTOR NEURON DISEASE (MND)/APHASIA

There is growing evidence that a full-blown aphasia can be associated with MND (Bak & Hodges, 2001; Mitsuyama, Kogoh, & Ata, 1985; Tscuchiya et al., 2000). In a few rare cases, primary progressive aphasia evolves to ALS. Caselli et al. (1993) reported 7 patients in whom articulatory and language impairment preceded rapidly progressive motor neuron disease. They suggest that rapidly progressive aphasic

TABLE 1.7

Summary of Group Studies of Neuropsychological Function in ALS

Reference	Type of ALS	Measures	Findings
Gallassi, Montagna, Giardulli, Lorusso, & Mussuto, 1985	22 patients with sporadic ALS without articulatory impairment and controls	Neuropsychologic testing	Impaired reasoning, response generation, initiation, abstraction, planning and organization, and new learning
Poloni, Capitani, Mazzini, & Ceproni, 1986	21 male patients with ALS and 21 with other nondementing diseases	Short neuropsychologic battery; CT scans	ALS group did not differ from controls, but 2 ALS patients had definitely low intelligence test scores; no relation between cognitive impairment and CT findings; cognitive impairment in ALS is discrete and rare
Gallassi et al., 1989	35 patients with sporadic motor neuron disease without dementia	Neuropsychologic testing, EEG and brain CT	Slight but definite and stereotyped cognitive impairment, temporal slow EEG activity, no differences in CT
Iwasaki, Kinoshita, Ikeda, Takamiya, & Shiojima, 1990	18 patients with ALS and controls	Selected neuropsychologic tests	Significant negative correlation between upper motor symptoms and mini-mental state examination and memory tests
Ludolph et al., 1992	18 patients with ALS with both upper and lower motor neuron signs and controls	Neuropsychologic testing and positron emission tomography	Glucose metabolism significantly reduced in frontal and entire context compared with controls; mild frontal dysfunction in neuropsychologic testing
Kew et al., 1993	16 nondemented patients with ALS and controls	Neuropsychologic testing and positron emission tomography	Impaired verbal fluency and picture recall in ALS group; abnormalities in regions along the limbo-thalamo-cortical pathways in ALS
Caselli, Smith, & Osbourne, 1995	9 patients with primary lateral sclerosis	Neuropsychologic test	Deficits associated with frontal lobe dysfunction
Massman et al., 1996	146 patients with typical, sporadic ALS	Neuropsychologic testing battery	35.6% performed at or below the 5th percentile on at least two of the eight measures; impairments most prevalent in dysarthric patients
Chari, Shaw, & Sahgal, 1996	50 individuals with motor neuron disease (MND) and controls	Cambridge Neuropsychological Test Automated Battery	MND group showed impairment of a visual search task, but no deficits in memory or learning
Frank, Haas, Heinze, Stark, & Munte, 1997	74 patients with sporadic ALS and controls	Neuropsychologic testing, magnetic resonance imaging	Deficits in visual attention, inhibition of response alternatives, visual memory, and word generation with associated change in MRI parameters
Abrahams et al., 1997	24 patients with ALS and pseudobulbar palsy; 28 patients with ALS and no pseudobulbar palsy	An extensive neuropsychologic battery	Cognitive deficits predominately in executive process, more prominent with pseudobulbar palsy
Cobble, 1998	9 patients with MND	Standardized language assessment	A subgroup showed deficits in naming, auditory comprehension of complex sentences, semantic tests, and spelling
Munte et al., 1998	8 patients with ALS and controls	Memory test and event-related potentials (ERP)	The ERP pattern suggested abnormal memory pattern in ALS
Strong et al., 1999	13 patients with ALS and 5 spousal controls	Word generation, recognition memory, motor-free visual perception	Bulbar onset patients showed greater impairment
Abrahams et al., 2000	22 patients with ALS	Verbal fluency and executive function	Significant impairment on some tests

dementia and motor neuron disease are a distinctive clinical entitity whose nosology is poorly understood. See Bak and Hodges (2001) for a complete review of this topic.

What Is Emotional Lability and Why Is It Associated with ALS?

Emotional lability is literally unsteadiness of emotions. Individuals may experience bouts of laughter and crying that are not in proportion to the stimuli. Often these episodes are not associated with the underlying mood or emotion. For example, individuals with emotional lability may cry uncontrollably even when they do not feel particularly sad. Emotional lability is a distressing and unfortunately common feature of ALS. Estimates suggest that as many as half of individuals with ALS experience emotional lability (Miller et al., 1999; Newson-Davis, Abrahams, Goldstein, & Leigh, 1999). About one fourth of individuals with ALS experience episodes of both laughing and crying. Another quarter of the ALS population experiences either bouts of laughter or crying (Gallagher, 1989). Emotional lability is not typically considered a psychologic, mood, or cognitive impairment. Rather, it is consistent with bilateral corticobulbar lesions that result in loss of pyramidal tract inhibitory control over the behavioral–expressive responses of an emotion (Montgomery & Erickson, 1987). Because it occurs commonly in individuals with pseudobulbar symptoms, it is also called pseduobulbar affect. Emotional lability also correlates with bulbar symptoms (Newson-Davis et al., 1999).

A variety of brief screening instructions are available for clinical use. For example, the Center for Neurologic Study–Lability Scale (CNS–LS) (Moore, Gresham, Bromberg, Kasarkis, & Smith, 1997) contains seven items that comprise both a labile laughter and labile tearfulness subscale. Individuals with ALS are asked to respond on a 5-point scale ranging from *never applies* to *applies most of the time* to items such as "I find that even when I try to control my laughter I am often unable do so" or "I find myself crying very easily." Management of the lability involves explaining to the patient and family that this is not a psychologic or mood problem, but rather a part of the motor involvement. Most patients prefer to be distracted or to have the subject changed rather than to dwell on the uninhibited expression of emotion. Drugs are also available to reduce emotional lability (Iannaccone & Ferini-Strambi, 1996; Miller et al., 1999; Schiffer, Cash, & Herndon, 1983; Schiffer, Herndon, & Rudick, 1985).

What Respiratory Problems Are Associated with ALS and Why Are These Problems So Critical?

The muscles of the respiratory system are weakened and later paralyzed as ALS progresses. The following is a description of the problems, how they progress, and how they are managed.

CHARACTERISTICS OF RESPIRATORY PROBLEMS

Failure of the respiratory system is the most common cause of death in ALS. Weakening of the respiratory muscles causes a number of complications, including respiratory muscle fatigue, respiratory failure, ineffective cough, and failure to protect the lungs from aspiration (Braun, 1987; Polkey, Lyall, Green, Nigel Leigh, & Moxham, 1998; Tidwell, 1993). Changing respiratory status in individuals with ALS can be measured in a number of ways (Annoni, Chevrolet, & Kesselring, 1993). Both maximum inspiratory pressure and maximum expiratory pressure decrease in ALS. As a consequence, the reduced effectiveness of their cough may place these individuals at particular risk for bronchial obstruction caused by secretions during respiratory infections. Respiratory risk is especially high for individuals with bulbar symptoms who are experiencing the cumulative effects of respiratory and swallowing problems. Lung volume measures such as vital capacity also decrease in ALS, whereas residual volumes increase. Because a reduction in vital capacity to as low as 50% of normal predicted values is frequently missed by clinical examination, spirometry is a useful means for detecting early respiratory problems (Fallat, Jewitt, Bass, Kamm, & Norris, 1979).

PROGRESSION OF RESPIRATORY PROBLEMS

Breathing problems are typically not one of the presenting symptoms in ALS. The typical rate of decline in respiratory muscle strength, as measured by vital capacity, was 3.5% per month in a series of 36 individuals followed by Schiffman and Belsh (1993). Also of clinical note in their series was that whereas 86% had evidence of respiratory muscle weakness, only 7% complained of respiratory symptoms. This suggests that monitoring of respiratory status should begin at initial evaluation rather than postponed until the person is experiencing symptoms. See Table 1.8 for a list of respiratory symptoms associated with ALS.

Understanding declining respiratory status is critical to the management of speech and swallowing disorders (Yorkston, Strand, & Miller, 1996). Poor respiratory support exaggerates the oral movement problems of individuals with bulbar symptoms and contributes to vocal changes in individuals with spinal symptoms. Respiratory decline must also be considered in management of swallowing disorders. Optimal timing of surgical feeding tube or percutaneous endoscopic gastrostomy placement is dependent not only on swallowing status but also on respiratory status (Strand, Miller, Yorkston, & Hillel, 1996). Finally, patients who opt for invasion mechanical ventilation must be followed closely to ensure that their communication needs are met.

MANAGEMENT OF RESPIRATORY PROBLEMS

Current medical management has a variety of life-prolonging technologies to offer individuals with ALS. Patients and their families are particularly interested in this topic. When asked what type of information they wished to have about a variety of topics—including respirators, wheelchairs, hospital beds, and communication systems—individuals with ALS ranked information about ventilation as the most important (Silverstein et al., 1991). Topics of greatest interest were kinds of ventilators, nursing care with ventilators, and insurance coverage for ventilators. Because many of the respiratory devices used affect communication, they are briefly described in the following section. A more complete description of respiratory management can be found elsewhere (Bach, 1998; Benditt, 1998; Hardiman, 2000; Kapadia, 1998).

TABLE 1.8	Symptoms of Early Indicators of Respiratory Insufficency in ALS

- Dyspnea (shortness of breath) on exertion
- Supine dyspnea
- Marked fatigue
- Disturbed sleep
- Morning headaches
- Daytime fatigue and sleepiness, concentration problems
- Nervousness, tremor, increased sweating, tachycardia

- Depression, anxiety
- Visible efforts of auxiliary respiratory muscles
- Reduced appetite, weight loss, recurrent gastritis
- Recurrent or chronic upper respiratory tract infections
- Cyanosis, edema
- Vision disturbances, dizziness
- Diffuse pain in head, neck, and extremities

Note. Adapted from "Palliative Care in Amyotrophic Lateral Sclerosis," by G. D. Borasio and R. Voltz, 1997, *Journal of Neurology, 244*(Suppl. 4), pp. S11–S17, and "Practice Parameters: The Care of the Patient with Amyotrophic Lateral Sclerosis," by R. G. Miller et al., 1999, *Neurology, 52*, pp. 1311–1323.

Assistive Ventilatory Devices

Generally, devices that compensate for weakness in the respiratory muscles are divided into two categories, noninvasive and invasive. A variety of noninvasive respiratory assistance devices are available, including intermittent positive pressure ventilation by mouth, by nose, or by both. Perhaps the most commonly used device is the Bilevel Positive Air Pressure (BiPAP) system (Pinto, Evangelista, Carvalho, Alves, & Sales Luis, 1995). The system is small, lightweight, portable, and easy to maintain. It delivers two levels of pressure: one pressure during inspiration and a lower pressure during expiration. It is worn for periods of time each day, typically during the night so that muscles of respiration recover from fatigue. Noninvasive ventilation has been associated with improving quality of life and increasing survival for periods of several months (Aboussouan, Khan, Banerjee, Arroliga, & Mitsumoto, 2001; Aboussouan, Khan, Meeker, Stelmack, & Misumoto, 1997; Cazzolli & Oppenheimer, 1996; Kleopa, Sherman, Neal, Romano, & Heiman-Patterson, 1999; Pinto et al., 1995).

Devices to assist coughing are also available (Hanayama, Ishikawa, & Bach, 1997). These devices supply a large tidal volume via positive pressure followed by a rapid negative pressure. This rapid change in pressure mimics a forceful cough and aids in clearing pulmonary secretions.

Ventilation via tracheostomy is an option selected by some individuals with ALS when noninvasive devices are no longer effective. These devices are considered invasive because they provide a small, secure connection with the airway when bulbar impairment makes noninvasive ventilation difficult. Because air is delivered via a surgical opening in the neck, the face is free of masks, headgear, and straps that are associated with many of the noninvasive devices. Individuals with ALS may survive for extended periods of time using such devices (Cazzolli & Oppenheimer, 1996). However, assisted ventilation does not alter the progress of other neurology symptoms. Only a minority of individuals with ALS require and receive ventilatory support (Goldblatt & Greenlaw, 1989). Information about the bulbar function of individuals on ventilators is critical because of the importance of effective communication in their lives. Bach (1993) studied communication status and survival of individuals with ALS who were receiving ventilatory support. Results suggested that maintenance of effective communication was associated with patients' ability to remain at home in the community while receiving ventilatory support. Effective communication was not shown to influence length of survival, but was associated with increased quality of life.

Decisions About Ventilatory Assistance

Although precise estimates are not available, it is clear that the use of ventilatory assistance has increased substantially in the last decade (Adams, Shapiro, & Marini, 1998). Decisions about ventilatory assistance are critical. In the American Academy of Neurology Practice Parameters, Miller and colleagues (1999) suggest using an algorithm for respiratory management. Using this algorithm, either respiratory symptoms or a forced vital capacity of less than 50% is the signal to initiate counseling regarding noninvasive ventilation. For those who decline or do not tolerate noninvasive ventilation, tracheostomy ventilation is discussed. If this is declined, symptom management and palliative care is put into place. For those who wish to have and are able to tolerate noninvasive ventilation, treatment options including tracheostomy ventilation are discussed to establish a plan for proceeding when noninvasive ventilation is no longer sufficient. Patients who use noninvasive ventilation may or may not choose to use invasive ventilation. The literature suggests that experience with noninvasive ventilation may assist the patient and family in deciding whether to choose a more invasive option. Plans for invasive ventilation include a discussion of withdrawal conditions (Borasio & Voltz, 1998).

Although patient satisfaction tends to be higher for noninvasive than invasive ventilation, studies suggest that patients on invasive ventilation are no more depressed than patients without ventilation (McDonald, Hillel, & Wiedenfeld, 1996; Pinto et al., 1995). Miller and colleagues (1999) reinforce the caveat that outsiders cannot accurately assess a patient's quality of life; only the individual living with the disorder can make that judgment. In a prospective study of individuals with ALS, patients who accepted this intervention tended to be recently diagnosed, to express a greater attachment to life, and to show greater decline in pulmonary function than those who did not (Albert, Murphy, Del Bene, & Rowland, 1999).

There are a variety of ethical issues relating to ventilator use in individuals with progressive neuromuscular diseases such as ALS. Many individuals with ALS will choose not to prolong their lives by artificial means. Moss et al. (1993) reported that fewer than 10% of individuals with ALS in their study chose home ventilation. Of those who chose this option, 90% were satisfied with the choice and would choose it again. Family caregivers, however, reported that ventilation was a major burden, and only half would choose home ventilation for themselves. The financial burden of home ventilation is also high. In 1993 the mean yearly cost of home ventilation was $153,252.

Speech Disorders

The dysarthria associated with ALS is described in this section. Next, a protocol for a complete speech and swallowing evaluation is presented. The examination is generally applicable to all the neurological diseases discussed in this manual. Finally, approaches to speech treatments are outlined for each stage of progression of the disease.

What Speech Characteristics Are Associated with ALS?

The motor speech impairment associated with ALS is classified as a mixed dysarthria showing features associated with both spasticity (lack of fine control) and flaccidity (weakness). The speech characteristics of individuals with ALS are well described. Darley, Aronson, and Brown (1975, p. 235) summarized the general features of moderate dysarthria in ALS in the following way:

1. Grossly defective articulation of both consonants and vowels, often rendering speech unintelligible

2. Laborious, extremely slow production of words in very short phrases

3. Marked hypernasality coupled with severe harshness and strained-strangled squeezing out of low-pitched tones

4. Complete disruption of prosody, with monotony suppressing meaningfulness and intervals between words and phrases becoming excessive

The characteristics of mild dysarthria in ALS are variable, depending on whether spasticity or flaccidity predominates. Severe dysarthria in ALS, on the other hand, is characterized by profound weakness, lack of oral movement, and reduced phonatory production.

Dysarthria in ALS can be viewed as a combination of features arising from spasticity and those arising from flaccidity. Table 1.9 lists, in order from most to least deviant, the perceptual features identified by Darley et al. (1975) in a group of 30 individuals with ALS. Also noted for each feature is whether it is present in spastic dysarthria (pseudobulbar palsy) and flaccid dysarthria (bulbar palsy). A review of the table indicates that many features are present in both spastic and flaccid dysarthria, and some are present in either spastic or flaccid dysarthria. For example, *low pitch*, *reduced stress*, and *strained-strangled quality* occur in spastic dysarthria as well as ALS. *Audible inspiration* and *nasal emission* occur in flaccid dysarthria as well as ALS. Three features common in ALS are not consistent with either spastic or flaccid dysarthria: *prolonged intervals*, *prolonged phonemes*, and *inappropriate silences*. These features may result from either the combination of spasticity and flaccidity or the respiratory changes common in ALS.

The pattern of prominent features of the dysarthria in 6 speakers was examined over time as they progressed from mild to moderate severity (Klasner, Yorkston, & Strand, 1999). Although the pattern of perceptual features tended to be consistent within each speaker over time, the speakers tended to exhibit a number of different patterns. For half of the speakers, pressure consonant and nasality differences were the most prominent perceptual feature. This pattern may indicate the supralaryngeal system, including the velopharyngeal and oral articulatory systems, may be most impaired. For other speakers, voice quality and voicing features were judged to be most prominent, indicating that the laryngeal system may be most impaired.

Since the mid-1970s, when Darley and colleagues published their classic work, investigation of the speech characteristics of individuals with ALS has continued. Many of the studies in the late 1970s and 1980s implicate the tongue as a major contributing component in ALS dysarthria. A variety of changes in tongue structure and function have been identified, including reductions in range and velocity of movements (Hirose, Kiritani, Ushijima, & Sawashima, 1978), changes in tongue strength (DePaul, Abbs, Caligiuri, Gracco, & Brooks, 1988; Dworkin, 1980), and changes in size, shape, position, and internal structure (Cha & Patten, 1989). Studies also suggest that changes in tongue function are highly associated with changes in speech production. For example, a high negative correlation was found between tongue force and severity of articulatory defect (Dworkin & Aronson, 1986). In other words, as the tongue weakens, articulation becomes increasingly impaired.

TABLE 1.9 Most Deviant Speech Dimensions in ALS Ordered from Most to Least Deviant

Rank of Dimension	Dimension	Present in Other Types of Dysarthria
1	Imprecise consonants	Spasticity/Flaccidity
2	Hypernasality	Spasticity/Flaccidity
3	Harsh voice quality	Spasticity/Flaccidity
4	Slow rate	Spasticity
5	Monopitch	Spasticity/Flaccidity
6	Short phrases	Spasticity/Flaccidity
7	Distorted vowels	Spasticity
8	Low pitch	Spasticity
9	Monoloudness	Spasticity/Flaccidity
10	Excess and equal stress	Spasticity
11	Prolonged intervals	
12	Reduced stress	Spasticity
13	Prolonged phoneme	
14	Strained-strangled quality	Spasticity
15	Breathiness	Spasticity/Flaccidity
16	Audible inspiration	Flaccidity
17	Inappropriate silences	
18	Nasal emission	Flaccidity

Note. Adapted from *Motor Speech Disorders*, by F. L. Darley, A. E. Aronson, and J. R. Brown, 1975, Philadelphia: Saunders.

R. D. Kent and his colleagues conducted a series of studies of articulatory error patterns in ALS dysarthria (J. F. Kent et al., 1992; R. D. Kent et al., 1990; R. D. Kent et al., 1991; R. D. Kent, Weismer, Kent, & Rosenbek, 1989). These studies suggested that the proportion and type of phonetic contrast errors in single words varied with the severity of dysarthria. The phonetic features most affected as intelligibility declined were voicing contrasts, place and manner of lingual consonants, and stop versus nasal consonants. Results of these perceptual studies are complemented by a growing number of studies using acoustic analysis techniques to study both vowel and consonant production in ALS. These studies are summarized in Table 1.10. A number of these acoustic studies have identified changes in speech production such as vowel formant trajectories, particularly flattening of the slope of the F_2 trajectories (J. F. Kent et al., 1992; R. D. Kent et al., 1990; Weismer, Kent, Hodge, & Martin, 1988; Weismer, Martin, Kent, & Kent, 1992).

Acoustic analysis techniques have also been applied to the study of phonatory features of ALS (see Table 1.10 for a summary). Important changes in phonatory instability and phonatory limits have been identified (Aronson, Ramig, Winholtz, & Silber, 1992; R. D. Kent et al., 1994; Ramig, Scherer, Klasner, Titze, & Horii, 1990). These phonatory abnormalities increase over time. The nature of phonatory characteristics in ALS is not consistent from one speaker to another. Strand, Buder, Yorkston, and Ramig (1994) reported perceptual and acoustic data for 4 women, all with bulbar-onset ALS. Voice quality and phonatory function were different for each of these women. Voice quality was described as breathy for one woman, strained-strangled for another, inconsistently harsh with flutter for a third, and inconsistently harsh with consistent flutter for the fourth. This variability may be associated with differences in the relative contribution of vocal weakness and vocal spasticity. Recently the complex relationships with acoustic measures and speech intelligibility have also been reported (Weismer, Jeng, Laures, Kent, & Kent, 2001; Weismer, Laures, Jeng, Kent, & Kent, 2000).

How Rapidly Do Speech Changes Occur in ALS?

Information about rate of symptom progression is critical in treatment planning. For example, it is important to begin planning for augmentative communication system funding, acquisition, and learning before use of the system is mandatory. Therefore, the methods, findings, and implications of a study tracking changes in speech function over time in a group of individuals with ALS will be presented in considerable detail (Yorkston et al., 1993).

A total of 44 individuals with ALS were followed for an average of 9 months. During each outpatient clinic visit, speech function was rated on the 10-point Speech Subscale of the ALS Severity Scale that appears in Chapter Appendix 1.2. This scale will be described in more detail later in this chapter when approaches to clinical assessment are discussed. The purpose of the scale is to assign a numerical value to speech function, with a score of 10 or 9 indicating generally normal speech function, a score of 8 or 7 indicating early speech problems, a score of 6 or 5 indicating behavioral compensations such as slowing of rate and repetition, a score of 4 or 3 indicating the need for augmentative communication devices, and a score of 2 or 1 indicating complete loss of function.

TABLE 1.10

Studies of the Acoustic Aspects of Dysarthria in ALS

Reference	Subjects	Measures	Findings
Speech Production			
Weismer, Kent, Hodge, & Martin, 1988	18 speakers with ALS	Acoustic analysis of the word *wax*	Formant trajectory and segment duration varied with the level of severity of the dysarthria
Weismer, Martin, Kent, & Kent, 1992	25 men with ALS; 15 controls	Acoustic analysis of formant trajectories	(1) Formant transitions slopes are shallow, (2) exaggerated formant trajectories at the onset of vocalic nuclei, (3) greater variability than control, and (4) less intelligible speakers were more aberrant
J. F. Kent et. al., 1992	10 women with ALS	Perceptual assessment using word identification test, acoustic analysis of F_2 trajectories	(1) Disrupted phonetic features include velopharyngeal valving, lingual function for consonant contrasts of place and manner and syllable shape; (2) F_2 slope reduction; and (3) some gender differences in ALS speech
Turner, Tjaden, & Weismer, 1995	5 men and 4 women with ALS and controls	Vowel space in a passage read at habitual, fast and slow rate	Speakers with ALS exhibited smaller vowel space and less systematic changes in vowel space as a function of speaking rate
Tjaden & Turner, 1997	3 women and 4 men with ALS	Spectral characteristics of word-initial fricative	Differences between speakers with ALS and controls in the coefficient of the first moment coefficients
Turner & Tjaden, 2000	9 speakers with mild to moderate dysarthria and ALS, 9 controls	F_1 and F_2, vowel space and duration in paragraph	A tendency for the difference in vowel space area for content and function words to be smaller for speakers with ALS
Bunton, Kent, Kent, & Rosenbek (2000)	Males with ALS and mild or more severe impairment	Acoustic measures pertaining to the regulation of duration F_o, intensity with tone units of conversation	Decrease in overall duration of tone units, fewer words in a tone unit, and smaller variation in F_o
Phonatory Function			
Ramig, Scherer, Klasner, Titze, & Horii, 1990	69-year-old man with ALS seen 5 times in 6 months	Acoustic measures of phonatory instability, phonatory limits, and nasal–oral amplitude ratio	Case showed increased phonatory instability and reduced phonatory limits over time
Aronson, Ramig, Winholtz, & Silber, 1992	4 men and 4 women with ALS and 8 matched controls	Acoustic analysis of sustained phonation	Amplitude and frequency modulations more prominent in ALS speakers
Strand, Buder, Yorkston, & Ramig, 1994	4 women with ALS	Acoustic analysis of phonatory function	Phonatory characteristics varied greatly among the cases
Robert, Pouget, Giovanni, Azulay, & Triglia, 1999	63 women with ALS (with and without bulbar symptoms) and 40 controls	8 acoustic parameters of sustained phonation	Differences found for jitter coefficient of variation for frequency, shimmer, number of harmonics, and maximum phonatory frequency range

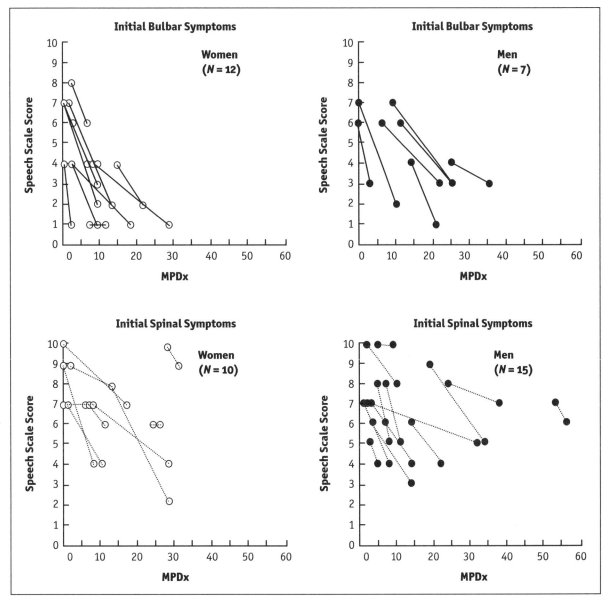

Figure 1.1. ALS Severity Scale scores for the initial and most recent visits for individuals with ALS who were followed for at least three clinic visits. Speech Subscale scores are plotted as a function of months postdiagnosis (MPDx) for women with initial bulbar symptoms, for men with initial bulbar symptons, for women with initial spinal symptoms, and for men with initial spinal symptoms. *Note.* From "Speech Deterioration in Amyotrophic Lateral Sclerosis: Implications for the Timing of Intervention," by K. M. Yorkston, E. Strand, R. Miller, A. Hillel, and K. Smith, 1993, *Journal of Medical Speech-Language Pathology, 1*(1), pp. 35–46. Copyright 1993 by Thomson Learning. Reprinted with permission.

Figure 1.1 summarizes the results of this longitudinal group study and illustrates the speech scale scores for first and last visits as a function of months postdiagnosis. Patients are grouped by gender and type of initial symptoms. Note that in each group there is a consistent pattern of decline in speech function, with some variability in the slope of progression. Visual inspection of the data suggests little relationship between the length of time since diagnosis and the severity of speech symptoms. In other words, some individuals have severe speech impairment at the

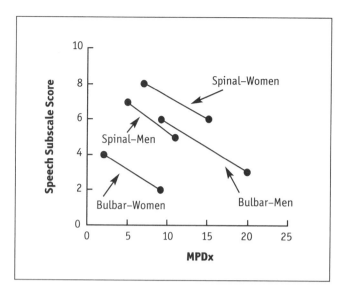

Figure 1.2. Median Speech Subscale scores versus months postdiagnosis (MPDx) for the groups by initial symptom and gender. Plotted are initial and most recent clinic visits. *Note.* From "Speech Deterioration in Amyotrophic Lateral Sclerosis: Implications for the Timing of Intervention," by K. M. Yorkston, E. Strand, R. Miller, A. Hillel, and K. Smith, 1993. *Journal of Medical Speech-Language Pathology, 1*(1), pp. 35–46. Copyright 1993 by Thomson Learning. Reprinted with permission.

time of diagnosis whereas others who are years postdiagnosis may exhibit relatively mild speech problems. As might be expected, individuals with initial bulbar symptoms tend to exhibit more severe speech problems than those with initial spinal symptoms. Many of the individuals followed in this study progressed to the point at which they needed an augmentative communication system (with a speech scale score of 4 or less) by their last outpatient clinic visit. A number of clinical implications can be drawn from these longitudinal data. Although rapid decline of speech function is certainly not inevitable, it occurs frequently enough that sound clinical management dictates early preparation. Although some individuals progress slowly, for others the rate of progress is rapid. The timing of augmentative communication intervention will be discussed in detail later.

In a disease in which individual rates of progression vary substantially, display of individual data (as in Figure 1.1) is helpful. However, it is also important to appreciate "typical" rates of progression for groups of individuals. To obtain an indication of central tendency for each group, median data are illustrated in Figure 1.2. Note that women with initial bulbar symptoms tend to be more severely impaired in speech function and tend to visit our clinic earlier than do men with initial bulbar symptoms.

What Information Is Obtained in a Clinical Examination of Speech and Swallowing ?

The following examination is carried out during a patient's initial clinic visit, and an abbreviated form is conducted on follow-up visits. We have organized the evaluation into three general areas:

1. *History,* in which information is obtained about the nature and course of the disorder, as well as about how the disorder is being managed

2. *Physical examination,* in which the physiologic abnormalities in the speech and swallowing mechanism are described

3. *Assessment of speech and swallowing function*, in which impact of the impairment is assessed with regard to the patient's ability to communicate efficiently and understandably, to maintain adequate nutrition and hydration, and to handle oral secretions adequately

The "Clinical Examination for ALS" form in Chapter Appendix 1.1 summarizes the information obtained during the clinical examination. During the course of the clinical examination, be cautious not to attribute all of the individual's problems to the neurologic disorder. Unfortunately, degenerative neurologic diseases are not an antidote to other disorders or conditions that might be present.

THE HISTORY

Taking the patient's history sets the stage for the remainder of the clinical examination. We are interested in the nature of the illness, its length, and specific details concerning its onset and diagnosis. We are also interested in how patients and their families are handling the speech and swallowing problems.

PATIENT INFORMATION

The standard patient information contained in the Clinical Examination form is obtained. Patient information includes not only demographic data, but also the referral source. It is important to know from whom the referral came. In the case of our clinic, referrals come primarily from neurologists, physiatrists, specialty clinics such as the muscular dystrophy clinic, and community agencies such as Home Health Care. We seek to know why the referral was made from two perspectives—that of the referring health-care specialist and that of the patient.

MEDICAL HISTORY

In obtaining the past medical history, we are interested in the neurologic disease, when it was diagnosed, and by whom. With many diseases such as ALS, diagnosis is at times complex. Therefore, if the individual has not sought a second opinion, we encourage doing so. Again, because of the complexity of the diagnosis, it is not unusual for the diagnosis to be made months and even years after the onset of first symptoms. Therefore, we want to know the approximate date of onset of the symptoms. What were the first symptoms? When did they begin? How have they progressed? We take particularly detailed information about the onset and progression of the speech and swallowing symptoms. Finally, when discussing the symptoms associated with degenerative neurologic diseases, it is important to obtain an understanding of the patient's level of knowledge of the disease process. This can range widely from individuals and families who are well read and conversant with the "statistics" of the disorder, to patients and families with little or no knowledge of the disease. The patient's desire to understand the disease process also varies widely: Some patients wish to read all they can about the disorder, whereas others wish to know no further information about it.

When taking the history, we are interested not only in the current illness, but also in the person's history of other disorders. Although the disease cannot be cured, care should be taken not to overlook other potentially treatable disorders (such as esophageal webs, esophageal masses, or gastroesophageal reflux) and not to wrongly attribute all symptoms to the known degenerative process.

A psychosocial history is also critical in assisting the individual with a degenerative disorder to make plans for the future. We need to know, for example, the person's employment status and how the disease has affected it. Information related to the person's living situation and household members is also obtained.

CURRENT HEALTH-CARE MANAGEMENT

During a discussion of the patient's current health-care management, we first review the medications that the patient is taking. Combinations of medications and their side effects may have important impacts on speech, swallowing, and saliva management. When considering saliva management, we often suggest that this is a good time to review with the primary-care physician all of the medications currently being taken and to consider the elimination of potentially unnecessary ones. With a diagnosis of ALS, the priority of health-care issues may change. Medications such as diuretics used to treat a cardiac condition may not be required, given this new life-threatening disease and may even complicate management of ALS symptoms. The review of current health-care management also allows us to evaluate how effectively the patient is using the health-care delivery system. We are interested in the following types of information:

1. What community resources is the person aware of or interested in exploring?

2. What adaptive equipment does the person currently have? When was it obtained? From whom was it obtained?

3. Does the person make use of attendant care to assist in activities of daily living?

For people who are difficult to understand because of severe dysarthria, we are interested in knowing whether an emergency communication system is in place. For those with swallowing difficulties, we are interested in knowing whether the patients and family members have been given instruction in administering first aid for choking and whether an emergency plan in case of choking is in place.

Many individuals with ALS establish a "living will," in which they make known their medical management wishes. These instructions regarding the level of medical care they wish to receive are implemented in cases in which patients are unable to make their wishes known to the health-care management team. Thus, it is important to know whether the patient has established a living will and the specific wishes of the person in case of emergency.

THE PHYSICAL EXAMINATION

During the physical examination, the impairment or physiologic abnormalities of the speech and swallowing mechanisms are evaluated. The physical examination is organized into general groups according to components of the speech and swallowing mechanisms.

Group 1: Tongue and Lips

Lip weakness can be detected by asking the patient to suck on a gloved finger (i.e., a suckling movement) or evaluated by asking the patient to blow out the cheeks. (Note that velopharyngeal competency is also required for the latter activity.) Lip weakness is also associated with the following progression: inability to whistle, food spillage, inability to use a straw, dysarthria, and lastly, drooling.

	Subjects	Minimum	25th	50th	75th	Maximum
			Percentile			
Subjects		**Minimum**	**25th**	**50th**	**75th**	**Maximum**
Normal	**/p/**					
	Males	4.5	6.2	6.5	6.9	7.5
	Females	4.6	5.8	6.1	6.4	8.6
	/t/					
	Males	4.4	6.0	6.5	7.0	8.2
	Females	4.3	5.6	6.0	6.5	8.5
	/k/					
	Males	4.4	5.5	6.1	6.4	7.5
	Females	4.3	5.2	5.7	6.2	7.9
ALS	**/p/**					
	Males	2.3	3.3	4.5	5.4	6.6
	Females	0	2.7	3.7	5.0	6.4
	/t/					
	Males	2.0	3.2	4.2	4.9	6.4
	Females	0	3.0	3.5	4.7	6.4
	/k/					
	Males	1.8	2.8	4.0	4.5	6.2
	Females	0	2.7	3.2	4.6	6.4

TABLE 1.11   Alternate Motion Rates (Syllables/Second) in Normal Subjects and Subjects with ALS

We use diadochokinetic rates or alternate motion rates in order to obtain an "objective" measure of the impairment of the lips, anterior and posterior tongue, and mandible (Darley et al., 1975). Alternate movement rates give an indication of the speed and regularity of reciprocal muscle movements. Normative data for alternate movement rates have been reported by a number of researchers (Dworkin & Aronson, 1986; Kreul, 1972; Lass & Sandusky, 1971; Ptacek, Sander, Mahoney, & Jackson, 1966). Generally, the mean syllable repetition rates for normal adults range from 5.8 to 6.9 syllables per second for repetitions of /p/ and /t/. Repetition rates for /k/ range from 5.2 to 6.2 for adults. Table 1.11 contains data taken from Dworkin and Aronson (1986) that may be useful as a measure against which to compare the clinical population. The table contains alternate motion rates (in syllables per second) for the syllables /p/, /t/, and /k/ obtained from a group of individuals without neurologic impairment and from a group of individuals with ALS. Normal males ($N = 67$) had a mean age of 38.5 years, and normal females ($N = 58$) had a mean age of 37 years, with a range from 20 to 72 years. The individuals with ALS (11 men and 8 women) had both flaccid and spastic components and represented various degrees of speech impairment.

Alternate motion rates may be measured in a number of ways. For example, the number of syllables produced by the speaker within a specified time period can be counted, or the speaker can be asked to produce a specified number of syllables and the time for that production measured. In a population in which generalized weakness is a problem, the combination of poor respiratory support and an inefficient velopharyngeal valve may make the production of long syllable sequences impossible. Therefore, we give the following instructions when asking a patient to perform the alternate movement rate tasks:

I am going to ask you to say a series of syllables as rapidly and precisely as you can. Go as fast as you can but make each syllable as distinct as you can. Be sure to take a deep breath before you start.

We obtain alternate movement rates for /p/, /t/, /k/, and /pataka/ and measure the time required to produce a sequence of five syllables. When the person has insufficient respiratory support to produce five syllables on one breath, we measure the time required to produce however many syllables the person can say on a single breath. Although alternative motion rates give some useful information related to tongue and lip impairment, results should be interpreted with some caution. A severely impaired speaker must compromise between the precision with which the syllable is produced and the rate of production. In other words, rate can be increased if precision is sacrificed and vice versa. As with any of the measures we obtain as part of the physical examination, alternate movement rates cannot be interpreted apart from other measures.

During the physical examination of swallowing, dysfunction of the lips is most easily seen by food spillage from the corners of the mouth. The earliest symptom of this dysfunction is an increased use of napkins during meals. Dysfunction of the lips may also be noted and described as the inability of the lips to constrict around the contour of the spoon to strip the food out of the bowl and retain it in the oral cavity. Dysfunction of the tongue is indicated by food debris sitting in the gingival sulcus of the mouth after swallowing, as well as by the need for extensive mastication. This dysfunction is due to the inability of the tongue, in conjunction with the buccal muscles, to gather the food on the lingual side of the teeth to form a bolus prior to the initiation of a swallow.

Group 2: Palate, Pharyngeal Constrictors, and Muscles of Mastication

Palatal function can be assessed by visual examination as well as by articulation testing. By observing a gag reflex, you can find out whether the oral pharyngeal muscles constrict and the palate elevates symmetrically and completely, elevates to Passavant's pad but weakly, or fails to meet Passavant's pad. Palatal impairment may result in a number of speech production problems, including the following:

1. Inability to produce accurately many of the speech sounds that require a buildup of intraoral air pressure, such as /p/, /b/, /t/, /s/, or /tʃ/

2. Nasalization of vowel production

3. Escape of air through the nose (nasal emission) rather than oral airflow

To test for more advanced palatal dysfunction, check for nasal air escape when the patient puffs out the cheeks. Progressive symptoms associated with palatal dysfunction are hypernasal speech, inability to use a straw, and lastly, nasal reflux. In our clinical experience, nasal reflux is not common in ALS (less than 5%) despite total palatal dysfunction in some patients. Individuals with ALS, even those with near-total palatal dysfunction, often cannot generate enough oropharyngeal constrictor pressure to cause the reflux that occurs in other patients with palatal dysfunction. Weakness of the soft palate may also cause ineffective transport of the food bolus from the anterior to the posterior part of the oral cavity. The palate must function in concert with the tongue in positioning the bolus and acting as a scaffold against which the tongue can propel the food bolus posteriorly. Pharyngeal constrictor weakness may be most evident in the patient's swallowing dysfunction. Specifically, the person may have difficulties clearing leafy vegetables, such as lettuce or cabbage; liquids may penetrate the airway before a swallow is triggered; and pooling in the hypopharynx may be evident due to inadequate pharyngeal stripping.

The deterioration of the muscles of mastication is difficult to assess clinically. Palpation of the masseter and temporalis muscles during biting movements can demonstrate muscle wasting. The pterygoid muscles can be assessed grossly by asking the patient to move the jaw from side to side. Few symptoms are noted early in the development of weakness in the muscles of mastication. Usually there are parallel developments in the oral cavity and pharynx that limit other aspects of swallowing ability. These simultaneous impairments may mask decreased ability to chew. In advanced bulbar ALS, weakness of the muscles of mastication may cause the jaw to be pulled downward by gravity, which leaves the mouth open. The pattern of airflow during rest breathing is changed from nasal to oral breathing, with the resultant problems of dry lips, dry mouth, and tenacious oral secretions.

Group 3: The Buccal/Frontal/Orbital Muscles (Facial Nerve), Sternocleidomastoid/Trapezius Muscle (Accessory Nerve), and the Vocal Folds (Vagus Nerve)

While the lower branches of the facial nerve (lips) are affected early in the course of bulbar disease, the upper branches of the facial nerve become involved later, with the result that the orbital and frontal muscles are affected least and latest. The sternocleidomastoid and trapezium muscles vary in the degree to which they are affected and, unlike the other cranial nerves, are often asymmetrically involved. Sternocleidomastoid involvement is manifested in an inability to keep the head from falling forward, and involvement of the trapezium in an inability to raise the arms—both symptoms being found in classical 11th nerve syndrome.

Examination of the vocal folds shows that most patients are able to adduct their vocal folds and phonate, even with rather advanced disease. In our experience, however, vocal fold abduction is impaired in 30% of patients and is usually symmetrically affected. Some patients, even on their initial indirect examination, are found to have the vocal folds nearly paralyzed in the midline. This finding may not be correlated with audible stridor if the respiratory muscles are too weak to generate sufficient negative pressures and the narrowed glottis does not present a functional restriction of the airway. In advanced cases, passive paradoxical movements of the vocal folds can be noted.

Our assessment of vocal fold function includes a prolonged phonation task in which the patient is asked to take a breath and say "ah" as long, steadily, and clearly as possible. This task is a good indicator of respiratory support for speech as well as vocal fold function. We listen for the following features:

- *Voice quality.* Does the voice sound smooth and clear in quality or does it lack full tonal clarity? Two general categories of dysphonic voices have been identified in neurologic disease (Darley et al., 1975). *Breathiness* is defined as a lack of fullness of voice associated with excess air wastage. Breathiness is frequently associated with flaccid paralysis. *Hoarseness* is the term used to describe a variety of noisy voices. Among the most important voice changes in ALS is the "strained-strangled" voice quality associated with spasticity, and the "wet" or "gurgly" voice quality associated with the accumulation of secretions in the larynx.
- *Duration.* Maximum sustained phonation is related to vital capacity, pitch, loudness, the function of the vocal folds, and the degree of effort used by the speaker during each trial. Phonation time was found to be a reliable predictor of vital capacity in a group of individuals with ALS (Hillel, Yorkston, & Miller, 1989). In a study

of 41 individuals with ALS, variation in sustained phonation time predicted almost 50% of the variability in vital capacity. Abnormal muscle tone of the vocal folds may also affect maximum phonation time. Generally, the greater the breathiness, the shorter the duration of phonation. Phonation times may also be shortened in severe cases of strained-strangled harshness (Darley et al., 1975).

  • *Pitch and steadiness.* Although pitch and steadiness alterations in voice quality are found in many neurologic disorders, they are relatively uncommon in the ALS population.

  • *Loudness.* Because of the close relationship between respiratory support and voice loudness, voices that are inadequately loud should be noted. Patients with reduced voice loudness will also frequently complain of fatigue after extended periods of speaking.

  • *Ability to initiate a quiet voice.* This task is a good indication of fine control of the laryngeal musculature because it removes some of the respiratory demands involved in the production of louder phonation.

  • *Alternate movement rates for phonation.* We also obtain alternate motion rates for the vowel /a/ versus no phonation. This task is particularly sensitive to problems in respiratory and phonatory control.

Group 4: The Muscles of Respiration

Although respiratory deterioration does not appear to have a clear pattern of progression in relation to other physical findings (Braun, 1987; Fallat & Norris, 1980), it usually occurs as bulbar/spinal symptoms progress (Griggs, Donohoe, Utll, & Goldblatt, 1980). Respiratory function can be measured clinically by assessing the depth and volume of respiration, as well as cough force and phonation time (Hillel, Yorkston, et al., 1989). However, other factors (vocal fold dysfunction and secretions) can obscure the accuracy of these measurements.

Early respiratory weakness is most sensitively measured by pulmonary function tests. A limited but simpler measurement uses a handheld respirometer to assess vital capacity (VC) (Fallat et al., 1979). Normal values for VC range from 2 to 7 liters, with the peak of the distribution curve at about 4 liters. The "expected" VC for an individual is affected by weight, height, age, sex, race, ethnic background, and altitude (Clausen, 1982). In more advanced stages of bulbar ALS, respirometers become difficult to use, as the patient cannot make a good seal around the mouthpiece, and laryngeal abductor weakness may restrict expired airflow. The formulas for predicted vital capacity based on age and height are as follows:

$$\textit{Men: NVC} = (-38 \times \text{age}) + (121 \times \text{height in inches}) - 2100 = \text{VC} \pm 970 \text{ cc}$$

$$\textit{Women: NVC} = (-22 \times \text{age}) + (110 \times \text{height in inches}) - 2980 = \text{VC} \pm 790 \text{ cc}$$

ASSESSMENT OF SPEECH AND SWALLOWING FUNCTION

The final phase of the clinical examination involves the documentation of the speech and swallowing functions. In other words, how has the impairment in the speech and swallowing mechanisms affected the person's ability to communicate understandably and efficiently, to maintain adequate fluid and nutritional intake, and to manage oral secretions in an acceptable manner? Studies suggest that there is a moderate to strong correlation between measures of speech function, as measured using intelligible words per minute, and motor function, as measured by the physical examination (Yorkston, Strand, & Hume, 1998). Factors such as cognition and rate of disease progress may contribute the lack of one-to-one relationships between these two measures of function.

Speech Function

A number of measures of overall speech function have been proposed (Yorkston, Beukelman, Strand, & Bell, 1999), including speech intelligibility, speaking rate, articulation adequacy, and speech naturalness. Of these measures, speech intelligibility is perhaps the most important in developing a communication management plan for an individual with degenerative neurologic disorders. In our clinic, we use sentence intelligibility along with speaking rate (Yorkston, Beukelman, & Tice, 1996) as a measure of speech function. Because fatigue is a concern, we shorten the standard test length by half, requiring the speaker to produce only one sentence at each sentence length. This results in a sample that is 110 words in length.

As the severity of the dysarthria increases, the sentence production task becomes increasingly fatiguing for the speaker, and little clinically useful information can be derived from it. Therefore, once sentence intelligibility has fallen below 30%, we begin to document the level of speech disability using a single-word production task. We developed a series of sets of semantically related words—for example, numbers from 1 to 20, colors, holidays, items of clothing, and others. The single words produced by the individual with ALS are audiotaped and judged both with and without context. We have found that single-word intelligibility within semantic context provides a useful indicator of how functional natural speech is in the severely dysarthric individual (Hammen, Yorkston, & Dowden, 1991; Yorkston, Hammen, & Dowden, 1991).

Swallowing Function

Perhaps the best overall measure of severity of dysphagia is obtained by comparing the current weight of the patient with previously recorded weights. The clinical examination should include a test swallow in order to evaluate the oral pharyngeal components of swallowing and assess the appropriateness of the patient's current swallowing technique. For example, has the person learned to tuck the chin to the chest when attempting to initiate a swallow?

Motion radiographic studies of swallowing (videofluoroscopic barium swallows) are used to evaluate swallowing in individuals with symptoms that cannot be explained on the basis of the physical examination. Because this population has previously diagnosed disease, most of the symptoms of swallowing impairment are predictable and consistent with the physical findings. In a small percentage of cases, however, when the complaints do not match the physical findings or the complaints and history suggest multiple problems—such as specific cricopharyngeal dysfunction, esophageal webs, diverticuli, esophageal dysmotility, or gastroesophageal reflux—radiographic studies are helpful. Because aspiration is evident on the basis of the physical examination and history, radiographic studies generally should not be used for the detection of aspiration alone. One exception is when the clinician is willing to recommend discontinuing oral intake and the patient is willing to accept this recommendation if airway penetration is evident. When motion radiographic swallows are indicated and ordered, the studies should include a complete assessment of all stages of swallowing to allow evaluation of oral function, pharyngeal contractions, laryngeal airway protection, esophageal motility, and gastroesophageal function, as well as the morphology of all these mechanisms.

In addition to the physical findings, detailed questions about the patient's swallowing complaints provide useful information regarding the severity of the swallowing disability. In progressive degenerative disorders, swallowing problems often have a slow onset. Thus, it is important to identify the early warning signs of progressive disorders so they can be managed effectively in order to avert further complications. The following are a series of complaints that can be viewed as early warning signs of a swallowing problem:

- *Complaints of difficulty with speech.* Dysphagia usually parallels or shortly follows the development of speech problems. If a patient is complaining of speech difficulty but not a swallowing problem, question him or her carefully to detect the possibility of an early swallowing disorder.
- *Decrease of food intake or alteration in diet.* Weight loss is often wrongly attributed to other symptoms (such as depression, malaise, or loss of muscle mass) but is often due to dysphagia.
- *Food spillage from the oral cavity.* Food spillage from the oral cavity results from discoordination and weakness of the lips, buccal muscles, and tongue, and is a strong indication of difficulty during the early oral phases.
- *Dehydration.* Dehydration is the most difficult finding to determine because its insidious onset causes a chronic condition. A generalized feeling of malaise, low-grade fever, decreased urine output, dry mouth, thick mucus, inability to clear pulmonary secretions, and decreased skin turgor are all symptoms of chronic dehydration.
- *Problems at isolated, specific sites along the swallowing mechanism.* The specific sites of dysphagia often can be determined early in the course of the disorder. As the disorder progresses, the problems usually become multiple and more generalized.

ALS SEVERITY SCALE

In addition to the measures of speech and swallowing functions just described, we use the ALS Severity Scale (see Chapter Appendix 1.2) as a staging system to rate the level of functional performance of the patient. This scale is an important part of the clinical examination of individuals with ALS. The use of the scale is to assign numerical values in each of four areas—speech (SP), swallowing (SW), lower extremity function (LE), and upper extremity function (UE)—so that data regarding a patient's clinical condition can be reported. Information regarding the reliability with which the scale can be used in the clinical setting can be found elsewhere (Hillel, Miller, et al., 1989; Yorkston et al., 1993). We have found that the ALS Severity Scale provides a degree of consistency when evaluating individuals with ALS. This consistency allows for evaluation of disease progression and rate of progression, as well as for designation of disease levels for which specific treatment guidelines can be recommended.

Each of the four subscales provides a choice of 10 scores based on progressive decline of function. The subscales are similar, in that scores of 9 or 10 indicate essentially normal functioning, 7 or 8 indicate detectable abnormalities, 5 or 6 indicate a need for behavioral modification, 3 or 4 indicate a need for technical modifications, and 1 or 2 indicate a loss of function. This scale is designed for use with the ALS population and is based on the progression of that disease. The scale should not be used with other disorders.

It is important to note that the ALS Severity Scale should not be completed based on interview alone. Acquire information for rating an individual by taking a history from the patient and performing a limited physical examination. In addition, information gathered from family members is not only allowed but encouraged. Use clinical judgment in interpreting the relative accuracy of conflicting statements from the patient and a family member. In some cases, you will have to estimate what a patient can do or *should be able to do* rather than what the patient *actually does*. The following are some general guidelines for using the ALS Severity Scale:

1. When rating someone, first identify the major heading under which the person falls. Once you have chosen the appropriate major heading, choose one of the two minor headings. The text provides a gen-

eral description of the minor headings, and single specific items in the text should not cause you to change the rating from one major heading to another.

2. In each case, when choosing a major or minor heading, look at one heading below your preliminary choice before making a final decision.

3. If you absolutely cannot decide between two choices even after examining the test supplement, choose the less severe (higher) scale score.

4. It is recommended that you use the scale openly in front of the patient so you can refer to the text and ask the necessary specific questions.

5. When using the rating scale during follow-up visits, refer to previous ratings and use those ratings as a starting point for questioning.

6. It is recommended that you rate the individual's skills in the order they are described in this chapter: speech, swallowing, lower extremity, and upper extremity.

The Speech Subscale

Normal Speech Processes. Normal speech is uncommon in bulbar ALS. A score of 10 (Normal Speech) would indicate that the patient has noticed no change in speech function and that you judge speech rate, precision, and loudness to be within normal limits. A score of 9 (Nominal Speech Abnormality) indicates that only the patient or spouse notices or suspects that speech has changed. The speaker in this category would maintain normal speaking rate and loudness but may indicate the need to "pay more attention" or "work harder" when speaking.

Detectable Speech Disturbance. Speech characteristics in this category can range from mild speech changes noticed during stress and fatigue to speech that is consistently impaired. As articulation and respiratory support problems increase, most people compensate unconsciously by decreasing their speaking rate and reducing the loudness of their speech. As symptoms progress during this stage, speech remains easily understood but develops a deliberate and, eventually, labored quality. Vocal fold spasticity can cause the voice to become harsh, and weakened respiratory effort can cause phrase lengths to diminish (Dworkin & Hartman, 1979). Specific speech characteristics will differ depending on the relative involvement of the upper motor neurons, lower motor neurons, and respiratory muscles (Darley et al., 1975). A speaker in this category is assigned a score of 8 if speech changes are perceptually obvious but speech rate remains normal. The most common early perceptual change is in voice quality. A speaker is assigned a score of 7 if speech remains understandable but rate, articulation, and resonance are impaired.

Behavioral Modifications. As symptoms progress, speakers may begin to make conscious behavioral modifications. Modifications may range from the need to repeat oneself only occasionally or only in adverse situations, such as noisy environments, to the need to repeat oneself frequently regardless of the environment. These speakers often use a spokesperson or "translator" (usually the person's spouse). This heralds the onset of communication isolation as the speaker, out of fatigue and frustration, begins to limit the complexity and length of messages. A speaker in this category is assigned a score of 6 if repetition is needed only in adverse situations. Speakers receiving this score do not limit the complexity or length of their messages. Speakers receive a score of 5 if they appear to limit the complexity and length of messages because of increasing speech difficulty.

Use of Augmentative Communication.

This category indicates that speech must now be combined with augmentative communication approaches. Speakers in this category almost always need a spokesperson in situations that require speech. Their natural speech is often limited to one-word responses or highly predictable messages such as greetings. For people who can write, writing is the most efficient means of augmentative communication. Intelligibility of natural speech can be enhanced by writing or pointing to the first letter of each word, or by writing out single key words to set the context for the listener. As symptoms worsen, patients will initiate most communication by writing and in later stages will vocalize only in response to specific questions. A speaker in this category is assigned a score of 4 if natural speech is or should be supplemented by augmentative techniques such as first-letter pointing. Communication breakdowns need to be resolved by spelling out the word or using a spokesperson. A speaker is assigned a score of 3 if speech can be understood only within a very narrow context, such as responses to simple questions. Speakers in this category usually initiate communication nonvocally.

Loss of Useful Speech.

People with advanced bulbar ALS have lost useful speech. Some individuals in this category can vocalize for emotional expression or with extreme effort. A speaker is assigned a score of 2 if vocalization is used to express emotion, affirmation, and negation. A score of 1 is assigned if vocalization is rarely attempted but may occur for crying or pain.

Tracheostomy.

Anyone who has a tracheostomy is given a score of X.

In each decision for the Speech Subscale, remember to consider what the person can do as well as what the person does. For example, a patient with a spouse who is hard of hearing might need to repeat more often than a similar patient whose spouse has normal hearing. Similar adjustments in rating should be made when the spouse is talkative or domineering rather than quiet and patient.

The Swallowing Subscale

Normal Eating Habits.

People with early bulbar ALS will effectively manage a normal diet and a normal rate of eating. These individuals might notice occasional difficulty with food becoming lodged in the gingivo-buccal sulcuses but generally function entirely normally and need no intervention. Patients in this category are assigned a score of 10 if they deny any difficulty chewing or swallowing and the physical examination reveals no abnormalities. They are assigned a score of 9 if they note some slight changes such as food lodging in the recesses of the mouth or sticking in the throat.

Early Eating Problems.

People with early swallowing difficulties will often complain first of swallowing difficulties with solid foods. As the disorder progresses, they will also complain of prolonged mealtimes and the need to take smaller bites of food than previously. Occasionally at this point, some foods such as steak, crackers, and leafy salads are avoided. Individuals in this category are assigned a score of 8 if they complain of swallowing difficulty but maintain a regular diet. Eating time for patients in this group has not increased substantially. Patients are assigned a score of 7 if eating time has increased significantly and smaller bites are required.

Dietary Consistency Changes. The initial dietary change is usually to a soft diet, but some people may be placed on a blenderized or liquid diet. These people have difficulty maintaining adequate liquid intake. Late in this stage, a critical nutritional event occurs—the person loses the sense of enjoyment associated with eating. This loss of enjoyment and the need for special food preparation heralds the onset of significant weight loss and failure to thrive. Individuals in this category are assigned a score of 6 if they have made the change to a soft diet, and a score of 5 if the change to a liquefied diet has been made.

Needs Tube Feeding. This group includes not only people who use a tube for feeding but also those who *should* be using a tube. Usually the need for tube feedings corresponds to a dread of meals. Aspiration events, food spillage, prolonged mealtimes, and respiratory fatigue during meals all contribute to an aversion to eating. Patients in this category are assigned a score of 4 if they continue to take greater than half of their nutrition by mouth, and a score of 3 if they take less than half of their nutrition by mouth.

Nothing by Mouth. The last stage of dysphagia is comprised of those people who can take nothing by mouth (NPO). All ingestion by mouth is unsafe. Most can manage their oral secretions, although some are helped by medications or devices such as aspirators. The most advanced patients in this group are those who aspirate their own secretions. Fortunately, bulbar ALS rarely progresses to this point. We have found that surgical aspiration procedures are almost never needed and should be reserved for individuals who are completely NPO, are aspirating their secretions, and have a reasonable respiratory prognosis. Patients in this category are assigned a score of 2 if they are able to handle secretions safely, and a score of 1 if secretions are aspirated.

In each decision related to the Swallowing Subscale, consider not only what the person *does* but what he or she *needs*. For example, someone who takes all nutrition by mouth but is failing to thrive probably needs a tube supplement and should be rated accordingly (a rating of 4 or less). In the Swallowing Subscale, a tube is defined as any kind of feeding tube (nasogastric, intermittent orogastric, esophagostomy, or gastrostomy).

Upper and Lower Extremities

A word of caution is appropriate regarding the subscales measuring upper extremity function and lower extremity function. These scales were not designed to be comprehensive indicators of overall function in these areas. Rather, they are meant simply to give an indication of selected aspects of performance that assist in planning the management of speech and swallowing disorders. For example, the Lower Extremity Subscale gives an indication of the person's ability to walk. When attempting to select an appropriate augmentative communication device, you will need rather specific information about mobility. An 8- to 10-pound augmentative communication device may be portable for someone with a lower extremity score of 10 (normal ambulation), but not for someone with a lower extremity score of 6 (walks with a mechanical device). The Upper Extremity Subscale is important in making a number of decisions related to the management of swallowing disorders. For example, good hand function is required in order to use an intermittent orogastric tube, and the team would need to consider the upper extremity scale score before making such a recommendation.

When using the subscale for lower extremity function, rate the best level of performance. This would represent the person's ability at the best time of day, when fatigue is minimal and when plenty of time is allowed to perform the task. Assign scores based on the following progression:

- *Normal ambulation.* Patient denies any weakness or fatigue. Examination detects no abnormality.

- *Fatigue suspected.* Patient suspects weakness or fatigue in lower extremities during exertion.

- *Difficulty with uneven terrain.* Patient notices difficulty and fatigue when walking long distances, climbing stairs, or walking over uneven ground (even thick carpet).

- *Observed changes in gait.* Noticeable changes in gait are present. Patient pulls on railing when climbing stairs and may use leg brace.

- *Walks with mechanical device.* Patient needs or uses cane, walker, or assistant to walk. Patient probably uses wheelchair away from home.

- *Walks with mechanical device and ascendant.* Patient does not attempt to walk without an attendant. Ambulation is limited to less than 50 feet. Avoids stairs.

- *Able to support weight.* At best, patient can shuffle a few steps with the help of an attendant for transfers.

- *Purposeful leg movements.* Patient is unable to take steps, but can position legs to assist an attendant in transfers. Moves legs purposefully to maintain mobility in bed.

- *Minimal movement.* Patient has minimal movement of one or both legs. Cannot reposition legs independently.

- *Paralysis.* Flaccid paralysis is present. Patient cannot move lower extremities (except perhaps to close inspection).

When rating upper extremity function, exclude the shoulder muscles; in other words, a shoulder shrug does not qualify as movement of the upper extremity. Rate the patient based on the estimated level of function, not simply on the reported level. This is necessary to control for the variability of help available to patients. For example, a patient with an extremely supportive spouse will get more assistance than a similar patient who lives alone. When evaluating dressing, judge only those aspects of dressing that rely solely on the upper extremities; for example, the inability to put on pants due to paralysis of the legs should not lower the UE rating. Assign scores based on the following progression:

- *Normal function.* Patient denies any weakness or unusual fatigue of upper extremities. Examination demonstrates no abnormality.

- *Suspected fatigue.* Patient suspects fatigue in upper extremities during exertion. Cannot sustain work for as long as normal. Atrophy not evident on examination.

- *Slow self-care performance.* Dressing and hygiene are performed more slowly than previously.

- *Effortful self-care performance.* Patient requires significantly more time (usually double or more) and effort to accomplish self-care. Weakness is apparent on examination.

- *Mostly independent.* Patient handles most aspects of dressing and hygiene alone. Adapts by resting, modifying (using electric razor), or avoiding some tasks (buttoning, tying).

- *Partial independence.* Patient handles some aspects of dressing and hygiene alone. However, patient routinely requires assistance for many tasks, such as applying makeup, combing, and shaving.

- *Attendant assists patient.* Attendant must be present for dressing and hygiene. Patient performs the majority of each task with the assistance of the attendant.

- *Patient assists attendant.* Attendant must participate in almost all tasks. Patient moves in a purposeful manner to assist the attendant. Patient does not initiate self-care tasks.

- *Minimal movement.* Minimal movement of one or both arms is present. Patient cannot reposition arms.

- *Paralysis.* Flaccid paralysis is present. Patient is unable to move upper extremities (except perhaps to close inspection).

What Approaches to Speech Treatment Are Available to Individuals with ALS?

Before describing the staging of specific approaches to intervention, we will outline the philosophy and principles that guide our clinical management decisions. The handout "Ways You Can Compensate for Dysarthria" offers information for managing speech treatment and is found in the Appendix at the back of the book.

PRINCIPLES OF INTERVENTION

Loss of the ability to communicate or even the prospect of that loss is one of the most distressing aspects of ALS. There are few aspects of adult lives that are not affected by reduced communication capabilities. Basic communication functions, such as the expression of wants and needs and the provision of information, may not be affected unless communication disorders are severe, but difficulty maintaining social closeness may arise at any level of communication impairment. We work aggressively to maintain ALS patients' ability to communicate, either in the form of natural speech or with assistive technology. We believe that maintenance of communication is essential to preserve some sense of control for individuals with ALS. Communication competence and the control it brings ensures that patients will maintain the ability to guide, direct, and influence the management of both medical and personal aspects of their lives.

Intervene Early

The first principle of management is early intervention. Attempts to manage the communication and swallowing needs of individuals with end-stage ALS are often frustrating. Although these people's needs are urgent and profound, intervention is often inadequate because of factors such as untreated secondary complications, patients and families who are unable to make informed decisions during times of crisis, lack of time or energy to implement intervention, and increasing emotional lability. Since establishing an outpatient clinic where early intervention is a primary goal, we have found this approach to be beneficial in a number of ways:

1. Early intervention allows the team to develop relationships with the patient and family.

2. The team can provide information regarding the disorder and how to deal with it at a pace at which the family can assimilate it and at the times when it is needed.

3. One of our chief goals is to help the patient and family become informed consumers of medical and technological services. This task can be accomplished only through education.

4. Early intervention also allows for the gradual introduction of technology, usually beginning with "light-tech" solutions for specific communication needs and, as the disorder progresses, gradually more compensation and perhaps more technologically sophisticated solutions.

The insidious decrease of motor control characteristic of ALS results in gradually changing communication needs, with a shift from reliance on natural speech to more and more dependence on technological and human assistance. In the early stages of the communication disorder, individuals with ALS tend to rely on their residual speech for most communication purposes. As their impairment becomes more severe, they may begin to use multiple communication approaches, depending on their communication partner, the context, and the communicative intent.

Focus on Communication Function
Rather Than on Speech Impairment

The focus of our intervention is on the maintenance of functional communication rather than on the reduction of the speech impairment. Unfortunately, we currently have no way to halt the progressive weakness and loss of function in the muscles of the speech mechanism. Intervention whose goal is to stabilize the speech impairment may be doomed to fail. For example, strengthening exercises may be counterproductive in a number of ways. There is some evidence that exercising to fatigue hastens neurological deterioration. Drills and exercise may so fatigue the person that the adequacy of speech production in natural settings may suffer. Finally, drills and exercise in which maximum performance is attempted and measured may serve as a demoralizing yardstick to monitor symptom progression. If, on the other hand, your intervention goals are to maintain communication function, compensatory techniques or alternative modes of communication can be employed to successfully accomplish your goals.

Acknowledge the Emotional and
Psychosocial Aspects of the Disease

Communication problems in ALS are part of a complex of physical and psychosocial problems. Because ALS is a disorder that ultimately results in generalized weakness, communication disorders must not be viewed apart from other medical, physical, and psychosocial consequences of the impairment. Individuals with ALS and their family members often face decisions about wheelchairs, beds, vans, aspirators, and ventilators in addition to communication devices. In many cases, we provide intervention when patients and their families are making difficult decisions regarding issues of death and dying. These multiple decisions can be overwhelming, especially if they are delayed until a crisis point.

Intervene at Critical Periods

The final principle of our approach to communication management is intervention at critical periods. Although we monitor our patients at regular intervals of from 1 to 3 months depending on the progression of the disorder, our goal is that intervention occurs promptly and briefly at critical points. These critical points are periods when the person's capabilities have changed and communication needs are not being met, but before fatigue and weakness are overwhelming. Identification and anticipation of these critical periods require that individuals with ALS be monitored, but it is rare to see an individual with ALS for speech therapy sessions over extended periods of time.

STAGING OF INTERVENTION

Earlier in this chapter, we outlined use of the Speech Subscale of the ALS Severity Scale to describe the progression of speech deficits. We also use the subscale as a means of staging intervention and defining critical periods. The major subheadings of the scale correspond nicely with the critical periods of intervention. The first critical period may occur at the time of diagnosis, even when motor speech capabilities are within normal limits (a scale score of 9 or 10). The intervention here is primarily to provide information and confirm the normalcy of speech. The second critical period corresponds to a Speech Subscale score of 7 or 8, when speech becomes noticeably impaired. At the point where a speech disorder is detectable, we advise the person to use strategies and techniques to modify the environment so that communication is as easy as possible. Again, provision of information is critical; in particular, we provide techniques to maximize practical interaction skills as well as techniques to maintain the best possible speech production. The next critical period occurs at a Speech Subscale score of 5 or 6, when we assist patients to develop behavioral techniques for modifying speech production. For example, we might teach energy-conservation techniques that modify respiratory patterns for speech. Other techniques involve selection of the most appropriate speaking rate and development of skills for resolving communication breakdowns. The final critical period of communication intervention occurs when natural speech is not sufficient to meet the person's communication needs. At this point, with a Speech Subscale score of 4 or less, alternative means of communication must be identified and implemented. The staging of speech intervention in ALS is summarized in Table 1.12. The following sections provide details of each intervention stage.

Stage 1. Normal Speech Processes

Symptoms. Individuals who receive a rating of 10 or 9 on the Speech Subscale of the ALS Severity Scale are functionally normal communicators. In the case of a rating of 9, only the patient or spouse may note some change from premorbid levels.

With the encouraging developments in course-altering drugs, the neurology community is increasingly interested in early diagnosis of bulbar symptoms. The speech–language pathologist can contribute important information in this area. Early changes in speech production have been investigated with a variety of research approaches. Studies of articulatory errors suggest that certain phonetic contrasts are particularly vulnerable to degeneration in ALS (Riddel, McCauley, Mulligan, & Tandan, 1995). A relatively high frequency of errors involving voicing may indicate that laryngeal involvement is an early sign of speech changes. Studies using acoustic analysis techniques have also suggested early changes in the periodicity of vocal fold diadochokinesis (Renout, Leeper, Bandur, & Hudson, 1995), consonant production (Tomik et al., 1999), and several parameters of voice including jitter and coefficient of variation for frequency (Robert, Pouget, Giovanni, Azulay, & Triglia, 1999). Changes in frequency range and phonatory stability have been shown to occur even before perceptual changes in voice can be identified (Silbergleit, Johnson, & Jacobson, 1997). Subtle changes in speaking rate may also signal early bulbar involvement (Ball, Beukelman, & Pattee, 2000; Nishio & Niimi, 2000). In a study of 218 individuals with ALS, Ball, Willis, Beukelman, and Pattee (2001) identified a series of early

TABLE 1.12

Summary of Speech Intervention in ALS

	Normal Speech Processes	Detectable Speech Disturbance	Behavioral Modification	Use of Augmentative Communication (AAC)	Loss of Useful Speech
Presenting Features	No changes or minimal changes are detected Changes are noticed by unfamiliar partners	Symptoms worsen with fatigue	Some reduction in speech intelligibility	Needs AAC system as primary or secondary system	No functional natural speech
Intervention	Confirm normalcy Answer questions	Minimize environmental adversity Establish context of message Maximize hearing of partners Teach strategies for coping with groups	Maintain slow speaking rate Conserve energy Fit with palatal lift Develop breakdown resolution strategies Increase the precision of speech production	Begin alphabet supplementation Suggest changing mode in different situations Set up alerting systems Teach strategies for telephone communication Introduce portable writing systems Introduce multi-purpose commu-nication systems	Develop adequate yes/no system Develop eye-gaze systems Enable communication for patients on ventilators

predictors of speech change including laryngeal control as reflected in voice quality, speaking rate, and listener ratings of communication effectiveness.

Intervention. At this point, behavioral intervention is, of course, not necessary. The "expert" providing the "good news" that all is going well in terms of speech is, however, usually appreciated by patients. They will often comment that this is the only good news they have heard recently. The major role of a speech–language pathologist at this point is the provision of information. We find that patients vary tremendously in their understanding of the disease and need for information. Some clearly indicate that they do not wish further information. Others will ask pointed questions about the likelihood of future speech problems. Still others will request technology long before their level of speech function dictates the need for it. Our general policy is to give patients the opportunity to ask questions but to provide only the information they request. At times, patients will begin to ask pressing questions only after the initial visit, when a relationship of trust has been established.

When patients request technology prematurely, we respond that we are unable to predict whether they will ever need it. We also share with them our hope that it will not become necessary. Should technology become necessary, we are unable to predict the specific characteristics of the device the person will need. Thus, prematurely prescribed technology is unlikely to be useful. We provide early "informational" visits to our Assistive Technology Center for patients interested in seeing a variety of communication technologies. These visits communicate a number of messages. The first is that many options are available that can be used regardless of residual motor capabilities. Second, light-tech solutions may meet needs in certain areas that families may not previously have identified—for example, simple alerting systems to gain the attention of someone in another room. Finally, patients and their families are reassured that expertise is available and that intervention will be available at the appropriate time. The handout "Augmentative Communication" found in the Appendix at the back of the book provides helpful information for patients and their families.

Stage 2. Detectable Speech Disturbance

Symptoms. Individuals who receive a rating of 7 or 8 report noticeable changes in speech which are made worse by fatigue or stress. Despite obvious changes, speech remains intelligible.

Intervention. Management of speech symptoms at this stage of the disorder involves what Berry and Sanders (1983) call "environmental education." They suggest that the intelligibility of dysarthric speakers can be improved by applying the principles traditionally used in aural rehabilitation to assist people with hearing impairments. Intervention at this stage involves optimizing the "signal-independent" information in the communication environment (Yorkston, Strand, & Kennedy, 1996). In other words, speakers can often compensate for their highly distorted speech signals by supplementing them with information from a variety of sources including semantic and syntactic context, situational cues, alphabet supplementation, and the use of gestures or illustrators. The following is a list of some techniques that may facilitate communication in natural communication settings.

Minimize Environmental Adversity. Some communication situations are difficult even for those with normal speech. Consider how tiring it can be to carry on a conversation in noisy, dimly lit, or crowded surroundings. Our advice to people with intelligible but dysarthric speech is to modify the environment to make communication as easy and effortless as possible. Noise is the first factor to evaluate. This is particularly troublesome to dysarthric speakers with ALS because there is a natural tendency to try to "talk over" the noise. For individuals with poor respiratory support, efforts to increase speech loudness can be extremely fatiguing. Instead, we suggest that, when possible, the noise be reduced. When the patient is engaged in conversation, the television and radio should be turned off. When possible, put the patient in control of setting TV and radio loudness levels. One husband reported that in the evening when they were watching television, his wife with ALS was "in charge" of the TV's remote control. Lowering the volume was the signal that she was about to say something and that he should pay attention.

If noise cannot be reduced in a particular situation, dysarthric speakers and their communication partners should move away from the source of the noise. The visual aspects of the environment may also influence the ease of communication. A well-lighted, face-to-face conversation promotes speech intelligibility. We advise our patients with ALS, "If your communication partner is too far away, don't try to talk louder. Rather, move closer to your listener."

Establish the Context of the Message. When the speech signal is degraded, as it is in dysarthria, predictable messages are more easily understood than unpredictable ones. It is wise, therefore, to introduce the topic if it is not predictable from the situation. For example, the speaker might introduce a topic with the phrase, "I want to talk about the holidays." This draws the listener's full attention to the topic. Dysarthric speakers should confirm their partners' understanding of the topic before proceeding. A speaker with severe dysarthria may need to use the most intelligible mode of communication to deliver the topic introduction. This may either be the person's "best" speech, delivered as clearly and distinctly as possible, or an alternative mode such as oral spelling or writing. Setting the context of the message should be done whenever a topic is changed abruptly within a conversation.

Maximize the Hearing of Frequent Communication Partners. Because ALS typically occurs in an older population, hearing loss in spouses of individuals with ALS is not uncommon. Even mild hearing loss may compound speech intelligibility problems in dysarthria, and individuals with a hearing loss may experience difficulty understanding dysarthric speech when others do not. Therefore, we ask about the hearing status of the people who frequently communicate with our patients. If there is any suggestion of hearing impairment, we refer them for audiologic evaluation and management.

Teach Strategies for Coping with Groups. Individuals with ALS at this level of severity frequently complain that communication in a group is difficult. Apparently, any reduction in the clarity or rating of communication interferes with the ability to function in groups, where success is dependent on the quickness of the speaker. Many aspects of group conversation are dependent on rapid pacing of exchanges. When important issues are being discussed, the group size should be small. When communication in a large group is necessary, we recommend that speakers with ALS position themselves so that all members of the group can see them. In this way, the communication partners can not only watch them as they speak but also watch for nonverbal signals that they wish to speak.

Many individuals with ALS also find it useful to talk with their friends and frequent communication partners about techniques to facilitate communication. An individual with ALS might tell a friend, "Even though I'm slow, let me finish what I have to say" or "It takes me a minute to get started talking, so give me a little extra time when I look like I have something to say" or "If you haven't understood what I have said, be sure to let me know." Openly discussing the communication problem and specifying the "rules of the game" for communication partners has at least two advantages. First, the guidelines suggested by the dysarthric speaker will probably improve intelligibility. Second, they may also be of benefit in making the communication partners more comfortable with their new communicative role.

Stage 3. Behavioral Modifications

Symptoms. Individuals who receive a rating of 5 or 6 are experiencing some reduction in speech intelligibility, especially in adverse listening conditions. They frequently will need to repeat portions of a message in order to resolve communication breakdowns.

Intervention. In addition to the environmental management techniques described earlier, intervention may involve some of the following procedures. Extensive behavior training usually is not necessary because of preserved cognition, gradual onset of symptoms, and good compensatory skills.

Maintain a Slow Speaking Rate. Individuals at this stage of ALS have already experienced a slowing of their speaking rate. They should be encouraged not to try to normalize their rate by speaking as fast as they previously did. Encourage them instead to maintain a slowed rate and attempt to exaggerate their speech, especially important words that they wish to stress or make prominent. They should be counseled that weak or spastic muscles in the speech mechanism cause the slow rate. Attempts to increase rate most typically have the negative consequence of articulatory undershooting; that is, articulators simply do not reach their intended targets.

Conserve Energy. Individuals with ALS at this stage of severity often indicate to us that fatigue has a significant impact on the quality of their speech. Therefore, we discuss with them a number of energy-conservation techniques. Perhaps the most obvious way to conserve energy and avoid fatigue is to discourage the person from exercising in the hope of strengthening weakened speech muscles. Patients frequently ask for exercise routines. We indicate to them that there is no evidence to suggest that exercising will improve the speech of individuals with ALS; rather, it appears that exercise to the point of fatigue may increase the rate at which motor function is lost.

One of the most fatiguing aspects of speech production for individuals with ALS is developing sufficient respiratory support to speak loudly. By avoiding noisy communication situations or situations where the listener is at a considerable distance from the speaker, individuals with ALS can reduce some of the energy demands associated with speech production.

As the disease progresses, it may be difficult for speakers to maintain a normal breath group pattern. If this is the case, counsel them to reduce the length of breath groups rather than to attempt to speak at inappropriately low lung volumes. Speech produced at low lung volumes requires considerably more effort than speech produced at more appropriate levels. If a speaker attempts to talk as long as possible on one breath, the last several words are usually "squeezed out" only with excessive effort.

If muscles continue to weaken, such behavioral compensations as shortening breath groups may no longer be effective. At this time, amplification may be considered. Portable amplifiers are available and may lessen fatigue associated with speaking, especially for individuals with relatively preserved phonatory and oral articulatory function in the presence of reduced respiratory support.

Fit with a Palatal Lift. People with Stage 3 ALS may exhibit a number of symptoms related to inadequate velopharyngeal function. These may include excessively hypernasal speech, difficulty producing consonants requiring buildup of intraoral air pressure, and fatigue in speaking associated with the extra respiratory effort needed to compensate for loss of air through the nose. A palatal lift prosthesis is a well-documented technique to compensate for poor velopharyngeal valving (Yorkston et al., 2001). Recent reports indicate successful fitting of palatals in individuals with ALS (Esposito, Mitsumoto, & Shanks, 2000). Case studies have also been reported in which palatal lift fitting was associated with marked improvement in speech intelligibility, as well as beneficial changes in consonant production and intraoral air pressure (Roth, Roburka, & Workinger, 2000). Because of the degenerative nature of dysarthria in ALS, we use the following guidelines to evaluate candidacy for palatal lift fitting in this population:

1. Poor velopharyngeal function in the presence of relatively preserved lip and tongue movement

2. Preserved ability to swallow saliva

3. Adequate dentition to support the prosthesis

4. A relatively slow progression of the disorder, suggesting that the person will continue to rely on natural speech as the primary mode of communication for at least several months

Develop Strategies to Resolve Communication Breakdowns. Although natural speech remains a functional mode of communication for individuals at this stage of ALS, intelligibility is frequently compromised, and resolution of communication breakdowns is often necessary. Counsel patients to pay close attention to their communication partners and to learn to read the signals that their message has not been understood. Frequent communication partners should be encouraged to develop a signaling system they can use to indicate to the dysarthric speaker that some portion of the message is not being understood. It is usually more difficult to resolve communication breakdowns if the listener waits until the end of the entire message before alerting the speaker to the problem. The need to repeat an entire message may be not only frustrating but also fatiguing for a person with ALS.

People with severe dysarthria and their frequent communication partners may adopt the following sequence as they resolve communication breakdowns:

1. The listener alerts the speaker to the problem. Most people prefer to use a nonverbal rather than a verbal signal.

2. The listener waits for the speaker to stop. At times, the speaker may wish to continue if he or she feels the message will be understood when the complete message is produced.

3. The listener tells the speaker what was understood. In this way, the speaker need not repeat the entire message, just the part that has not been understood.

4. The speaker repeats the message as distinctly as possible using the same wording as in the first attempt.

5. If this fails, the speaker rewords the message.

6. If this fails, an alternative communication mode is used—for example, orally spelling the misunderstood word or writing a portion of the message.

Increase the Precision of Speech Production. We have indicated before that speakers with ALS frequently are functioning as well as possible in light of their physiologic impairment. Therefore, formal speech training is rarely necessary. However, in our clinic we do spend some time helping patients develop techniques that will allow them to "switch into high gear" when necessary. These techniques encourage the production of "clear speech" (Picheny, Durlach, & Braida, 1986, 1989) and may include increasing precision by slowing articulatory rate, exaggerating oral articulatory movements, paying special attention to inclusion of final consonants, and, as much as possible, increasing the overall forcefulness with which speech is produced. Individuals at this level of severity do not usually use these techniques all the time but call them into play when listeners have failed to understand a message or when they must communicate with an unfamiliar partner.

Stage 4. Use of Augmentative Communication

Symptoms. Individuals who receive a rating of 3 or 4 must rely on augmentative systems, either as their primary means of communication or to supplement natural speech when it is not understood.

Intervention. The transition to reliance on augmentative communication approaches is one of the major critical periods in the management of individuals with

ALS. Acceptance of technology is influenced by a number of factors including previous experience with technology (Doyle & Phillips, 2001). The issue of acceptance is receiving increasing attention in the research literature (Lasker & Bedrosian, 2001; Zeitlin, Abrams, & Shah, 1995). The following section describes several basic types of augmentative communication.

Alphabet Supplementation. Alphabet supplementation is a transitional technique that may bridge the gap between total reliance on natural speech and dependence on augmentative communication technology. Speakers with dysarthria can be encouraged to point to the first letter of each word as they speak. This technique is useful for individuals whose natural speech is difficult to understand but may still be functional for some types of communication, with some communication partners, or in particular communication settings.

First-letter pointing has a number of advantages. First, it allows the individual to continue to use natural speech longer than would be possible without it. Second, pointing to the initial letter of each word slows the person's speaking rate, separating words and allowing weakened muscles more time to achieve articulatory targets. Finally, it provides a ready means of resolving communication breakdowns, as the user can simply spell messages that have not been understood. In our clinic, we have alphabet boards in several sizes. All are arranged in alphabetic order. We use the enlarging/reduction feature of a copy machine to create the display size that each individual prefers. We find that most people prefer a small size that they can carry in a purse or pocket. A small alphabet board may also avoid the fatigue associated with larger movements.

Alerting Systems. Natural speech serves so many purposes so easily that we tend to overlook some of its most basic functions. One such basic function is calling attention or alerting. Frequently, individuals with ALS will not have the respiratory drive to generate a voice loud enough to call their partner in the next room. Among the most popular devices in the lending library of equipment are alerting systems. These can take the form either of simple buzzers or of devices such as baby monitors that transmit signals to distant locations within the house.

Telephone Communication. The perceived need for telephone communication varies considerably among individuals with ALS. For some, there is little perceived need because they are rarely without an attendant or family member to assist them. For others, occasional telephone use is necessary for periods of time when the person is alone. This need is especially important because the telephone may serve to summon help in an emergency. In many areas, the location of every caller to 911 is automatically identified for the emergency response team. For individuals in rural areas, loop tape systems may be used to prepare emergency messages. Services that help speakers with dysarthria communicate on the telephone are also available. Finally, one of the features that leads some individuals to select multipurpose augmentative communication equipment is the feature of synthesized speech that may be employed for telephone as well as face-to-face communication. It has been our experience that speech output devices are most successful when the listener is familiar with their use. The length of time required to prepare a message, along with speech that is often less than perfectly intelligible, makes telephone communication with the naive public difficult.

Portable Writing Systems. A large proportion of our patients at this stage use portable writing systems to augment natural speech. These systems are typically introduced as backup systems to resolve communication breakdowns when natural speech has not been understood. They can also be used to introduce communicative topics when natural speech is difficult to understand. As the dysarthria progresses, patients may depend more and more heavily on writing. Portable writing systems fall into two broad categories: paper-and-pencil systems and the small handheld systems that print a "hard copy." It has been our experience that individuals with ALS who have the hand function to hold a pencil and write prefer to do so rather than using an electronic system. They report that handwriting is usually faster than typing and that the convenience of needing only a pad of paper and pencil outweighs the potential benefits of whole message retrieval available in some handheld electronic systems.

Multipurpose Systems. A number of computer-based multipurpose augmentative and alternative communication (AAC) systems are commercially available. We will not review these systems in detail because technology is changing so rapidly that today's systems will no doubt be replaced by more efficient and effective ones in the near future. Rather, readers are referred to a comprehensive Web site that provides links to vendors of AAC systems, device tutorials, and other current information (University of Nebraska, AAC Center, http://aac.unl.edu/). Readers are also referred to the nonprofit organization called Communication Independence for the Neurologically Impaired (CINI; http://www.cini.org/). This organization disseminates information about communication technology to individuals with ALS and their families (Kazandjian, 1997).

Classification of Functional Capabilities. Selection of appropriate augmentative communication systems depends on a variety of factors. Among the most important of these factors in the ALS population is the user's level of mobility and hand function. For example, can the person access an augmentative communication system via a keyboard? Is handwriting an acceptable means of resolving communication problems in face-to-face situations? Is the person walking normally or with assistance of devices such as walkers or canes? Is the person wheelchair dependent?

The functional capabilities of individuals with ALS vary along a number of dimensions. Speech adequacy, hand function, and mobility are critical when considering augmentative communication intervention. One way of providing an overview of augmentative communication needs in the ALS population is to divide the population into six groups based on these critical factors. For purposes of the following discussion, Speech Subscale scores of 5 and above are considered adequate, in that natural speech remains a functional means of communication. Thus, poor speech is defined as a Speech Subscale Score of 4 or less. Similarly, poor hand function is defined as an Upper Extremity Subscale score of 4 or less. In contrast, poor mobility is defined as a Lower Extremity Subscale score of 6 or less, thus including people who are still walking but who are in need of assistive devices such as canes and walkers. We have placed these individuals in the poor mobility category because augmentative equipment must be both lightweight and portable to be functional for them. Individuals with ALS can be divided into six groups based on their functional capabilities (Yorkston et al., 1993). Descriptions of these groups follow.

Group 1: Adequate Speech and Adequate Hand Function. The largest group (approximately half of our clinic patients) are individuals who have both adequate speech and adequate upper extremity function. For these people, augmentative communication intervention involves monitoring their status and providing them with whatever information they request.

Group 2: Adequate Speech and Poor Hand Function. The next largest group (approximately 20%) are those who have adequate speech but poor upper extremity function. Depending on their lifestyles and communication needs, these individuals may need access to an augmentative communication system other than handwriting to supplement speech.

Group 3: Poor Speech, Adequate Hand Function, and Adequate Mobility. Severe dysarthria but adequate upper and lower extremity functions characterize the next largest group. Many of these individuals continue to speak using alphabet supplementation (first-letter pointing). Many resolve communication breakdowns by writing. More sophisticated means of augmentative communication, perhaps utilizing speech synthesis or loop tapes, are necessary if independent telephone communication is an urgent need. Attention-getting devices such as buzzers are often a priority for people in all capability groups where speech is rated as poor.

Group 4: Poor Speech, Adequate Hand Function, and Poor Mobility. Severe dysarthria and poor mobility but adequate hand function characterize approximately 10% of our clinic population. In many ways, the augmentative communication needs of this group are similar to those of Group 3 except that selecting highly portable, lightweight systems is often not as critical because the equipment can be mounted on the person's wheelchair.

Group 5: Poor Speech, Poor Hand Function, and Good Mobility. The smallest group is probably also the most difficult to serve adequately in terms of technology. A small proportion of our clinic population (2%–5%) is made up of individuals with severe dysarthria and poor hand function, but adequate mobility. Thus, in selecting their augmentative communication systems, we need to take into account both the feasibility of alternative access and also the need for it to be lightweight and highly portable, because the system frequently needs to be carried rather than mounted on a wheelchair.

Group 6: Poor Speech, Poor Hand Function, and Poor Mobility. Severe dysarthria may also be present along with poor hand function and poor mobility. For these individuals, alternative access to augmentative systems often is necessary, and frequently consists of switches and scanning systems. Augmentative communication systems used by this group do not need to be extremely lightweight because they are typically mounted on a wheelchair.

Patterns of System Use. Reports of patterns of AAC system use in ALS are beginning to appear in the literature. Users generally report employing a collection of systems at any given time (Mathy, Yorkston, & Gutmann, 2000). They tend to use their unassisted and low-technology systems (e.g., alphabet boards) for communicating in conversation and to indicate quick needs and wants, and their high-technology systems for communicating detailed needs and wants, written communications, and stories. Familiarity with the communication partner influences the selection of the AAC system. Individuals generally reported great satisfaction with their collection of methods with the exception of conversation, which was rated much less satisfactory than written communication. This result may be explained by the fact that written communication is a solitary activity that proceeds at one's own pace, while conversation is a rapid exchange of ideas, opinions, and information.

Patterns of AAC system use also change over time for individuals with ALS. Doyle and Phillips (2001) followed the AAC usage patterns of 4 individuals. They found that individuals with ALS relied more heavily on unaided or low-technology approaches in the early stage. In the middle stages they relied increasingly on high-technology options, whereas in the late stages they returned to low-technology approaches. The authors suggest that individuals do not abandon high-technology options in late stages; rather, they appear to reserve the use of electronic devices for specific activities and communication partners.

A small proportion of individuals with ALS wish to continue to work despite severe functional limitations. AAC systems are particularly critical for these individuals. McNaughton, Light, and Groszyk (2001) conducted an Internet focus group discussion with 5 individuals with ALS who continued to work. The participants who clearly described the benefits of work also identified a series of barriers to employment including physical, technological, attitudinal, and policy barriers. Most felt there were also important information barriers with one participant stating, "nearly everything I have learned [about AAC] I have learned on my own" (p. 188). The comments of these participants were summarized in a list of recommendations to policy makers, employers, service providers, technology developers, and individuals with ALS (see Table 1.13).

Funding of AAC Systems. Important changes in the funding of AAC systems have recently occurred. As of January 2001, Medicare covers and provides reimbursement for some AAC devices called "speech generating devices." These devices are now classified as "durable medical equipment." They are available to Medicare beneficiaries when the beneficiary (a) is enrolled in Medicare Part B; (b) lives in his or her family home or an assisted living facility (but not in a hospital, skilled nursing facility, or hospice); and (c) is determined, following an assessment by a speech–language pathologist, to require an AAC device to meet daily functional communication needs, and has a physician prescribe the AAC device. Readers are referred to the Rehabilitation Engineering Research Center on Communication Enhancement Web site (http://aac-rerc.com/) for a complete description of the process for applying for this funding.

Stage 5. Loss of Useful Speech

Symptoms. Individuals who receive a rating of 1 or 2 have lost natural speech as a functional means of communication. Therefore, they must rely entirely on alternative communication technology and techniques.

Intervention. Many of the issues and communication techniques just described for individuals in Stage 4 (Use of Augmentative Communication) are also appropriate for individuals in Stage 5.

Yes/No Systems. Establishing a nonfatiguing and reliable means of indicating yes or no is a mandatory element of communication management plans for individuals with ALS who no longer have functional natural speech. The development of an adequate yes/no system typically involves a series of tasks. The first is to identify a reliable motor response. Natural gestures such as head nods and shakes are preferred. Some individuals with ALS no longer have the ability to move their heads or use their hands, however. Fortunately, eye movements are usually preserved in even the most severe cases of ALS.

The second task is to train individuals with ALS and their frequent communication partners in the use of the system. Effectively asking and answering yes/no questions is more challenging than it might initially appear. We suggest a question-

TABLE 1.13	Recommendations To Facilitate Employment for Individuals with ALS Who Use AAC	

Audience	Recommended Actions
Policy makers	Enforce laws that support the rights of people with disabilities
	Increase prevalence of long-term care insurance
	Increase funding of assistive technologies
	Provide options for leasing of equipment
	Support equipment exchange programs
	Guarantee access to medical insurance for all
	Ensure availability of personal care service
	Ensure availability of transportation services
Employers	Learn about ALS
	Facilitate changes in job responsibilities
	Provide training for new jobs that are more appropriate
	Support appropriate benefits for employees
Service providers	Provide ongoing technical support
	Provide ongoing services as needs and skills change
	Introduce AAC options early, before decline of natural speech
	Provide computer training for Internet access and communication
	Increase training of service providers in ALS and AAC
Technology developers	Decrease learning demands
	Provide instruction/documentation on the Internet
	Improve quality of speech output
	Develop lighter, smaller, more portable systems
	Design more attractive systems
	Increase diversity of functions in systems (e.g., cellular phones)
	Increase battery life
People with ALS	Seek out and share information about ALS; educate employers and coworkers regarding ALS
	Be knowledgeable; know and understand legislation
	Recognize that ALS will require changes in job and lifestyle
	Propose accommodations to facilitate continued employment
	Advocate for yourself and others with ALS
	Accept AAC; learn AAC technologies early on
	Make decisions based on personal preferences and needs

Note. Adapted from "Don't Give Up: Employment Experiences of Individuals with Amyotrophic Lateral Sclerosis," by D. McNaughton, J. Light, and L. Groszyk, 2001, *Augmentative and Alternative Communication, 17*(3), pp. 179–195. Copyright 2001 by the International Society for Augmentative and Alternative Communication. Adapted with permission.

asking strategy in which general questions about the topic are asked first, and then more and more specific information is sought. Many of our patients prefer to have four responses available rather than just two, so they can respond "yes," "no," "I don't know the answer to that question," or "Choose a new line of questioning." If the person with ALS is in a setting in which communication with many people is necessary, documentation of the system needs to be written and posted in places where communication typically occurs.

Eye-Gaze Systems. Because eye gaze is usually preserved in individuals with ALS, eye pointing or eye gaze can frequently be used as a selection technique when head and hand movements are no longer functional. The person with ALS looks at a selected item (word or letter) long enough for the partner to identify the direction of the gaze and confirm the selected item. Eye-gaze systems can be quite complex and incorporate encoding strategies, so partner training is critical. More complete descriptions of selection techniques and encoding strategies are available (Beukelman & Mirenda, 1998).

Communication for Patients on Ventilators. The majority of individuals on ventilators also experience significant cranial nerve involvement. Because many of these individuals have poor oral movement, use of natural speech via a modified tracheostomy tube or electrolarynx is not possible. For these people, the eye-gaze augmentative communication system described earlier may be appropriate.

Swallowing Disorders

Swallowing difficulties generally parallel speech difficulties, but there is tremendous variability in individual rates of progression. It is important to be prepared for a sudden, rapid decline in skills.

What Is the Rate of Progression of Swallowing Problems in ALS?

As noted earlier, the rate of symptom progression in ALS is extremely variable. Although the disease is often described as relentlessly progressive, some individuals will stabilize or gradually progress over extended periods of time. Although the rate of progression of bulbar symptoms is difficult to predict, the sequence of symptom appearance is fairly predictable. In order to stage and deliver intervention in a timely fashion, one needs to understand this sequence of symptom appearance. Our clinical experience suggests that the time postdiagnosis has little value in predicting the extent of swallowing problems in individuals with ALS (Strand et al., 1996). There is, however, a strong relationship between swallowing symptoms and other bulbar functions such as motor speech. This relationship is illustrated in Figure 1.3, a scatterplot of Swallowing versus Speech Subscales on the ALS Severity Scale for approximately 200 consecutive patient visits. Note that for 71% of these individuals, swallowing and speech scores were within 1 point of one another. Thus, clinicians who work with individuals with ALS who have speech difficulties can expect to see swallowing disorders as well and vice versa.

It has been our experience that the best predictor for the immediate future of the swallowing status of someone with ALS comes from an understanding of that person's clinical history, including both current and previous speech and swallowing symptoms and the rates of progression of those symptoms. Because the ALS Severity Scale is an ordinal one, the progression of symptoms is built into the scale. Thus, we attempt to prepare individuals for the intervention that will be necessary for the difficulties described at 1 or 2 scale points lower than their current level. In our clinic population, there is a consistent pattern of decline if patients are followed for extended periods of time. However, considerable variability in rate of progression is also present. Thus, clinicians need to be prepared for change and for the possibility that the change may be relatively rapid.

How Is Swallowing Function Assessed in Individuals with ALS?

In addition to the physical examination described earlier, we use the Swallowing Subscale of the ALS Severity Scale and a detailed history as indicators of swallowing function. With

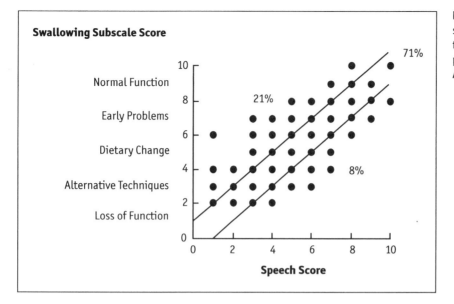

FIGURE 1.3. Swallowing versus Speech Subscale scores on the ALS Severity Scale for approximately 200 consecutive ALS patient visits.

all patients but those who have severe swallowing problems (those below a scale score of 4), we also observe them drinking water. In this way we can observe the behavioral modifications each person adopts and confirm the patient's report of presence or absence of difficulty with drinking thin liquids. The rate at which the person is able to swallow safely is also an excellent indicator of the general effort required to maintain fluid intake. Although we routinely ask about the occurrence of aspiration pneumonia, it is remarkably infrequent in individuals with ALS. Perhaps this low rate of occurrence is due to the gradual onset of the disease and intact sensation and cognitive function.

The patient interview related to swallowing disorders is summarized in the "Swallowing Disorders Interview Worksheet" in Chapter Appendix 1.3. This form contains the clinic visit data, Swallowing Subscale scores, and a checklist of patient complaints in the areas of saliva management, oral stage difficulty, pharyngeal stage difficulty, and general problems. This form allows one to track complaints over time and as a function of interventions, which are also noted on the worksheet. A weight-loss history is also documented on the worksheet. A careful dietary history, including estimates of total calorie intake and liquid intake per day, is part of the interview. We ask the patient to estimate time required for a typical meal. A record is maintained of all the patient's medications that have a potential effect on swallowing and nutritional management.

Understanding respiratory status is critical in management of swallowing disorders for a number of reasons. First, because respiration is momentarily interrupted during the pharyngeal phase of swallowing, individuals with severely compromised respiratory support may experience fatigue with eating that is unrelated to oral or pharyngeal weakness. Second, adequate respiratory support is needed for a productive cough, one of the primary defense mechanisms against aspiration. Finally, adequate respiratory status is critical when undergoing the surgical interventions described later in this chapter.

Impaired respiratory function is a progressive feature throughout the course of ALS. It is typically found earlier in the bulbar form of ALS than in the spinal form. Frequently, patients are unaware of a respiratory problem until it is relatively severe because their relative inactivity due to other muscle weakness makes them asymptomatic. A decline in respiratory function, as measured by vital capacity, parallels the decline in the Swallowing Subscale score. In our clinic population, vital capacity progressively declines with decreasing Swallowing Subscale scores (Strand et al., 1996).

When vital capacity is less than 50% of predicted (a percentage based on an individual's height and age), patients generally complain of respiratory fatigue. Vital capacities of less than 25% to 30% of predicted leave patients symptomatic and without sufficient respiratory reserve (Miller et al., 1999). Problems of secretion management, ineffective cough, and reduction in speech loudness become evident. In people with respiratory insufficiency, shortness of breath while eating may be evident. Because swallowing requires a momentary pause in respiration, and the duration of the swallow of individuals with ALS is prolonged, it is an ominous sign when the patient's respiratory reserve is inadequate to compensate for the required pause in breathing.

Monitoring of respiratory status is also necessary when attempting to stage surgical intervention for alternative means of feeding. Individuals with poor respiratory support are not good surgical candidates, even for procedures such as percutaneous endoscopic gastrostomy (PEG) that can be carried out under local anesthetic. In our clinic, we categorize respiratory status in three gross levels. Generally, we find individuals with a vital capacity greater than 75% to 80% of predicted to be asymptomatic. We place individuals with vital capacities between 75% and 50% of predicted into a marginal category, especially if surgical intervention is being considered. Finally, individuals with vital capacities of less than 50% are usually considered poorer candidates for surgical intervention. Note that individuals who need alternative means of feeding also are likely to exhibit marginal or poor respiratory status. Thus, at times, we recommend placement of an alternative feeding tube prior to the time when it is mandatory in terms of swallowing status. Such surgery needs to be performed before poor respiratory status makes the surgical risks too high.

Weight is measured at each clinic visit. Weight loss in ALS may be associated with failure to take in sufficient calories and fluids and, therefore, may be a useful indicator of the effectiveness of the management of swallowing disorders. Even when nutritional needs and hydration are managed adequately, however, weight loss may occur as a consequence of muscle loss or atrophy, a cardinal feature of the disorder. It has been demonstrated that survival time for patients with ALS is worse for those who are malnourished and those with reduced vital capacity. In one study, malnourished patients had a 7.7-fold increased risk of death (Desport et al., 1999). In some instances, malnutrition may develop in the absence of clinically significant dysphagia (Hardiman, 2000).

Specialists in radiology, gastroenterology, neurology, and pulmonary medicine are frequently consulted to assist in the management of specific needs of individuals with swallowing problems. For example, when swallowing complaints are inconsistent with the diagnosis of ALS or the complaints suggest problems in addition to those caused by the primary disease, videofluoroscopy of swallowing is performed.

What Approaches to Management Are Available for Swallowing Disorders in ALS?

Swallowing management in ALS can be staged according to the broad headings of the Swallowing Subscale previously described. A summary of this intervention can be found in Table 1.14.

STAGE 1. NORMAL EATING HABITS

Symptoms

People with spinal ALS or early bulbar ALS generally describe normal chewing, swallowing, and rate of eating. Some patients, when they receive the diagnosis of ALS and understand the implications of it, will experience sensations of obstruction or "gagging" for which there is no physical basis. These people should be reassured regarding the relationship between swallowing dysfunction and physical findings. Individuals with nominal abnormalities will often report food lodging in the gingivo-buccal sulcuses or food sticking in the throat. In most cases, detectable speech changes coincide with the first reports of swallowing difficulty, and Speech and Swallowing Subscale ratings tend to parallel each other throughout the course of the disease.

Intervention

Management during this stage involves education. This education includes confirming the normalcy of the swallowing function and alerting the person to symptoms that may occur as progression continues. Although no intervention is typically necessary at this stage of the disorder, patients and their families need to know when to return and seek further assistance. At this stage we may also provide patients and their families with factual material. (See "Amyotrophic Lateral Sclerosis (ALS)" in the Appendix at the back of the book.) This material describes the normal swallowing process and outlines some swallowing symptoms that may be expected in ALS.

TABLE 1.14	Summary of Swallowing Interventions in ALS			
	Early Swallowing Problems	**Dietary Consistency Changes**	**Unable To Meet Needs by Mouth**	**Salivary Problems**
Presenting Features	Solid foods difficult to eat Longer mealtimes Need for smaller bites	Weight loss Chronic dehydration Loss of enjoyment	Decline in calorie intake Decline in fluid intake Food spillage from mouth Respiratory fatigue	Complaints of too much saliva Complaints of drooling
Intervention	Use chin tuck position Maintain liquid intake Try drinking through a straw Eliminate caffeine Use double swallow Learn choking first aid Avoid washing food down with liquids	Change to soft diet Maintain liquid intake Eat calorie-dense foods Increase taste, temperature (colder), and texture sensations of liquids	Insert percutaneous endoscopic gastrostomy (PEG)	Maintain adequate hydration Use aspirator Use medication Surgically relocate salivary ducts

STAGE 2. EARLY EATING PROBLEMS

Symptoms

The second stage of swallowing difficulty is described as early eating problems. In people with early tongue, facial, and masticatory muscle weakness, prolonged mealtimes, chewing fatigue, and oral transport problems lead to difficulty eating solid foods. Foods with dry, crumbly textures (such as crackers and chips) present problems. Foods that require lengthy mastication and oral preparation (such as steak and leafy salads) may be difficult to manage. When tongue involvement, particularly spasticity, is combined with pharyngeal weakness, coughing with the ingestion of thin liquids often occurs early in disease progression. The first complaint is most frequently difficulty with drinking water or similar thin liquids. In many instances, patients consciously reduce their fluid intake because of difficulty in swallowing, and they present with mild chronic dehydration. This confounding condition produces changes in salivary consistency that the person describes as a thickening of secretions or even dryness of the mouth. Additionally, the person may suffer from excessive fatigue and malaise, which is associated with a chronic state of dehydration. In some cases, patients without signs of dysphagia will limit fluid intake because of the difficulty they experience in transferring to a toilet.

Intervention

At this stage, intervention involves behavioral compensations for swallowing difficulty. Patients should be trained in a number of swallowing techniques. For example, postural adjustments may decrease the instances of choking.

Use Chin Tuck Position. Because of the anatomic relationship between the deglutitory and respiratory tracts, the likelihood of aspiration into the airway is increased when the head and neck are in an extended posture, that is, when the head is back. Conversely, when the neck is flexed with the chin down toward the chest, the airway is practically blocked by the epiglottis, and the risk of aspiration is lessened. (See the illustration of proper and improper head positions on the "Ways You Can Compensate for Swallowing Difficulties" handout in the Appendix at the back of this book.)

Maintain Liquid Intake. At all stages of management of swallowing disorders in ALS, we recommend that patients drink at least 2 quarts of liquid per day. Included in this amount are all fluids that are liquid or that melt to a liquid. Caffeinic beverages do not count in liquid intake because of their diuretic properties. Some people find it helpful to use a straw for drinking. Use of a straw encourages proper head position but may be difficult for individuals with severe velopharyngeal or lip incompetence.

Use Double Swallow. Patients with early swallowing difficulties can be helped by increasing their concentration on some of the mechanics of swallowing. For example, the cough reflex is the final protective mechanism for the airway. Just prior to coughing there must be a quick intake of breath. If a patient has partially aspirated and is about to cough, the quick intake of air will suck the debris deeper into the airway. In order to avoid this, teach the person to take a breath before swallowing, hold the breath, forcefully exhale or gently cough after the swallow, and then swallow again (double swallow). This routine must become habitual in order to be helpful.

Learn First Aid for Choking. Health-care providers and family should be trained in techniques to assist patients who experience complete airway obstruction. It is important for them to recognize, however, that a person who is in the act of coughing does not have a completely obstructed airway, as air is passing around the blockage. In this case, one should allow the person every opportunity to clear the material using an unassisted cough.

Avoid Washing Foods Down with Liquids. Care providers and family members should also avoid having patients attempt to "wash down" partially swallowed food with liquids, as this combination can increase the chance for aspiration. The mealtime environment should be free from unnecessary distractions, and the patient must avoid talking while eating.

At this stage of intervention, we provide patients and their families with information on first aid for choking, the "Emergency Plan" handout, and the "Ways You Can Compensate for Swallowing Difficulties" in the Appendix at the back of the book. The latter information sheet can be individualized for each patient by checking the items that are especially important.

STAGE 3: DIETARY CONSISTENCY CHANGES

Symptoms

The third stage of swallowing difficulty begins with a requirement to modify the consistency of the diet. At this point, the person has gone beyond eliminating certain foods that require excessive chewing or that have a tendency to stick because of dryness or leafy texture. The person begins to need special meal preparation—for example, adding sauces or gravies to the menu when they otherwise would not be included. In some cases, the person will use a blender to create puréed textures or even resort to a completely liquid diet. Most of these people will also experience difficulty maintaining an adequate fluid intake, and weight loss may be a prominent feature. Once the person enters this stage of dietary consistency changes and special food preparation, there is frequently a loss of enjoyment associated with eating.

Intervention

In addition to the suggestions appropriate for early swallowing problems, the following techniques may be applied as swallowing problems worsen.

Change to Soft Diet. Dietary modification in many cases can allow a person to continue an adequate oral intake despite increasing swallowing difficulty. Modification of food texture is a key strategy. Moist foods—such as puddings, fruits, sauces, and gravy-covered foods—are fairly easily handled. Foods that fall apart—such as puréed foods and applesauce—are not easily handled. In addition, the strategy of adding pills to applesauce to aid in their ingestion is usually not successful. Foods that do not fall apart are thick puddings, gelatin, and custards. It is advisable to avoid dry, sticky foods, such as mashed potatoes (although gravy helps), dry casseroles, unripe bananas, bakery goods, and ground meat (broth does not help, although gravy does). Constipation is a frequent complaint in individuals with ALS who have weakened abdominal musculature. Therefore, a high-fiber diet including such foods as chopped vegetables, shredded lettuce, and bran is recommended.

Maintain Liquid Intake. The biggest problem in terms of oral management of dysphagia is usually the adequate intake of fluid. Fluids that are effective in reducing the osmotic load are usually the most difficult to swallow. Fluids such as milk shakes and prepared formulas, although somewhat easier to swallow, do not provide adequate free fluid. Foods that increase liquid ingestion are gelatin, frozen flavored ice pops, frozen juices, sherbets, and fruit ices. It is advisable to record liquid intake and output for a person with dysphagia on an intermittent basis to ensure a consistent habit of adequate fluid intake. Chronic dehydration is insidious in onset, as the fluid deficit is created over a long period of time. Its symptoms, although masked, can be severe and life-threatening.

Eat Calorie-Dense Foods. As swallowing problems increase, it is important to modify the diet so that every bite counts. This typically involves changing to calorie-dense foods. Examples are whole milk rather than skim milk and rich sauces and gravies rather than thin broths. Preliminary reports suggest that some ALS patients have diets chronically deficient in carbohydrates and need to augment their intake of energy foods (Kasarskis, Berryman, Vanderleest, Schneider, & McClain, 1996).

Increase Taste, Temperature, and Texture Sensations of Liquids. Modifications in food preparation can also increase the likelihood of success in swallowing. These modifications apply especially to liquids and consist of techniques to enhance sensory stimulation during swallowing. Chilling liquids provides a temperature sensation that can aid in the detection of the fluid during swallowing. This temperature advantage is usually not achieved by serving hot liquids, as the tolerance for ingestion of hot liquids is limited. Most people handle hot liquids by cooling them significantly before ingestion and by further cooling them in the oral cavity before they reach the pharynx. Most people have a fair tolerance for cold liquids, however. The texture of liquids can also be modified to provide an increase in sensation by adding carbonation. Carbonated beverages have a quality of gentle irritation that can reinforce sensory input. Another factor that aids in the detection of fluids is taste. In effect, the most difficult fluid to swallow is room-temperature water, whereas the fluid that provides the greatest sensation is a chilled, carbonated soft drink.

At this stage of intervention, we provide patients and their families with the "Dietary Changes To Compensate for Swallowing Difficulties" handout found in the Appendix at the back of the book. This information sheet can be individualized for each patient by checking the items that are especially important.

STAGE 4. NEEDS TUBE FEEDING

Symptoms
Loss of enjoyment of meals often leads to a dread of mealtimes. It is at this point that most people enter the fourth stage of dysphagia, the need for tube feeding. This category includes all patients who use tubes for primary feeding, those who require tube feeding to supplement oral intake, and those who, in your judgment, should be using a tube. Choking episodes, food spillage, the need for special meal preparation, prolonged mealtimes, and respiratory or chewing fatigue all contribute to an aversion to eating in individuals at this stage.

Intervention
A variety of enteral accesses are available. These include intermittent orogastric tube passage, nasogastric tubes, cervical esphagostomy, percutaneous endoscopic gastrostomy (PEG), standard gastrostomy, and jejunostomy. Although all procedures may be used for specific patients, the PEG is most commonly used in our clinic.

The insertion of a percutaneous endoscopic gastrostomy tube is a way of placing a feeding tube while avoiding complicated surgery. Although there are several variations on the technique, generally patients are given a local anesthetic to the site at which the tube is placed. A surgeon places an endoscope through the patient's mouth and into the stomach. As the surgeon views the stomach lining to determine the insertion site, a small incision is made in the abdominal wall. The PEG tube then lies in the stomach and exits through the skin of the abdomen. The procedure generally lasts from 30 to 45 minutes.

Among the variations for placing a feeding tube, one involves placing the tube in the jejunum, a portion of the small intestine. This procedure is used for those patients who have significant gastroesophageal reflux. This can be performed either by placing the tube directly through an abdominal wall incision into the jejunum (PEJ), a procedure very similar to a PEG, or by threading a thinner tube through a PEG tube and advancing it into the jejunum (PEG/PEJ or jPEG). The "Gastroesophageal Reflux Disease (GERD)" handout found in the Appendix at the back of the book provides helpful information for patients and their families.

Timing of Intervention

It should be emphasized that therapy for dysphagia in ALS must be undertaken as early as possible to prevent significant weight loss, weakness, and chronic dehydration. The majority of people with neuromuscular diseases are resistant to alternative means of feeding because the therapy is seen as "giving in" or as a setback. This attitude can often be changed by compassion and counseling, emphasizing that surgical placement of a tube for feedings can actually prolong the person's ability to enjoy eating so that it does not become a chore and can also prevent the devastating secondary effects of severe weight loss and dehydration. Early surgical intervention is essential. It is ideal for surgical intervention to be completed before dehydration and significant weight loss occur.

Late surgical intervention is usually complicated by respiratory weakness, which often parallels the development of dysphagia and is often worsened by dehydration and significant weight loss. Studies have shown that patients who have PEG tubes live an average of 1 to 4 months longer than those who refuse or who are not candidates for a PEG (Miller et al., 1999). The survival advantage is greatest for those who have a PEG placed before developing respiratory symptoms. Patients who wait until their respiratory capacity falls below 50% of their predicted volume are at greater risk for developing respiratory complications. Recently, the use of bilevel positive pulmonary ventilation support during the PEG insertion procedure has been reported as a means of avoiding respiratory failure in more compromised patients (Boitano, Jordan, & Benditt, 2001). However, even considering that tube placement is possible for patients with severely compromised breathing, most reports recommend that the procedure should be undertaken before vital capacity falls to 50% of predicted volume and prior to the loss of 5% to 10% of body weight (Hardiman, 2000).

It is also preferable to provide surgical therapy before eating becomes a chore. None of the methods of surgical intervention inhibits a person's ability to take food and fluids orally. If a feeding procedure is done early in the course of the disease, the person can keep oral intake as an enjoyable process and eat only as much as is comfortable, reserving the alternative means of feeding as a supplement. Eating, therefore, effectively remains a pleasure. Emphasizing that surgical intervention will not alter the ability to eat can be most helpful in allaying the patient's fears of tube feeding and surgery.

It should be emphasized that patients who are able can supplement their tube feedings with a small amount of orally ingested food. This allows for participation in the feeding process, and although the contribution is often insignificant in terms of caloric or fluid intake, the psychological benefits can be tremendous.

The ethical considerations of prolonging a person's life by surgical techniques must be evaluated in each case. The surgical placement of a feeding tube is not very different from the placement of a nasogastric tube and can make the patient much more comfortable. Health-care workers often set their limits of support just short of surgery because of their desire to define a stopping point. One must realize that this is an arbitrary stopping point, however. The decision to perform surgery to improve a person's access to nourishment is conceptually no different than the decision to use a blender to prepare meals when the person can no longer swallow solid foods.

Management of Tube Feeding

Tube feedings, when instituted, should begin with quarter-strength feedings of 200- to 300-cc boluses. Bolus feedings are preferable to continuous drips because they allow the patient to be unfettered between feedings. After an initial trial period of two to three feedings at quarter strength, the diet should be advanced to half, and then to full strength. Feedings ideally should advance to 500 to 1,000 cc per feeding as tolerated. It is important always to flush the tube with clear water (or cranberry juice, which tends to wash the tube) at the end of each feeding. The tube-feeding diet should be a blenderized diet or a blenderized diet supplemented by commercially available formulas. The use of canned formulas as a complete diet is not necessary for tube feedings. These canned formulas should be used only as a convenience for increasing caloric intake. Canned supplements with added fiber may be considered for individuals with constipation.

The patient's liquid intake must be monitored closely with tube feedings. Because the person is not experiencing oral sensations, perception of thirst is unlikely to be useful as a sign of dehydration. Unless the person with ALS has an additional history of cardiac or renal disease, there is relatively little risk of fluid overload. A 1,000-cc daily minimum of free water is essential to augment a blenderized or canned formula diet. On a warm day or if the patient has a fever, more fluids are needed. Basically, too much liquid is almost never a problem. Because dehydration has such serious consequences, it is advisable to keep a daily intake record for patients undergoing tube feeding.

STAGE 5. NOTHING BY MOUTH

The final stage of dysphagia is reached when the patient cannot safely manage any oral intake. At this point, many patients require assistance with the management of secretions in the form of aspirators, medications, or both, to decrease salivary flow. Although initially a swallow reflex can still be elicited, the frequency with which the person spontaneously swallows secretions diminishes. The most advanced patients can no longer manage their own secretions. Intervention for individuals who have difficulty with salivary management is described in the following section.

What Problems with Saliva Management Are Common for Individuals with ALS?

In the later stages of bulbar disease, the patient can have such difficulty handling his or her own saliva that continuous drooling occurs, increasing the difficulty of caring for the person and decreasing the person's self-respect. In the very late stages of this difficulty, usually in conjunction with dysphagia, patients may aspirate and, effectively, drown in their own saliva. Salivary problems in ALS are almost never caused by an actual excess in salivation, although many patients report this to be the case. Rather, a problem with salivary transport, dehydration, or both, results in a thickening of secretions. Although there is some speculation that in some neuromuscular diseases salivary secretion is increased, the clinical symptoms in ALS are not due to the amount of saliva, but instead to the management of it. Normal salivary flow can vary up to an increase of almost tenfold the resting rate, but normal individuals can handle this high volume of secretions without drooling and without aspiration because the transport systems are working.

SALIVA TRANSPORT PROBLEMS

The problems of salivary transport in neuromuscular diseases result from dysfunction in the oral phases of deglutition. The patient loses the ability to gather the saliva in the oral cavity and move it to the back of the mouth. This failure is usually due to incoordination of the buccal muscles, the tongue, and the palate. There is also failure to initiate propulsive deglutition in the oropharynx, which would transport the bolus downward past the larynx and into the esophagus. The problems of salivary management usually parallel the development of eating difficulties because the same swallowing mechanisms are employed with both functions.

THICKENED SALIVA

Another factor that causes increased difficulty with handling secretions is thickened saliva. Thickened saliva is caused by three major factors:

1. In advanced bulbar disease, the respiratory pathways can change. Normal breathing occurs primarily through the nasal passages, which causes humidification of the air before it reaches the lungs. The mouth usually remains closed except during times of increased respiratory need, when mouth breathing is done. In advanced neuromuscular disease, the muscles that keep the jaw and lips closed are weakened to the extent that the mouth may hang open. The airway path of least resistance is then through the oral cavity. The flow of unhumidified air through the oral cavity causes evaporation, which then thickens the saliva.

2. The second factor, which increases the problem of evaporation, is the pooling of saliva in the oral cavity due to poor mechanisms of oral transport. This large volume of saliva resting in the oral cavity is susceptible to evaporation and effectively results in a large volume of thickened saliva.

3. The third factor is related to the patient's difficulty in deglutition. When swallowing problems occur, the most difficult materials to swallow are liquids. Solids that tend not to break apart are usually swallowed successfully, while liquids, which do not hold together, are more difficult to manage. Therefore, there is a tendency for people with dysphagia to become dehydrated. This chronic dehydration is insidious and often not recognized. Dehydration is a major cause of thickened salivary secretions.

How Are Problems with Saliva Managed in Individuals with ALS?

In assessment, a determination must be made whether the difficulties are due to the transport of the secretions, the consistency of the secretions, or both. The treatment of thickened secretions involves a combination of fluid management and drug management. Treatment of salivary transport problems varies depending on the degree of difficulty. Simple mechanical measures can be effective in some cases. Surgical management is required in other cases.

TREATMENT OF THICKENED SECRETIONS

The first evaluation must be the individual's state of hydration. Simple examination of skin turgor can give a general impression of this. A daily measurement of urine output can give quantified results, and a simple urine-specific gravity can be helpful. It should be noted, however, that in a chronic state of dehydration, the urine-specific gravity might be normal. Other clinical factors that indicate dehydration are increasing weakness, malaise, and low-grade fever.

Perhaps the simplest method to evaluate chronic dehydration is an empirical one. Because most individuals with ALS do not have concomitant cardiac or renal problems, it is safe to administer a large volume of clear liquid. Liquids in the form of a "liquid diet" or "blenderized meal" do not provide free water because they have significant osmotic loads. Apple juice, sodas, gelatin, and ice pops do fall in the category of clear liquids, and 3,000 cc per day will reverse a state of chronic dehydration. Over the course of several days of such hydration, urine output should increase, urine specific gravity should decrease, and low-grade fevers and malaise, if present, should resolve. It is useful during this period of time to keep records of intake and output.

Drug management of thickened secretions can be helpful, but as with any drug management, some side effects can be expected. Over-the-counter guaifenesin (pure expectorant cough medicine) can be helpful by causing an increase in salivary flow to thin the saliva. Potassium iodide (SSKI) acts as a mild irritant of mucosal surfaces and can cause an increase and, therefore, a thinning of secretions. Generally, a response to potassium iodide is not noted until about 2 weeks after beginning its administration. The third pharmaceutical that can be helpful is papase, an enzyme present in papaya. Although it can be obtained at some drugstores, it is also available in the supermarket as an ingredient in meat tenderizer. Papase on a cotton swab applied to the mouth causes dissolution of thickened secretions and allows for easier transport. Drinking papaya juice has the same benefit for many patients. Apple juice, tea with lemon, and club soda have all been anecdotally reported to be beneficial.

TREATMENT OF TRANSPORT PROBLEMS

The simplest treatment of saliva transport problems is the use of a suction device or aspirator. Ideally, the suction tube would be employed by the patient, but if this is not possible, it can be applied by an assistant. If lip function is adequate, the most effective technique is for the patient to apply his or her lips around the suction tube as though it were a straw. Suctioning does not provide a very effective long-term solution as it is labor intensive and the removal of the saliva can cause electrolyte imbalances. We caution our patients not to use an aspirator as a means of dealing with choking emergencies. Its use may move the obstruction further into the trachea.

A towel or bib can be used to absorb secretions. Although simple and not labor intensive, it is unsightly and can cause some maceration of the skin where the wet towel lies. Drugs for drying up secretions have been used for saliva management with varying results. The goal is to diminish the volume of secretions while minimizing undesired side effects. Drugs of the atrophine family, transdermal patches for motion sickness, and over-the-counter medications used for colds and allergies dry the mouth, but may have undesired side effects. Small doses of an antidepressant like amitriptyline have achieved the goal of reducing saliva flow with a minimum number of undesired side effects. When this has not been effective, glycopyrrolate, a stronger medication used to block acetylcholine, has been successful. Although the treatment is as yet unproven, some doctors have prescribed beta-blockers like propranolol in an attempt to diminish the production of mucus secretions. A final experimental approach has involved the injection of botulinum toxin type B into the parotid gland. This procedure reportedly provides temporary benefit in reducing saliva flow, but requires repeat injections for lasting effect.

Radiation treatments for cancer have been noted to have a side effect of decreasing salivary flow. A change in salivary flow has been seen after a single dose of irradiation (7.0–7.5 Gy) directed at the parotid and submandibular glands (Andersen, Gronberg, Franzen, & Funegard, 2001). This radiation side effect can be used to advantage as a treatment for salivary management, although the response can be variable and temporary.

Surgical management has been employed with considerable success in experienced hands. There are a number of procedures, and the appropriateness of each depends on the patient's condition and symptoms. One surgical management approach is to address the neural control of the major salivary glands. Sectioning the chorda tympani and tympanic nerve interrupts the parasympathetic innervation of the submandibular and parotid glands, thus significantly decreasing oral secretions. The easiest access to these two nerves is through the middle ear, and this approach, known as a tympanic neurectomy, can easily be done under local anesthesia. Severing the parasympathetic supply can decrease salivary flow by about 50%, but this decrease is often only temporary.

Ligation of the ducts of major salivary glands is another technique that can lessen salivary flow and that may be performed in conjunction with tympanic neurectomy. Ligation of the ducts causes obstruction of flow, which then secondarily causes an inflammation of the gland, sometimes resulting in fibrosis. The subsequent atrophy of the glands lowers salivary output. Wharton's duct from the submaxillary gland and Stensen's duct from the parotid gland are amenable to this form of therapy. The sublingual gland has no single defined duct, and it is not amenable to duct ligation. Duct ligation can be performed under local anesthesia. Problems with duct ligations are (a) the obstructed duct can sometimes form a new opening into the oral cavity at another point and (b) there is some pain and discomfort during the inflammation that follows a duct ligation. The weaknesses and strengths of duct ligation and tympanic neurectomy are complementary, and these procedures should be performed together. The neurectomy will temporarily decrease the salivary flow, which will reduce the inflammation when the ducts are ligated and also lessen the likelihood that a new duct opening to the oral cavity will develop.

The submaxillary glands can be excised under local anesthesia, and excision of these two glands can provide a significant lessening of salivary flow in the resting state. The procedure requires a neck incision below the jaw on each side but generally has a low complication rate.

Duct transpositions are procedures that directly address the problem of salivary transport. Both Wharton's duct from the submaxillary gland and Stensen's duct from the parotid gland can be surgically rerouted to open into the oropharynx. These procedures effectively route the saliva posteriorly so that transport from the oral cavity to the oropharynx is not a problem. A limitation of these procedures is that the saliva still must be managed in the oropharynx, so to some degree the swallowing mechanism must be intact.

Salivary reduction and diversion procedures are usually not necessary if medical management is vigorously pursued (Hillel & Miller, 1989). It is imperative that adequate hydration be maintained while attempting to address saliva management.

How Is Aspiration in ALS Managed?

Individuals with ALS only rarely develop significant problems with aspiration during the course of their disease. When aspiration occurs as a symptom, however, it can have serious consequences, and if left unattended, it can lead to the rapid deterioration or demise of the patient. The deterioration in the functioning of the oral cavity, oropharynx, and esophagus can be viewed as a progression in terms of difficulty in speaking, in swallowing liquids, in swallowing solids, in managing saliva, and in preventing aspiration. The occurrence of aspiration is usually the last event in a longer series of events of decreasing bulbar function. When one examines the occurrence of aspiration pneumonia in general, it is most often precipitated by a single event with a rapid onset such as a stroke, surgery to the upper respiratory system, or trauma. Because of the relatively slow onset of dysphagia in ALS, the person is often able to compensate, and aspiration is not a common occurrence. When aspiration does occur, however, it is usually a devastating event because of the usual concomitant severe lack of pulmonary reserve in these individuals. Because aspiration is usually a result of decreasing function of the muscles in the oral cavity and oropharynx, its presence is indicative of complete dysphagia. Vocal fold weakness is also present. The person is usually unable to achieve adequate glottic closure for a strong cough, which is a protective mechanism against aspiration. In addition, if there is respiratory or abdominal wall muscle weakness, the ability to generate a strong protective cough is diminished.

MANAGEMENT OF MILD ASPIRATION

If the person is still able to speak understandably and to eat when symptoms of aspiration are first noted, management of aspiration can be conservative. It is important to determine whether the person can clear aspirated material by coughing, and it is probably advisable to document this with a chest X-ray. If the person is in a dehydrated state, which is frequently the case with the dysphagic stage of ALS, a pneumonia is unlikely to show on a chest X-ray. With mild aspiration, dietary tricks can be helpful. Moist foods, such as puddings, fruit sauces, and gravies, are more easily handled than foods that fall apart, such as puréed foods and applesauce. Liquid intake can be increased using foods such as gelatin, frozen flavored ice pops, frozen juices, sherbets, and fruit ices.

In addition, mild aspiration can be helped by instructing the individual in swallowing techniques. The person should be in an upright position while eating. Small manageable portions of food should be taken into the oral cavity. During the initiation of swallowing, the neck should be flexed so the chin is in a downward position. The person can also be counseled to double swallow before proceeding to the next morsel of food.

If aspiration becomes clinically significant, oral intake of food and liquids should be halted. Significant aspiration is defined as the entrance of food or liquid into the trachea without it being effectively cleared by coughing. The diagnosis of significant aspiration is a clinical decision, although a chest X-ray in a well-hydrated person can be very helpful in determining the extent of aspiration. The discontinuance of oral intake should be immediate and should last until the aspiration pneumonia is resolved and measures have been taken to correct the problem. Intravenous fluid administration is recommended for rehydration of the patient but does not supply any significant nutrient value and should not be relied upon for more than a day or two. Temporal placement of a nasogastric tube should be considered to provide caloric and liquid intake.

SURGICAL MANAGEMENT OF ASPIRATION

If, after adequate investigation and management trials by conservative methods, aspiration remains a problem, surgical intervention needs to be considered. The decision-making process regarding surgery is a difficult one that hinges most importantly on an evaluation of the patient's swallowing. If the person can significantly enjoy oral intake of liquids and solids aside from the problem of aspiration, then a surgical procedure addressing aspiration might be indicated. If, however, the oral, oropharyngeal, and esophageal phases of swallowing are debilitated to the point that oral intake of liquids and solids is not effective, surgical management should address a feeding procedure. The surgical management of aspiration is indicated only when one of the following conditions exists:

1. It is desirable that the patient continue taking foods and liquids orally but the person cannot do so only because of the occurrence of aspiration; or

2. In spite of being alimented nonorally, the patient experiences aspiration secondary to the management of saliva.

The surgical management of feeding and saliva control have been discussed. There are a number of additional procedures that are used specifically to address problems in aspiration.

Tracheostomy

Tracheostomy is often the first resort chosen for surgical management of aspiration. The most important thing to note about tracheostomy is that it does not prevent aspiration. A tracheostomy tube with a balloon cuff, while it impedes the flow of material into the lungs, does not prevent it. The junction of the balloon cuff and the tracheal wall cannot be tight enough to prevent the passage of liquids around the cuff without being so tight as to cause significant injury to the tracheal wall. Tracheostomy, however, does provide excellent access for pulmonary toilet and is important as an airway when combined with other procedures that directly deal with aspiration. Basically, procedures that are directed toward preventing aspiration do so by closing the airway in the hypopharynx so that liquids and solids cannot get into the tracheobronchial trees. This closure ends the person's ability to breathe orally and therefore requires a tracheostomy. Tracheostomy is usually easily performed under local anesthesia. The complications of tracheostomy are bleeding, infection, pneumothorax, obstruction of the tracheostomy tube, and tracheostenosis. Although these complications can occur, they are rare with a well-managed tracheostomy. Tracheostomy is also used for individuals with ALS who have significant abductor vocal fold paralysis with functional airway obstruction.

Vocal Fold Closure

Vocal fold closure is a procedure that approximates the true vocal folds in such a fashion that closure of the airway occurs. Vocal fold closure must be combined with a tracheostomy. In essence, the technique is to expose the vocal folds through the neck and to remove the epithelium overlying the edges of the vocal folds. The vocal folds are then sewn together and heal together. The procedure is done under general anesthesia. While some authors claim that the procedure is reversible, many others question the results obtained after attempting reversal. The risks of vocal fold closure are bleeding, infection, and anesthetic risk. Vocal fold closure is often unsuccessful due to failure of healing at the posterior commissure, and it can be technically difficult to perform. After successful vocal fold closure, however, a person who has adequate oral and pharyngeal phases of swallowing will be able to swallow without aspiration.

Tracheal Diversion

In tracheal diversion procedures, the trachea is separated from the larynx and brought directly out to the skin. Effectively, the connection between the oral cavity, oropharynx and hypopharynx, and tracheobronchial trees is severed. The lower end of the larynx is then sewn closed as a blind-ended pouch or anastomosed into the esophagus. The former approach is less complex and requires less operating time. Although some authors claim that the procedure is reversible, the success of reversibility is questionable. The risks of tracheal diversion are bleeding, infection, and anesthetic risk. The procedure is usually successful in experienced hands, although it is sometimes technically difficult depending upon the patient's anatomy (Lindeman, 1975). The tracheal diversion procedure is contraindicated when a previous tracheostomy has been performed.

Laryngectomy

In a narrow-field laryngectomy, the entire larynx is removed. The trachea is severed from the larynx and is brought to the skin. As in tracheal diversion procedures, the tracheobronchial tree is separated from the oropharynx and hypopharynx. Laryngectomy is not reversible but is always successful in preventing aspiration. Laryngectomy usually needs to be performed under general anesthesia and, although it is a more extensive procedure than a tracheal diversion, there is a higher rate of success and less likelihood that revision will be needed. The risks of laryngectomy are bleeding, infection, anesthetic risk, and the development of a fistula between the hypopharynx and the neck skin, which usually can be successfully managed conservatively. The greatest objection to laryngectomy, however, is an emotional one, and although the surgery provides no less functional ability than tracheal diversion or vocal fold closure, it is usually rejected by both physician and patient. As with vocal fold closure and tracheal diversion, the person with adequate swallowing function can eat without risk of aspiration.

Epiglottic Sew-Down Procedures

The epiglottic sew-down procedure also must be combined with tracheostomy. In this procedure, the epiglottis is rotated downward and sewn over the opening to the larynx. This procedure must be done under general anesthesia. The risks are bleeding, infection, and anesthetic risk. In experienced hands, the epiglottic sew-down procedure has a reasonable success rate, but it can be a difficult procedure to perform.

APPENDIX 1.1

Clinical Examination for ALS

PATIENT INFORMATION

Name: _____ Hospital Number: _____

Date of Visit: _____ Birth Date/Age: _____

Accompanying Person(s): _____

Referring Physician: _____

Reason for Referral: _____

_____

MEDICAL HISTORY

Primary Diagnosis/Date Made/By Whom: _____

_____

Date of Onset of Symptoms and Progression: _____

_____

_____

Date of Onset and Progression of Speech/Swallowing Symptoms: _____

_____

Knowledge of Disease Process: _____

_____

Other Medical History: _____

Smoking/Alcohol History: _____

_____

Allergies: _____

_____

Psychosocial History:

Employment Status: _____

Household Members: _____

Children (where residing): _____

(continues)

CURRENT HEALTH-CARE MANAGEMENT

Medications: _____

_____

Physicians Currently Following: _____

_____

Community Resources Agencies: _____

_____

Equipment:

Type: _____

Date Acquired: _____

From Whom: _____

Attendant Care: _____

_____

Emergency Communication System: _____

_____

First Aid Plan for Choking: _____

_____

Living Will: _____ Yes _____ No   Description of Wishes: _____

_____

_____

PHYSICAL EXAMINATION

Group 1: The Tongue and Lips

Graded Tongue Movement (Rate both right and left. Pick worse side.)

_____ Grade 5—Tongue protrudes forcefully and in the midline. Tongue can cross the alveolar ridge firmly at the level of the molars and exert force against the examiner's finger on the cheek.

_____ Grade 4—Tongue cannot cross the alveolar ridge at the molars, but can cross the alveolar ridge at the premolar/canine area and exert force against the examiner's finger on the cheek.

_____ Grade 3—Tongue can cross the alveolar ridge only in the midline. Midline is defined as the width of the lips.

_____ Grade 2—Effective tongue movement but cannot cross the alveolar ridge.

_____ Grade 1—No movement or minimal effective movement.

Alternate Motions Rates

/p/: _____   /k/: _____

/t/: _____   /pataka/: _____

(continues)

Fasciculations

Tongue:_____

Lips:_____

Group 2: The Palate, Muscles of Mastication, Pharyngeal Constrictors, and Buccinators

Symptoms Checklist:

_____ Nasal emission   _____ Chewing fatigue

_____ Hypernasal speech   Denture: _____ None

_____ Inability to use a straw   _____ Partial

_____ Nasal reflux   _____ Full

Group 3: The Buccal/Frontal/Orbital Muscles, Sternocleidomastoid/Trapezius Muscle and the Vocal Cords

_____ Reduced ability to abduct vocal folds

_____ Reduced ability to adduct vocal folds

_____ Vocal quality—breathiness

_____ Vocal quality—harshness

_____ Stridor

_____ Inability to hold head up

_____ Reduced loudness

Sustained Phonation Time: _____

Group 4: Respiratory Muscles

Vital Capacity (VC): _____   % Predicted VC: _____

Volitional Cough: _____ Normal   _____ Weak   _____ Absent

Comments: _____

_____

_____

ASSESSMENT OF SPEECH AND SWALLOWING FUNCTION

Speech Intelligibility

Sentence Intelligibility: _____   Speaking Rate: _____

Single Word Intelligibility

Without Context: _____   With Context: _____

Swallowing Complaints

Current Weight: _____   History of Weight Loss: _____

Length of Mealtimes: _____   _____

Glasses of Water per Day: _____

Saliva:

_____ Drooling

_____ Excessive saliva

_____ Dry mouth

_____ Thin saliva

_____ Choking on saliva

_____ Thick or sticky saliva

Pharyngeal Stage:

_____ Difficulty initiating

_____ Nasal regurgitation

_____ Food sticks in throat

_____ Coughing after swallow

_____ Immediate choking

ALS Scale Scores:

_____ Speech

_____ Swallow

_____ Lower Extremity

_____ Upper Extremity

Oral Stage Difficulty:

_____ Leakage from mouth

_____ Difficulty chewing

_____ Difficulty in transport

_____ Pocketing of food

General:

_____ Slow eating rate

_____ Lack of enjoyment

_____ Insufficient calories

_____ Insufficient fluids

_____ GE reflux

_____ History of pneumonia

APPENDIX 1.2

ALS Severity Scale

Speech

NORMAL SPEECH PROCESSES

10—**Normal Speech:** Patient denies any difficulty speaking. Examination demonstrates no abnormality.

9—**Nominal Speech Abnormality:** Only the patient or spouse notices that speech has changed. Maintains normal rate and volume.

DETECTABLE SPEECH DISTURBANCES

8—**Perceived Speech Changes:** Speech changes are noted by others, especially during fatigue or stress. Rate of speech remains essentially normal.

7—**Obvious Speech Abnormalities:** Speech is consistently impaired. Affected are rate, articulation, and resonance. Remains easily understood.

BEHAVIORAL MODIFICATIONS

6—**Repeats Messages on Occasion:** Rate is much slower. Repeats specific words in adverse listening situations. Does not limit complexity or length of message.

5—**Frequent Repeating Required:** Speech is slow and labored. Extensive repetition or a "translator" is commonly needed. Patient probably limits the complexity or length of messages.

USE OF AUGMENTATIVE COMMUNICATION

4—**Speech Plus Augmentative Communication:** Speech is used in response to questions. Intelligibility problems need to be resolved by writing or a spokesperson.

3—**Limits Speech to One-Word Response:** Vocalizes one-word response beyond yes/no; otherwise writes or uses a spokesperson. Initiates communication nonvocally.

LOSS OF USEFUL SPEECH

2—**Vocalizes for Emotional Expression:** Uses vocal inflection to express emotion, affirmation, and negation.

1—**Nonvocal:** Vocalization is effortful, limited in duration, and rarely attempted. May vocalize for crying or pain.

X—**Tracheostomy**

Note. From "Speech Deterioration in Amyotrophic Lateral Sclerosis: Implications for the Timing of Intervention," by K. M. Yorkston, E. Strand, R. Miller, H. Hillel, and K. Smith, 1993, *Journal of Medical Speech–Language Pathology, 1*(1), pp. 35–46. Copyright 1993 by the Journal of Medical Speech–Language Pathology. Reprinted with permission.

SWALLOWING

NORMAL EATING HABITS

10—**Normal Swallowing:** Patient denies any difficulty chewing or swallowing. Examination demonstrates no abnormality.

9—**Nominal Abnormality:** Only patient notices slight indicators such as food lodging in the recesses of the mouth or sticking in the throat.

EARLY EATING PROBLEMS

8—**Minor Swallowing Problems:** Complains of some swallowing difficulties. Maintains essentially a regular diet. Isolated choking episodes.

7—**Prolonged Time or Smaller Bite Size:** Mealtime has significantly increased and smaller bite sizes are necessary. Must concentrate on swallowing liquids.

DIETARY CONSISTENCY CHANGES

6—**Soft Diet:** Diet is limited primarily to soft foods. Requires some special meal preparation.

5—**Liquified Diet:** PO intake adequate. Nutrition limited primarily to liquified diet. Adequate thin liquid intake usually a problem. May force self to eat.

NEEDS TUBE FEEDING

4—**Supplemental Tube Feedings:** PO intake alone is no longer adequate. Patient uses or needs a tube to supplement intake. Patient continues to take significant (greater than 50%) of nutrition PO.

3—**Tube Feeding with Occasional PO Nutrition:** Primary nutrition and hydration accomplished by tube. Receives less than 50% of nutrition PO.

NPO

2—**Secretions Managed with Aspirator/Medication**: Cannot safely manage any PO intake. Secretions managed by an aspirator and/or medications. Swallows reflexively.

1—**Aspiration of Secretions:** Secretions cannot be managed noninvasively. Rarely swallows.

Note. From "Speech Deterioration in Amyotrophic Lateral Sclerosis: Implications for the Timing of Intervention," by K. M. Yorkston, E. Strand, R. Miller, H. Hillel, and K. Smith, 1993, *Journal of Medical Speech–Language Pathology, 1*(1), pp. 35–46. Copyright 1993 by the Journal of Medical Speech–Language Pathology. Reprinted with permission.

LOWER EXTREMITIES (WALKING)

NORMAL

10—**Normal Ambulation:** Patient denies any weakness or fatigue. Examination detects no abnormality.

9—**Fatigue Suspected:** Patient suspects weakness or fatigue in lower extremities during exertion.

EARLY AMBULATION PROBLEM

8—**Difficulty with Uneven Terrain:** Difficulty and fatigue when walking long distances, climbing stairs, and walking over uneven ground (even thick carpet).

7—**Observed Changes in Gait:** Noticeable change in gait. Pulls on railing when climbing stairs. May use leg brace.

WALKS WITH ASSISTANCE

6—**Walks with Mechanical Device:** Needs or uses canes, walker, or assistant to walk. Probably uses wheelchair away from home.

5—**Walks with Mechanical Device and Attendant:** Does not attempt to walk without an attendant. Ambulation limited to less than 50 feet. Avoids stairs.

FUNCTIONAL MOVEMENT ONLY

4—**Able To Support Weight:** At best can shuffle a few steps with the help of an attendant for transfers.

3—**Purposeful Leg Movements:** Unable to take steps, but can position legs to assist an attendant in transfers. Moves legs purposefully to maintain mobility in bed.

NO PURPOSEFUL LEG MOVEMENT

2—**Minimal Movement:** Minimal movement of one or both legs. Cannot reposition legs independently.

1—**Paralysis:** Flaccid paralysis. Cannot move lower extremities (except, perhaps, to close inspection).

Note. From "Speech Deterioration in Amyotrophic Lateral Sclerosis: Implications for the Timing of Intervention," by K. M. Yorkston, E. Strand, R. Miller, H. Hillel, and K. Smith, 1993, *Journal of Medical Speech–Language Pathology, 1*(1), pp. 35–46. Copyright 1993 by the Journal of Medical Speech–Language Pathology. Reprinted with permission.

UPPER EXTREMITIES (DRESSING & HYGIENE)

NORMAL FUNCTION

10—**Normal Function:** Patient denies any weakness or unusual fatigue of upper extremities. Examination demonstrates no abnormality.

9—**Suspected Fatigue:** Patient suspects fatigue in upper extremities during exertion. Cannot sustain work for as long as normal. Atrophy not evident on examination.

INDEPENDENT AND COMPLETE SELF-CARE

8—**Slow Self-Care Performance:** Dressing and hygiene performed more slowly than usual.

7—**Effortful Self-Care Performance:** Requires significantly more time (usually double or more) and effort to accomplish self-care. Weakness is apparent on examination.

INTERMITTENT ASSISTANCE

6—**Mostly Independent:** Handles most aspects of dressing and hygiene alone. Adapts by resting, modifying (using electric razor), or avoiding some tasks (e.g., buttoning, tying).

5—**Partial Independence:** Handles some aspects of dressing and hygiene alone. However, routinely requires assistance for many tasks such as applying make-up, combing, shaving, etc.

NEEDS ATTENDANT FOR SELF-CARE

4—**Attendant Assists Patient:** Attendant must be present for dressing and hygiene. Patient performs the majority of each task with the assistance of the attendant.

3—**Patient Assists Attendant:** The attendant assists the patient for almost all tasks. The patient moves in a purposeful manner to assist the attendant. Does not initiate self-care tasks.

TOTAL DEPENDENCE

2—**Minimal Movement:** Minimal movement of one or both arms. Cannot reposition arms.

1—**Paralysis:** Flaccid paralysis. Unable to move upper extremities (except, perhaps, to close inspection).

Note. From "Speech Deterioration in Amyotrophic Lateral Sclerosis: Implications for the Timing of Intervention," by K. M. Yorkston, E. Strand, R. Miller, H. Hillel, and K. Smith, 1993, *Journal of Medical Speech–Language Pathology, 1*(1), pp. 35–46. Copyright 1993 by the Journal of Medical Speech–Language Pathology. Reprinted with permission.

APPENDIX 1.3

Swallowing Disorders Interview Worksheet

Name: _____ Date: _____

Swallowing score: _____ Weight: _____ Estimated calories: _____

Estimated liquids: _____

SWALLOWING COMPLAINT CHECKLIST

Saliva Management

Drooling _____

Excessive saliva _____

Dry mouth _____

Thin saliva _____

Choking on saliva _____

Sticky saliva _____

Pharyngeal Stage Difficulty

Difficulty initiating _____

Nasal regurgitation _____

Food "sticks in throat" _____

Coughing after swallow _____

Oral Stage Difficulty

Leakage from mouth _____

Difficulty chewing _____

Difficulty in transport _____

Pocketing of food _____

General Problems

Slow eating rate _____

Lack of enjoyment _____

Insufficient calories _____

Insufficient fluids _____

INTERVENTION

Behavioral

General (positon, rate, amount) _____

Specific (supraglottic) _____

First aid for choking _____

Dietary changes _____

Consistency adjustments _____

Increase calories _____

Increase fluids _____

Saliva Medication

Reduce amount _____

Thin _____

Surgery

Salivary duct _____

Myotromy _____

Tracheostomy _____

PEG Placement _____

References

Aboussouan, L. S., Khan, S. U., Banerjee, M., Arroliga, A. C., & Mitsumoto, H. (2001). Objective measures of the efficacy of non-invasive positive pressure ventilation in amyotrophic lateral sclerosis. *Muscle Nerve, 24*(3), 403–409.

Aboussouan, L. S., Khan, S. U., Meeker, D. P., Stelmack, K., & Mitsumoto, H. (1997). Effect of noninvasive positive-pressure ventilation on survival in amyotrophic lateral sclerosis. *Annals of Internal Medicine, 127*(6), 450–453.

Abrahams, S., Goldstein, L. H., Al Chalabi, A., Pickering, A., Morris, R. G., Passingham, R. E., Brooks, D. J., & Leigh, P. N. (1997). Relation between cognitive dysfunction and pseudobulbar palsy in amyotrophic lateral sclerosis. *Journal of Neurology, Neurosurgery and Psychiatry, 62*(5), 464–472.

Abrahams, S., Goldstein, L. H., Brooks, D. J., Lloyd, C. M., Frith, C. D., & Leigh, P. N. (1996). Frontal lobe dysfunction in amyotrophic lateral sclerosis: A PET study. *Brain, 119*, 2105–2120.

Abrahams, S., Leigh, P. N., Harvey, A., Vythelingum, G. N., Grise, D., & Goldstein, L. H. (2000). Verbal fluency and executive dysfunction in amyotrophic lateral sclerosis (ALS). *Neuropsychologia, 38*(6), 734–747.

Adams, A. B., Shapiro, R., & Marini, J. J. (1998). Changing prevalence of chronically ventilator-assisted individuals in Minnesota: Increases, characteristics, and the use of noninvasive ventilation. *Respiratory Care, 43*(8), 643–648.

Albert, S. M., Murphy, P. L., Del Bene, M. L., & Rowland, L. P. (1999). A prospective study of preferences and actual treatment choices in ALS. *Neurology, 53*, 278–283.

Andersen, P. M., Gronberg, H., Franzen, L., & Funegard, U. (2001). External radiation of the parotid glands significantly reduces drooling in patients with motor neurone disease with bulbar paresis. *Journal of the Neurological Sciences, 191*(1–2), 111–114.

Annoni, J., Chevrolet, J., & Kesselring, J. (1993). Respiratory problems in chronic neurological disorders. *Critical Reviews in Physical and Rehabilitation Medicine, 5*(2), 155–192.

Appel, V., Stewart, S. S., Smith, G., & Appel, S. H. (1987). A rating scale for amyotrophic lateral sclerosis: Description and preliminary experience. *Annual of Neurology, 22*(3), 328–333.

Armon, C. (2001). Environmental risk factors for amyotrophic lateral sclerosis. *Neuroepidemiology, 20*(1), 2–6.

Aronson, A. E., Ramig, L. O., Winholtz, W. S., & Silber, S. R. (1992). Rapid voice tremor, or "flutter," in amyotrophic lateral sclerosis. *Annals of Otology, Rhinology & Laryngology, 101*(6), 511–518.

Bach, J. R. (1993). Amyotrophic lateral sclerosis. Communication status and survival with ventilatory support. *American Journal of Physical Medicine & Rehabilitation, 72*, 343–349.

Bach, J. R. (1998). Rehabilitation of the patient with respiratory dysfunction. In J. DeLisa (Ed.), *Rehabilitation medicine: Principles and practice* (3rd ed., pp. 1359–1384). Philadelphia: Lippincott.

Bak, T., & Hodges, J. R. (1999). Cognitive, language, and behavior in motor neuron disease: Evidence of frontotemporal dysfunction. *Dementia and Geriatric Cognitive Disorders, 10*(Suppl. 1), 29–32.

Bak, T. H., & Hodges, J. R. (2001). Motor neurone disease, dementia and aphasia: Coincidence, co-occurrence or continuum? *Journal of Neurology, 248*, 260–270.

Ball, L. J., Willis, A., Beukelman, D. R., & Pattee, G. L. (2001). A protocol for identification of early bulbar signs in amyotrophic lateral sclerosis. *Journal of the Neurological Sciences, 191*, 43–53.

Baumann, A. (1991). ALS–decision making under uncertainty: A positive approach. *Axone, 13*(2), 41–44.

Beisecker, A. E., Cobb, A. K., & Ziegler, D. K. (1988). Patients' perspectives of the role of care providers in amyotrophic lateral sclerosis. *Archives of Neurology, 45*, 553–556.

Belsh, J. M. (1999). Diagnostic challenges in ALS. *Neurology, 53*(8, Suppl. 5), S26–30, S35–36.

Belsh, J. M., & Schiffman, P. L. (1996). The amyotrophic lateral sclerosis (ALS) patient perspective on misdiagnosis and its repercussions. *Journal of the Neurological Sciences, 139*(Suppl.), 110–116.

Benditt, J. O. (1998). Management of pulmonary complications in neuromuscular disease. *Physical Medicine and Rehabilitation Clinics of North America, 9*(1), 167–185.

Bennett, R. L., & Knowlton, G. C. (1958). Overwork weakness in partially denervated skeletonal muscle. *Clinical Orthopedics, 12,* 22–29.

Bensimon, G., Lacomblez, L., & Meininger, V. (1994). A controlled trial of Riluzole in amyotrophic lateral sclerosis. *New England Journal of Medicine, 330*(9), 585–591.

Berry, W., & Sanders, S. (1983). Environmental education: The universal management approach for adults with dysarthria. In W. Berry (Ed.), *Clinical dysarthria* (pp. 203–216). Austin, TX: PRO-ED.

Beukelman, D. R., & Mirenda, P. (1998). *Augmentative and alternative communication: Management of severe communication disorders in children and adults* (2nd ed.). Baltimore: Brookes.

Boitano, L. J., Jordan, T., & Benditt, J. O. (2001). Noninvasive ventilation allows gastrostomy tube placement in patients with advanced ALS. *Neurology, 56*(3), 413–414.

Borasio, G. D., & Voltz, R. (1997). Palliative care in amyotrophic lateral sclerosis. *Journal of Neurology, 244*(Suppl. 4), S11–S17.

Borasio, G. D., & Voltz, R. (1998). Discontinuation of mechanical ventilation in patients with amyotrophic lateral sclerosis. *Journal of Neurology, 245*(11), 717–722.

Braun, S. R. (1987). Respiratory systems in amyotrophic lateral sclerosis. *Neurologic Clinics, 5*(1), 9–31.

Brooks, B. R. (1991). The role of axonal transport in neurodegenerative disease spread: Meta-analysis of experimental and clinical poliomyelitis compared with amyotrophic lateral sclerosis. *Canadian Journal of Neurological Sciences, 18*(Suppl. 3), 435–438.

Bunton, K., Kent, R. D., Kent, J. F., & Rosenbek, J. C. (2000). Perceptuo-acoustic assessment of prosodic impairment in dysarthria. *Clinical Linguistics & Phonetics, 14,* 13–24.

Caroscio, J. T., Mulvihill, M. N., Sterling, R., & Abrams, B. (1987). Amyotrophic lateral sclerosis: Its natural history. *Neurology Clinics, 5*(1), 1–8.

Carter, G. T., Bednar-Butler, L. M., Abresch, R. T., & Ugalde, V. O. (1999). Expanding the role of hospice care in amyotrophic lateral sclerosis. *American Journal of Hospice & Palliative Care, 16*(6), 707–710.

Caselli, R. J., Smith, B. E., & Osbourne, D. (1995). Primary lateral sclerosis: A neuropsychological study. *Neurology, 45*(11), 2005–2009.

Cazzolli, P. A., & Oppenheimer, E. A. (1996). Home mechanical ventilation for amyotrophic lateral sclerosis: Nasal compared to tracheostomy-intermittent positive pressure ventilation. *Journal of the Neurological Sciences, 139,* 123–128.

Cedarbaum, J. M., Stabler, N., Malta, E., Fuller, C., Hilt, D., Thurmond, B., & Nakanishi, A. (1999). The ALSFRS–R: A revised ALS functional rating scale that incorporates assessments of respiratory function. BDNF AALS Study Group (Phase III). *Journal of the Neurological Sciences, 169*(1–2), 13–21.

Cha, C. H., & Patten, B. M. (1989). Amyotrophic lateral sclerosis: Abnormalities of the tongue on magnetic resonance imaging. *Annals of Neurology, 25*(5), 468–472.

Chari, G., Shaw, P. J., & Sahgal, A. (1996). Nonverbal visual attention, but not recognition memory of learning processes are impaired in motor neurone disease. *Neuropsychologia, 34*(5), 377–385.

Chio, A. (1999). ISIS Survey: An international study of the diagnostic process and its implications in amyotrophic lateral sclerosis. *Journal of Neurology, 246*(15), S1–S5.

Clausen, J. L. (1982). *Pulmonary function testing guidelines and controversies.* New York: Academic Press.

Cobble, M. (1998). Language impairment in motor neuron disease. *Journal of the Neurological Sciences, 160*(Suppl. 1), S47–52.

Cwik, V. A. (2000). Pharmaceutical treatment of amyotrophic lateral sclerosis. *Newsletter: SID 2–Neurophysiology and Neurogenic Speech and Language Disorders, 10*(2), 11–16.

Dal Bello-Haas, V., Kloos, A. D., & Mitsumoto, H. (1998). Physical therapy for a patient through six stages of amyotrophic lateral sclerosis. *Physical Therapy, 78*(12), 1312–1324.

Darley, F. L., Aronson, A. E., & Brown, J. R. (1975). *Motor speech disorders.* Philadelphia: Saunders.

DeLisa, J. A., Mikulic, M. A., Miller, R. M., & Melnick, R. R. (1979). Amyotrophic lateral sclerosis: Comprehensive management. *American Family Physician, 19*(3), 137–142.

DePaul, R., Abbs, J. H., Caligiuri, M. P., Gracco, V. L., & Brooks, B. R. (1988). Hypoglossal, trigeminal, and facial motoneuron involvement in amyotrophic lateral sclerosis. *Neurology, 38,* 281–283.

Desport, J. C., Preux, P. M., Trunong, T. C., Vallat, J. M., Sautereau, D., & Couratier, P. (1999). Nutritional status is a prognostic factor for survival in ALS patients. *Neurology, 53*(5), 1059–1163.

Doyle, M., & Phillips, B. (2001). Trends in augmentative and alternative communication use by individuals with amyotrophic lateral sclerosis. *Augmentative and Alternative Communication, 17*(3), 167–178.

Drory, V. E., Goltsman, E., Goldman Reznik, J., Mosek, A., & Korczyn, A. D. (2001). The value of muscle exercise in patients with amyotrophic lateral sclerosis. *Journal of the Neurological Sciences, 191*(1–2), 133–137.

Dworkin, J. P. (1980). Tongue strength measurement in patients with amyotrophic lateral sclerosis: Qualitative vs. quantitative procedures. *Archives of Physical Medicine and Rehabilitation, 61*(9), 422–424.

Dworkin, J., & Aronson, A. (1986). Tongue strength and alternate motion rates in normal and dysarthric subjects. *Journal of Communication Disorders, 19,* 115–132.

Dworkin, J. P., & Hartman, D. E. (1979). Progressive speech deterioration and dysphagia in amyotrophic lateral sclerosis: Case report. *Archives of Physical Medicine and Rehabilitation, 60,* 423–425.

Eisen, A. (1999). How to improve the diagnostic process. *Journal of Neurology, 246*(Suppl. 3), III6–9.

Eisen, A., & Krieger, C. (1993). Pathogenic mechanism in sporadic amyotrophic lateral sclerosis. *Canadian Journal of Neurologic Sciences, 20*(4), 286–296.

Eisen, A., Schulzer, M., MacNeil, M., Pant, B., & Mak, E. (1993). Duration of amyotrophic lateral sclerosis is age dependent. *Muscle & Nerve, 16*(1), 27–32.

Esposito, S. J., Mitsumoto, H., & Shanks, M. (2000). Use of palatal lift and palatal augmentation prostheses to improve dysarthria in patients with amyotrophic lateral sclerosis: A case series. *Journal of Prosthetic Dentistry, 83,* 90–98.

Fallat, R. J., Jewitt, B., Bass, M., Kamm, B., & Norris, F. H. (1979). Spirometry in amyotrophic lateral sclerosis. *Archives of Neurology, 36,* 74–80.

Fallat, R. J., & Norris, F. H. (1980). Respiratory problems. In D. W. Mulder (Ed.), *The diagnosis and treatment of amyotrophic lateral sclerosis* (pp. 301–320). Boston: Houghton Mifflin.

Fischbeck, K. H. (1997). Kennedy disease. *Journal of Inherited Metabolic Disease, 20,* 152–158.

Francis, K., Bach, J. R., & DeLisa, J. A. (1999). Evaluation and rehabilitation of patients with adult motor neuron disease. *Archives of Physical Medicine and Rehabilitation, 80,* 951–963.

Frank, B., Haas, J., Heinze, H. J., Stark, E., & Munte, T. F. (1997). Relation of neuropsychological and magnetic resonance findings in amyotrophic lateral sclerosis: Evidence for subgroups. *Clinical Neurology and Neurosurgery, 99*(2), 79–86.

Gallagher, J. P. (1989). Pathologic laughter and crying in ALS: A search for their origin. *Acta Neurologica Scandinavica, 80*(2), 114–117.

Gallassi, R., Montagna, P., Ciardulli, C., Lorusso, S., & Mussuto, V. (1985). Cognitive impairment in motor neuron disease. *Acta Neurologica Scandinavica, 71,* 480–484.

Gallassi, R., Montagna, P., Morreale, A., Lorusso, A., Tinuper, P., Daidone, R., & Lugaresi, E. (1989). Neuropsychological, electroencephalogram and brain computed tomography findings in motor neuron disease. *European Neurology, 29,* 115–120.

Goldblatt, D., & Greenlaw, J. (1989). Starting and stopping the ventilator for patients with amyotrophic lateral sclerosis. *Neurology Clinics, 7*(4), 789–806.

Griggs, R. C., Donohoe, K. M., Utll, M. J., & Goldblatt, D. (1980). Pulmonary function testing. In D. W. Mulder (Ed.), *The diagnosis and treatment of amyotrophic lateral sclerosis* (pp. 291–299). Boston: Houghton Mifflin.

Gurney, M. E., Cutting, F. B., Zhai, P., Doble, A., Taylor, C. P., Andrus, P. K., & Hall, E. D. (1996). Benefit of vitamin E, Riluzole and Gabepentin in a transgenic model of familial amyotrophic lateral sclerosis. *Annals of Neurology, 39,* 147–157.

Hammen, V. L., Yorkston, K. M., & Dowden, P. A. (1991). Index of contextual intelligibility I: Impact of semantic context in dysarthria. In C. Moore, K. M. Yorkston, & D. R. Beukelman (Eds.), *Dysarthria and apraxia of speech: Perspectives on intervention* (pp. 43–54). Baltimore: Brookes.

Hanayama, K., Ishikawa, Y., & Bach, J. R. (1997). Amyotrophic lateral sclerosis: Successful treatment of mucous plugging by mechanical insufflation–exsufflation. *American Journal of Physical Medicine & Rehabilitation, 76*(4), 338–339.

Hardiman, O. (2000). Symptomatic treatment of respiratory and nutritional failure in amyotrophic lateral sclerosis. *Journal of Neurology, 247*(4), 245–251.

Hillel, A. D., & Miller, R. M. (1989). Bulbar amyotrophic lateral sclerosis: Patterns of progression and clinical management. *Journal of Head and Neck Surgery, 11,* 51–59.

Hillel, A. D., Yorkston, K. M., & Miller, R. M. (1989). Use of phonation time to estimate vital capacity in amyotrophic lateral sclerosis. *Archives of Physical Medicine and Rehabilitation, 70,* 618–620.

Hirose, H., Kiritani, S., Ushijima, T., & Sawashima, M. (1978). Analysis of abnormal articulatory dynamics in two dysarthric patients. *Journal of Speech and Hearing Disorders, 43*(1), 96–105.

Househam, E., & Swash, M. (2000). Diagnostic delay in amyotrophic lateral sclerosis: What scope for improvement? *Journal of the Neurological Sciences, 180*(1–2), 76–81.

Hudson, A. J. (1981). Amyotrophic lateral sclerosis and its association with dementia, parkinsonism and other neurologic disorders: A review. *Brain, 104*(2), 217–247.

Iannaccone, S., & Ferini-Strambi, L. (1996). Pharmacologic treatment of emotional lability. *Clinical Neuropharmacology, 19*(6), 532–535.

Iwasaki, Y., Kinoshita, M., Ikeda, K., Takamiya, K., & Shiojima, T. (1990). Neuropsychological dysfunction in amyotrophic lateral sclerosis: Relation to motor abilities. *International Journal of Neuroscience, 54*(2), 191–195.

Jackson, C. E., & Bryan, W. W. (1998). Amyotrophic lateral sclerosis. *Seminars in Neurology, 18*(1), 27–39.

Janiszewski, D. W., Caroscio, J. T., & Wisham, L. H. (1983). Amyotrophic lateral sclerosis: A comprehensive rehabilitation approach. *Archives of Physical Medicine and Rehabilitation, 64,* 304–307.

Kapadia, F. (1998). Mechanical ventilation: Simplifying the terminology. *Postgraduate Medical Journal, 74*(872), 330–335.

Kasarskis, E. J., Berryman, S., Vanderleest, J. G., Schneider, A. R., & McClain, C. J. (1996). Nutritional status of patients with amyotrophic lateral sclerosis: Relation to the proximity of death. *American Journal of Clinical Nutrition, 63,* 130–137.

Kazandjian, M. S. (1997). *Communication and swallowing solutions for the ALS/MND community.* San Diego, CA: Singular.

Kent, J. F., Kent, R. D., Rosenbek, J. C., Weismer, G., Martin, R., Sufit, R., & Brooks, B. R. (1992). Quantitative description of the dysarthria in women with amyotrophic lateral sclerosis. *Journal of Speech and Hearing Research, 35,* 723–733.

Kent, R. D., Hyang-Hee, K., Weismer, G., Kent, J. F., Rosenbek, J. C., Brooks, B. R., & Workinger, M. (1994). Laryngeal dysfunction in neurological disease: Amyotrophic lateral sclerosis, Parkinson disease, and stroke. *Journal of Medical Speech–Language Pathology, 2*(3), 157–176.

Kent, R. D., Kent, J. F., Weismer, G., Sufit, R. L., Rosenbek, J. C., Martin, R. E., & Brooks, B. R. (1990). Impairment of speech intelligibility in men with amyotrophic lateral sclerosis. *Journal of Speech and Hearing Disorders, 55*(4), 721–728.

Kent, R. D., Sufit, R. L., Rosenbek, J. C., Kent, J. F., Weismer, G., Martin, R. E., & Brooks, B. R. (1991). Speech deterioration in amyotrophic lateral sclerosis: A case study. *Journal of Speech and Hearing Research, 34,* 1269–1275.

Kent, R. D., Weismer, G., Kent, J. F., & Rosenbek, J. C. (1989). Toward phonetic intelligibility testing in dysarthria. *Journal of Speech and Hearing Disorders, 54,* 482–499.

Kew, J. J., Goldstein, L. H., Leigh, P. N., Abrahams, S., Cograve, N., Passingham, R. E., Frackowiak, R. S., & Brooks, D. J. (1993). The relationship between abnormalities of cognitive function and cerebral activation in amyotrophic lateral sclerosis: A neuropsychological and positron emission tomography study. *Brain, 116,* 1399–1423.

Kiernan, J. A., & Hudson, A. J. (1994). Frontal lobe atrophy in motor neuron diseases. *Brain, 117,* 747–757.

Klasner, E. R., Yorkston, K. M., & Strand, E. A. (1999). Patterns of perceptual features in speakers with ALS: Prominence and intelligibility considerations. *Journal of Medical Speech–Language Pathology, 7*(2), 117–126.

Kleopa, K. A., Sherman, M., Neal, B., Romano, G. J., & Heiman-Patterson, T. (1999). Bipap improves survival rate of pulmonary function decline in patients with ALS. *Journal of the Neurological Sciences, 164*(1), 82–88.

Klivenyi, P., Ferrante, R. J., Matthews, R. T., Bogdanov, M. B., Klein, A. M., Andreassen, O. A., Mueller, G., Wermer, M., Kaddurah-Haouk, R., & Beal, M. F. (1999). Neuroprotective effects of creatine in a transgenic animal model of amyotrophic lateral sclerosis. *Nature Medicine, 5,* 347–350.

Kreul, E. (1972). Neuromuscular control examination (NMC) for parkinsonism: Vocal prolongations and diadokokinetic and reading rates. *Journal of Speech and Hearing Research, 15,* 72–83.

Lasker, J. P., & Bedrosian, J. L. (2001). Promoting acceptance of augmentative and alternative communication by adults with acquired communication disorders. *Augmentative and Alternative Communication, 17*(3), 141–153.

Lass, N., & Sandusky, J. (1971). A study of the relationship of diadokokinetic rate, speaking rate, and reading rate. *Today's Speech, 19,* 49–54.

Lindeman, R. C. (1975). Diverting the paralyzed larynx: A reversible procedure for intractable aspiration. *Laryngoscope, 85*(1), 157–180.

Lloyd, C. M., Richardson, M. P., Brooks, D. J., Al-Chalabi, A., & Leigh, P. N. (2000). Extramotor involvement in ALS: PET studies with the GABA(A) ligand(11C) flumazenil. *Brain, 123*(11), 2289–2296.

Ludolph, A. C., Langen, K. J., Regard, M., Herzog, H., Kemper, B., Kuwert, T., Bottger, I. G., & Feinendegen, L. (1992). Frontal lobe function in amyotrophic lateral sclerosis: A neuropsychologic and positron emission tomography study. *Acta Neurologica Scandinavica, 85*(2), 81–89.

Massman, P. J., Sims, J., Cook, N., Haverkamp, L. J., Appel, V., & Appel, S. H. (1996). Prevalence and correlates of neuropsychological deficits in amyotrophic lateral sclerosis. *Journal of Neurology, Neurosurgery and Psychiatry, 61,* 450–455.

Mathy, P., Yorkston, K. M., & Gutmann, M. (2000). Augmentative communication for individuals with amyotrophic lateral sclerosis. In D. R. Beukelman, K. M. Yorkston, & J. Reichle (Eds.), *Augmentative and alternative communication for adults with acquired neurologic disabilities* (pp. 191–240). Baltimore.: Brookes.

McDonald, E. R., Hillel, A., & Wiedenfeld, S. A. (1996). Evaluation of the psychological status of ventilatory-supported patients with ALS/MND. *Palliative Medicine, 10*(1), 35–41.

McDonald, E. R., Wiedenfeld, S. A., Hillel, A., Carpenter, C. L., & Walter, R. A. (1994). Survival in amyotrophic lateral sclerosis: The role of psychological factors. *Archives of Neurology, 51*(1), 17–23.

McNaughton, D., Light, J., & Groszyk, L. (2001). "Don't give up": Employment experiences of individuals with amyotrophic lateral sclerosis who use augmentative and alternative communication. *Augmentative and Alternative Communication, 17*(3), 179–195.

Miller, R. G., Rosenberg, J. A., Gelinas, D. F., Mitsumoto, H., Newman, D., Dufit, R., Borasio, G. D., Bradley, W. G., Bromberg, M. B., Brooks, B. R., Kasarskis, E. J., Munsat, T. L., Oppenheimer, E. A., & ALS Practice Parameters Task Force. (1999). Practice parameter: The care of the patient with amyotrophic lateral sclerosis (an evidence-based review): Report of the Quality Standards Subcommittee of the American Academy of Neurology. *Neurology, 52,* 1311–1323.

Mitsuyama, Y., Kogoh, H., & Ata, K. (1985). Progressive dementia with motor neuron disease. An additional case report and neuropathological review of 20 cases in Japan. *European Archives of Psychiatry and Neurological Sciences, 235*(1), 1–8.

Montgomery, G. K., & Erickson, L. M. (1987). Neuropsychological perspectives in amyotrophic lateral sclerosis. *Neurologic Clinics, 5*(1), 61–81.

Moore, S. R., Gresham, L. S., Bromberg, M. B., Kasarkis, E. J., & Smith, R. A. (1997). A self report measure of affective lability. *Journal of Neurology, Neurosurgery and Psychiatry, 63*(1), 89–93.

Moss, A. H., Casey, P., Stocking, C. B., Roos, R. P., Brooks, B. R., & Siegler, M. (1993). Home ventilation for amyotrophic lateral sclerosis patients: Outcomes, costs, and patient, family and physician attitudes. *Neurology, 43*(2), 438–443.

Munte, T. F., Troger, M., Nusser, I., Wieringa, B. M., Matzke, M., Johannes, S., & Dengler, R. (1998). Recognition memory deficits in amyotrophic lateral sclerosis assessed with event-related brain potentials. *Acta Neurologica Scandinavica, 98*(2), 110–115.

Neary, D., Snowden, J. S., & Mann, D. M. (2000). Cognitive change in motor neurone disease/amyotrophic lateral sclerosis (MND/ALS). *Journal of the Neurological Sciences, 180*(1–2), 15–20.

Neatherlin, J. S. (1998). Management of amyotrophic lateral sclerosis with Riluzole. *Journal of Neuroscience Nursing, 30*(4), 257–261.

Newson-Davis, I. C., Abrahams, S., Goldstein, L. H., & Leigh, P. N. (1999). The emotional lability question: A new measure of emotional lability in amyotrophic lateral sclerosis. *Journal of the Neurological Sciences, 169*, 22–25.

Nishio, M., & Niimi, S. (2000). Changes over time in dysarthric patients with amyotrophic lateral sclerosis (ALS): A study of changes in speaking rate and maximum repetition rate. *Clinical Linguistics & Phonetics, 14*(7), 485–497.

Oliver, D. (1996). The quality of care and symptom control: The effects on the terminal phase of ALS/MND. *Journal of the Neurological Sciences, 139*(Suppl.), 134–136.

Oliver, D., Borasio, G. D., & Walsh, D. (Eds.). (2001). *Palliative care in amyotrophic lateral sclerosis: Motor neuron disease.* London: Oxford University Press.

Orrell, R. W., & Figlewicz, D. A. (2001). Clinical implications of the genetics of ALS and other motor neuron disease. *Neurology, 57*, 9–17.

Pasetti, C., & Zanini, G. (2000). The physician–patient relationship in amyotrophic lateral sclerosis. *Neurological Sciences, 21*, 318–323.

Picheny, M., Durlach, N., & Braida, L. (1986). Speaking clearly for the hard of hearing II: Acoustic Characteristics of clear and conversational speech. *Journal of Speech and Hearing Research, 29*(4), 434–446.

Picheny, M., Durlach, N., & Braida, L. (1989). Speaking clearly for the hard of hearing III: An attempt to determine the contribution of speaking rate to differences in intelligibility between clear and conversational speech. *Journal of Speech and Hearing Research, 32*(3), 600–603.

Pinto, A. C., Evangelista, T., Carvalho, M., Alves, M. A., & Sales Luis, M. L. (1995). Respiratory assistance with a non-invasive ventilator (BiPAP) in MND/ALS patients: Survival rates in a controlled trial. *Journal of the Neurological Sciences, 129*, 19–26.

Polkey, M. I., Lyall, R. A., Green, M., Nigel Leigh, P., & Moxham, J. (1998). Expiratory muscle function in amyotrophic lateral sclerosis. *American Journal of Respiratory Critical Care Medicine, 158*(3), 734–741.

Poloni, M., Capitani, E., Mazzini, L., & Ceroni, M. (1986). Neuropsychological measures in amyotrophic lateral sclerosis and their relationship with CT scan-assessed cerebral atrophy. *Acta Neurologica Scandinavica, 74*(4), 257–260.

Pradas, J., Finison, L., Andres, P. L., Thornell, B., Hollander, D., & Munsat, T. L. (1993). The natural history of amyotrophic lateral sclerosis and the use of natural history control in therapeutic trials. *Neurology, 43*(4), 751–755.

Ptacek, P. H., Sander, E. H., Mahoney, W. H., & Jackson, C. C. (1966). Phonatory and related changes in advanced age. *Journal of Speech and Hearing Research, 9*, 353–360.

Rakowicz, W. P., & Hodges, J. R. (1998). Dementia and aphasia in motor neuron disease: An under-recognized association? *Journal of Neurology, Neurosurgery and Psychiatry, 65*, 881–889.

Ramig, L. O., Scherer, R. C., Klasner, E. R., Titze, I. R., & Horii, Y. (1990). Acoustic analysis of voice in amyotrophic lateral sclerosis: A longitudinal case study. *Journal of Speech and Hearing Disorders, 55,* 2–14.

Renout, K. A., Leeper, H. A., Bandur, D. L., & Hudson, A. J. (1995). Vocal fold diadochokinetic function of individuals with amyotrophic lateral sclerosis. *American Journal of Speech–Language Pathology, 4*(1), 73–80.

Riddel, J., McCauley, R. J., Mulligan, M., & Tandan, R. (1995). Intelligibility and phonetic contrast errors in highly intelligible speakers with amyotrophic lateral sclerosis. *Journal of Speech and Hearing Research, 38*(2), 304–314.

Ringel, S. P., Murphy, J. R., Alderson, M. K., Bryan, W., England, J. D., Miller, R. G., Petajan, J. H., Smith, S. A., Roelofs, R. I., Ziter, F., et al. (1993). The natural history of amyotrophic lateral sclerosis. *Neurology, 43*(7), 1316–1322.

Riviere, M., Meininger, V., Zeisser, P., & Munsat, T. (1998). An analysis of extended survival in patients with amyotrophic lateral sclerosis treated with Riluzole. Archives of *Neurology, 55,* 526–528.

Robbins, R. A., Simmons, Z., Bremer, B. A., Walsh, S. M., & Fischer, S. (2001). Quality of life in ALS is maintained as physical function declines. *Neurology, 56,* 442–444.

Robert, D., Pouget, J., Giovanni, A., Azulay, J., & Triglia, J. (1999). Quantitative voice analysis in the assessment of bulbar involvement in amyotrophic lateral sclerosis. *Acta Oto Laryngologica, 119*(6), 724–731.

Rosen, A. (1978). Amyotrophic lateral sclerosis: Clinical features and prognosis. *Archives of Neurology, 35,* 638–642.

Rosen, D. R., Siddique, T., Patterson, D., Figlewicz, D. A., Sapp, P., Hentati, A., Donaldson, D., Goto, J., O'Regan, J. P., & Deng, H. X. (1993). Mutations in Cu/Zn superoxide dismutase gene are associated with familial amyotrophic lateral sclerosis. *Nature, 362,* 59–62.

Roth, C. R., Roburka, B. J., & Workinger, M. S. (2000). The effects of a palatal lift prosthesis on speech intelligibility in amyotrophic lateral sclerosis: A case study. *Journal of Medical Speech–Language Pathology, 8*(4), 365–370.

Rothstein, J. D., Martin, L., & Kuncl, R. W. (1992). Decreased glutamate transport by the brain and spinal cord in amyotrophic lateral sclerosis. *The New England Journal of Medicine, 326*(22), 1464–1493.

Sanjak, M., Reddan, W., & Brooks, B. R. (1987). Role of muscular exercise in amyotrophic lateral sclerosis. *Neurologic Clinics, 5*(2), 251–268.

Schiffer, R. B., Cash, J., & Herndon, R. M. (1983). Treatment of emotional lability with low-dosage tricyclic antidepressants. *Psychosomatics, 24,* 1094–1096.

Schiffer, R. B., Herndon, R. M., & Rudick, R. A. (1985). Treatment of pathologic laughing and weeping with amitriptyline. *New England Journal of Medicine, 312,* 1480–1482.

Schiffman, P. L., & Belsh, J. M. (1993). Pulmonary function at diagnosis of amyotrophic lateral sclerosis: Rate of deterioration. *Chest, 103*(2), 508–513.

Silbergleit, A. K., Johnson, A. F., & Jacobson, B. H. (1997). Acoustic analysis of voice in individuals with amyotrophic lateral sclerosis and perceptually normal vocal quality. *Journal of Voice, 11*(2), 222–231.

Silverstein, M. D., Stocking, C. B., Antel, J. P., Beckwith, J., Roos, R. P., & Siegler, M. (1991). Amyotrophic lateral sclerosis and life-sustaining therapy: Patients' desires for information, participation in decision making, and life-sustaining therapy. *Mayo Clinic Proceedings, 66,* 906–913.

Stone, N. (1987). Amyotrophic lateral sclerosis: A challenge for constant adaptation. *Journal of Neuroscience Nursing, 19*(3), 166–173.

Strand, E. A., Buder, E. H., Yorkston, K. M., & Ramig, L. O. (1994). Differential phonatory characteristics of four women with amyotrophic lateral sclerosis. *Journal of Voice, 8*(4), 327–339.

Strand, E. A., Miller, R. M., Yorkston, K. M., & Hillel, A. D. (1996). Management of oral-pharyngeal dysphagia symptoms in amyotrophic lateral sclerosis. *Dysphagia, 11,* 129–139.

Strong, M. J., Grace, G. M., Orange, J. B., & Leeper, H. A. (1996). Cognition, language and speech in amyotrophic lateral sclerosis: A review. *Journal of Clinical and Experimental Neuropsychology, 18*(2), 291–303.

Strong, M. J., Grace, G. M., Orange, J. B., Leeper, H. A., Menon, R. S., & Aere, C. (1999). A prospective study of cognitive impairment in ALS. *Neurology, 53*, 1665–1671.

Strong, M. J., Hudson, A. J., & Alvord, W. G. (1991). Familial amyotrophic lateral sclerosis, 1850–1989: A statistical analysis of the world literature. *Canadian Journal of Neurologic Science, 18*(1), 45–58.

Tarnopolsky, M., & Martin, J. P. (1999). Creatine monohydrate increases strength in patients with neuromuscular disease. *Neurology, 52*, 854–857.

Theys, P. A., Peeters, E., & Robberecht, W. (1999). Evolution of motor and sensory deficits in amyotrophic lateral sclerosis estimated by neurophysiological techniques. *Journal of Neurology, 246*(6), 438–442.

Tidwell, J. (1993). Pulmonary management of the ALS patients. *Journal of Neurologic Nursing, 25*(6), 337–342.

Tjaden, K., & Turner, G. S. (1997). Spectral properties of fricative in amyotrophic lateral sclerosis. *Journal of Speech, Language, and Hearing Research, 40*(6), 1358–1372.

Tomik, B., Krupinski, J., Glodzik-Sobanska, L., Bala-Slodowska, M., Wszolek, W., Kusiak, M., & Lechwacka, A. (1999). Acoustic analysis of dysarthria profile in ALS patients. *Journal of the Neurological Sciences, 169*(1–2), 35–42.

Tscuchiya, K., Ozawa, E., Fukushima, J., Yasui, H., Kondo, H., Nakano, I., & Ikeda, K. (2000). Rapidly progressive aphasia and motor neuron disease: A clinical, radiological, and pathological study of an autopsy case with circumscribed lobar atrophy. *Acta Neuropathologica (Berlin), 99*, 81–87.

Turner, G., & Tjaden, K. (2000). Acoustic differences between content and function words in amyotrophic lateral sclerosis. *Journal of Speech, Language, and Hearing Research, 43*(3), 769–781.

Turner, G. S., Tjaden, K., & Weismer, G. (1995). The influence of speaking rate on vowel space and speech intelligibility for individuals with amyotrophic lateral sclerosis. *Journal of Speech and Hearing Research, 38*(5), 1000–1013.

Weismer, G., Jeng, J. Y., Laures, J. S., Kent, R. D., & Kent, J. F. (2001). Acoustic and intelligibility characteristics of sentence production in neurogenic speech disorders. *Folia Phoniatrica et Logopaedica, 53*(1), 1–18.

Weismer, G., Kent, R. D., Hodge, M., & Martin, R. (1988). The acoustic signature for intelligibility test words. *Journal of the Acoustical Society of America, 84*(4), 1281–1291.

Weismer, G., Laures, J. S., Jeng, J., Kent, R. D., & Kent, J. F. (2000). Effects of speaking rate manipulations on acoustic and perceptual aspects of dysarthria in amyotrophic lateral sclerosis. *Folia Phoniatrica et Logopaedica, 52*(5), 201–219.

Weismer, G., Martin, R., Kent, R. D., & Kent, J. F. (1992). Formant trajectory characteristics of males with amyotrophic lateral sclerosis. *Journal of the Acoustical Society of America, 91*(2), 1058–1098.

World Federation of Neurology Research Group on Neuromuscular Disease. (1994). El Escorial World Federation of Neurology criteria for the diagnosis of amyotrophic lateral sclerosis. *Journal of the Neurological Sciences, 124*(Suppl.), 96–107.

World Health Organization. (1990). *Cancer Pain Relief. Report of the WHO Expert Committee* (Technical Report Series 804). Geneva, Switzerland: Author.

Yorkston, K. M., Beukelman, D. R., Strand, E. A., & Bell, K. R. (1999). *Management of motor speech disorders in children and adults.* Austin, TX: PRO-ED.

Yorkston, K. M., Beukelman, D. R., & Tice, R. (1996). *Sentence Intelligibility Test.* Lincoln, NE: Tice Technology Services.

Yorkston, K. M., Hammen, V. L., & Dowden, P. A. (1991). Index of contextual intelligibility II: A perceptual analysis of intelligible versus unintelligible productions in severe dysarthria. In C. Moore, K. M. Yorkston, & D. R. Beukelman (Eds.), *Dysarthria and apraxia of speech: Perspectives on intervention* (pp. 55–64). Baltimore: Brookes.

Yorkston, K. M., Spencer, K. A., Duffy, J. R., Beukelman, D. R., Golper, L. A., Miller, R. M., Strand, E. A., & Sullivan, M. (2001). Evidence-based practice guidelines for dysarthria: Management of velopharyngeal function. *Journal of Medical Speech–Language Pathology, 9*(4), 257–273.

Yorkston, K. M., Strand, E. A., & Hume, J. (1998). The relationship between motor function and speech function in amyotrophic lateral sclerosis. In M. Cannito, K. M. Yorkston, & D. R. Beukelman (Eds.), *Neuromotor speech disorders: Nature, assessment, and management* (pp. 85–98). Baltimore: Brookes.

Yorkston, K. M., Strand, E. A., & Kennedy, M. R. T. (1996). Comprehensibility of dysarthric speech: Implications for assessment and treatment planning. *American Journal of Speech–Language Pathology, 5*(1), 55–66.

Yorkston, K. M., Strand, E. A., & Miller, R. M. (1996). Progression of respiratory symptoms in amyotrophic lateral sclerosis: Implications for speech function. In D. A. Robin, K. M. Yorkston, & D. R. Beukelman (Eds.), *Disorders of motor speech: Assessment, treatment and clinical characterization* (pp. 193–204). Baltimore: Brookes.

Yorkston, K. M., Strand, E., Miller, R., Hillel, A., & Smith, K. (1993). Speech deterioration in amyotrophic lateral sclerosis: Implications for the timing of intervention. *Journal of Medical Speech–Language Pathology, 1*(1), 35–46.

Zeitlin, D. J., Abrams, G. M., & Shah, B. K. (1995). Use of augmentative/alternative communication in patients with amyotrophic lateral sclerosis. *Journal of Neurological Rehabilitation, 9*(4), 217–220.

2

PARKINSON DISEASE

Nature of the Problem

This section provides background information on Parkinson disease and the Parkinson plus syndromes that are often grouped with it. Topics covered include its nature, symptoms, and medical management. A summary of information is found in the "Parkinson Disease" handout in the Appendix at the back of the book.

What Is Parkinson Disease?

Parkinson disease (paralysis agitans or shaking palsy) is a relatively common, slowly progressive disease of the central nervous system, specifically the basal ganglia. The essential problem in Parkinson disease is the inability to automatically execute learned motor plans (Marsden, 1984). The hallmark features or classic triad of the motor impairment are resting tremor, bradykinesia, and rigidity, each of which will be discussed in detail. The disease is typically categorized into three etiologic groups. By far the largest is the *idiopathic* group, in which the origin of the disease is spontaneous or unknown. Another is the *secondary* or *acquired* group, in which the disease results from use of certain drugs, exposure to certain toxins, or vascular lesions such as repeated head trauma in boxers. Finally, there is a group of disorders collectively called *Parkinson Plus Syndromes*. Because signs of parkinsonism are among the primary clinical features, this group is frequently misdiagnosed as idiopathic Parkinson disease, especially early in the disease process. Collectively, however, they are not as responsive to levodopa therapy and have additional signs and symptoms (e.g., cortical and cerebellar) that are not commonly associated with parkinsonism. These diseases usually have a worse prognosis. Although these disorders all share signs of parkinsonism, they are different from one another and different from Parkinson disease. Two major categories of Parkinson plus syndromes are multiple system atrophy and progressive supranuclear palsy.

Idiopathic Parkinson disease is relatively common, with 1% of the population over the age of 50 exhibiting the disorder. The incidence of Parkinson disease varies as a function of age (Tanner & Aston, 2000). It is estimated that 50,000 Americans are diagnosed with Parkinson disease each year and that over a million individuals in the United States have the disease (*Parkinson's Disease*, 2001). Reports suggest that rates of occurrence are similar across countries and that these rates have not changed over the past century (Duvoisin, 1991). Men and women are affected in equal numbers.

What Changes in Neural Systems Are Associated with Parkinson Disease?

Parkinson disease may be described in biochemical terms as an imbalance between dopamine-activated and acetylcholine-activated neurons of the corpus striatum, and in neuropathologic terms as an imbalance between excitatory and inhibitory striatal influences. It is a disorder of the basal ganglia (caudate, lentiform, and subthalamic nuclei, the claustrum, substantia nigra, and the dopaminergic neurones of the ventral tegmental area) affecting motor control and cognition. A more detailed discussion of the basal ganglion system can be found elsewhere (Brown & Marsden, 1998; Graybiel, 1998; Obeso et al., 2000). It has been hypothesized that the basal ganglia operate to bind input to output, thus providing an automatic link between voluntary effort, sensory input, and the evoking and running of a sequence of motor programs or thoughts (Brown & Marsden, 1998).

What Symptoms Are Associated with Parkinson Disease?

The classic three symptoms associated with Parkinson disease are tremor, bradykinesia, and rigidity. A description of these terms along with the underlying neuropathologic mechanism are presented in Table 2.1. Perhaps the most common feature occurring in approximately two thirds of individuals is a *resting tremor* with a frequency of 3 to 6 Hz. A resting tremor or "pill-rolling" movement of the hand is frequently the initial symptom of parkinsonism. Later, the tremor may spread to the arms, trunk, neck, and lower extremities. The tremor is variable and is reduced during activity or sleep and intensified by fatigue, stress, and movement of the opposite limb.

Bradykinesia is literally translated as slowness of movement, but is more appropriately thought of as an inability to initiate or to perform voluntary movement sequences. When a movement is initiated, it is often performed more slowly than normal and with rapid fatigue. Many of the symptoms of parkinsonism are a consequence of bradykinesia. For example, a number of automatic movements are decreased, including eye blinking, swinging of the arms while walking, expressive gestures of the hands, expressive facial gestures, handwriting, and perhaps swallowing of saliva.

Rigidity is an increase in muscle tone that is present more or less constantly throughout the movement, as opposed to spasticity, which is present at the start of the movement. Cogwheel rigidity may be tested at the elbow or wrist joint. If the

TABLE 2.1   Classic Triad of Symptoms Associated with Parkinson Disease

Symptom	Description	Neuropathology
Tremor	Resting tremor with a frequency of 3–6 Hz. May involve hands, limbs, and trunk. Is suppressed by activity or sleep.	Loss of inhibitory input to the striatal cholinergic system, allowing excessive excitatory output and facilitating oscillatory loops in the thalamocortical system.
Bradykinesia	Slowness of movement, including difficulty initiating, executing, and halting a movement. Accounts for masklike face, decreased swallowing and drooling, micrographia, and some characterstics of dysarthria.	Delays in motor unit recruitment and greater amount of excitatory input from the cortex before movements are activated.
Rigidity	Increased tone of both antagonist and protagonist muscle groups.	Augmentation of alpha motor neuron activity.

joint is flexed and extended rapidly through its range of motion, the joint surface feels as if it consists of two cogwheels moving in stepwise relation to one another. The cogwheel pattern may be a superimposition of tremor on rigidity.

Postural instability is also a characteristic and debilitating feature of parkinsonism. The typical individual with parkinsonism has a flexed or stooped posture. The lack of postural reflexes leads to a tendency to fall to one side (lateral pulsion) or backward (retropulsion). The patient is unable to correct postural imbalances and therefore is at risk for falls.

Table 2.2 contains a listing of common signs and symptoms of parkinsonism. Many of these associated symptoms are consequences of tremor, rigidity, and bradykinesia. For example, loss of blinking, masklike face, and drooling may be associated with bradykinesia. Fatigue may be associated with excessive muscular activity resulting from tremor and rigidity.

How Is the Diagnosis of Parkinson Disease Made?

Diagnosis of Parkinson disease is complicated by the fact that early symptoms may be difficult to distinguish from the normal aging process and from other neurologic-conditions, particularly those known as parkinsonism plus. Diagnostic criteria are based on the relative sensitivity and specificity of clinical signs of disorder (Siderowf, 2001). *Sensitivity* is the proportion of individuals with Parkinson disease who have a positive test. For example, 99% of those with pathologically defined Parkinson disease have two of the three cardinal features (tremor, bradykinesia, or rigidity). *Specificity*, on the other hand, is the proportion of individuals without the disease who have

TABLE 2.2	Symptoms Associated with Parkinson Disease	
Classic Triad	**Other Physical Symptoms**	
Tremor	Expressionless face	
Rigidity	Loss of blinking	
Bradykinesia	Dysphagia	
	Micrographia	
Psychological	Dysarthria	
Cognitive slowness	Constipation	
Subcortical dementia	Postural instability	
Depression	Altered body posture	
Perceptual deficits	Fatigue	
	Gait disturbances	
	Hyperhidrosis (excessive sweating)	
	Orthostasis	
	Sialorrhea (excessive saliva)	
	Bladder dysfunction	
	Disturbances of eye movements	

a negative test. In other words, low specificity suggests that the symptom is not distinct to Parkinson disease; rather, it is found in other disorders as well. Ward and Gibb (1990) suggest the following criteria that balance good sensitivity with acceptable specificity:

1. Progressive disease

2. Presence of at least two of the three cardinal features

3. Presence of at least two of the following: markedly positive response to levodopa, asymmetric signs, asymmetry at onset, or initial symptom tremor

4. Absence of clinical characteristics of alternative diagnoses

5. Absence of etiology known to cause similar features

Diagnostic confusion may exist, particularly in early stages, between Parkinson disease and other disorders such as progressive supranuclear palsy (PSP) or multiple system atrophy. The following section describes these disorders.

How Do the Parkinson Plus Disorders Differ from Parkinson Disease?

Multiple system atrophy (MSA) is a heterogenous group of disorders characterized by atypical parkinsonism and relative unresponsiveness to antiparkinsonian medications. Varying degrees of cerebellar, pyramidal, autonomic, and cognitive problems occur in different types of MSA (Wenning, Seppi, Scherfler, Stefanova, & Puschba, 2001). Onset of MSA is usually between 50 and 70 years but it can be diagnosed as early as 30. Mean survival length is approximately 8 years. The three primary disorders associated with the MSA diagnostic category are olivopontocerebellar atrophy, striatonigral degeneration, and Shy-Drager syndrome.

Olivopontocerebellar atrophy (OPCA) is associated with degeneration of the pontine, arcuate, and olivary nuclei, but may also involve the middle cerebellar peduncles and the cerebellum. The disorder is also associated with degenerative changes in the basal ganglia, cerebral cortex, spinal cord, and peripheral nerves. OPCA is diagnosed by prominent cerebellar symptoms (ataxia, kinetic tremor). The clinical signs are variable, but primarily cerebellar. Other clinical findings include parkinsonism, movement disorders, and dementia. The dysarthria associated with OPCA is primarily described as a mixed spastic/ataxic, although there are few reports in the literature (Duffy, 1995).

Striatonigral degeneration (SND) is closely related to Parkinson disease in that is usually presents early with unilateral rigidity and akinesia. It will typically spread to the other side of the body and progress in severity. The symptoms include flexed posture, slow movement, and poor balance. Cerebellar signs and tremor are not usually present. Differential diagnosis of SND usually occurs in the presence of prominent anterocollis and pyramidal dysfunction. Although the dysarthrias accompanying SND have not been investigated, hypokinetic dysarthria would be expected. One might also expect a coexisting hyperkinetic or spastic dysarthria.

Shy-Drager syndrome (SDS) affects the motor components of the autonomic and the somatic divisions of the central nervous system. Early signs include orthostatic hypotension, incontinence, and decreased respiration. If autonomic signs go unrecognized, the disease may be misdiagnosed as cerebellar degeneration or Parkinson disease. The differential diagnosis is made when the dysautonomia outweighs other signs. Dysarthria occurs frequently in SDS. There may be a single dysarthria (ataxic or hypokinetic), but mixed types (hypokinetic–ataxic, ataxic–spastic, aspastic–ataxic–hypokinetic) may be present.

Progressive supranuclear palsy (PSP) is the most common among the Parkinson plus syndromes, and is often misdiagnosed as idiopathic Parkinson disease early in disease progression. PSP has recently been noted to be more common than previously considered and frequently misdiagnosed (Nathan et al., 2001; Schrag, Ben-Shlomo, & Quinn, 2000). There is usually involvement of the subthalamic nucleus, globus pallidus, superior colliculus, pretectal area, and substantia nigra, with possible involvement of a number of brain stem cranial nuclei. Cortical involvement is rare except for the frontal lobe. The clinical signs of PSP share some clinical features with Parkinson disease, including bradykinesia, rigidity, dysarthria, dysphagia, and dementia. Tremor is rarely seen, however. There is evidence of bilateral frontal lobe dysfunction (e.g., pseudobulbar affect), gait difficulty, and postural instability. Vertical-ocular gaze paresis is the most salient feature of PSP (Rehman, 2000). The patient frequently develops both dysarthria and dysphagia.

Similar to Parkinson disease, most patients develop symptoms of PSP in the sixth or seventh decade. The mean length of the disease, however, is 9 to 10 years. Santacruz, Uttl, Litvan, and Grafman (1998) reported that the course of PSP is dominated by motor symptoms, which affect every patient. Emotional, cognitive, and personality changes may occur, but are not seen with every patient. Medical management for PSP has been more difficult than for Parkinson disease. The use of antiparkinsonian medications as well as other neurotransmitter replacement therapies has been reported to be ineffective. Further, frequent adverse effects of these medications have been noted (Kompoliti, Goetz, Litvan, Jellinger, & Verny, 1998).

How Rapidly Does Parkinsonism Progress?

Parkinson disease is not considered fatal; however, there is an increase in both morbidity (sickness rate) and mortality (death rate). Morbidity is associated with a variety of functional limitations. Although Parkinson disease was often not listed as the cause of death in a community-based study, twice as many individuals with the disease died from pneumonia than the control group (Beyer, Herlofson, Arsland, & Larsen, 2001).

A number of scales are available to monitor progression of these limitations. For example, the Hoehn and Yahr Functional Rating Scale (1967) is widely reported in the literature as a general index of the severity of the disease. The scale (summarized in Table 2.3) ranges from mild, unilateral symptoms to severe disability and complete dependence. Note that the distinction between Stages 1 and 2 is unilateral versus bilateral involvement. Normal balance versus postural instability distinguishes Stages 2 and 3. In Stage 4 ambulation is no longer independent, and in Stage 5 the individual is wheelchair dependent. Disease progression has been studied in Parkinson disease and related disorders. Figure 2.1 illustrates the time between onset of symptoms and progression to each of the Hoehn and Yahr stages. Note that progression from stage to stage is much longer for Parkinson disease than for either PSP or MSA. Also, the rate of disease progression is not affected by drugs such as levodopa (Poewe & Wenning, 1998).

TABLE 2.3	Functional Rating Scale for Parkinson Disease

Stage 1: Unilateral disease. The disease in this stage is characterized by mild resting tremor, rigidity, bradykinesia, dysarthria, trunk tilt, fine motor incoordination, and facial immobility. These symptoms are noticeable but not disabling. Symptoms often present in unilateral or hemiparetic fashion.

Stage 2: Bilateral disease, without impairment of balance. The individual is mildly disabled as symptoms appear liberally and standing posture becomes stooped. Gait is a shuffle. Fatigue, bradykinesia, and weakness impair home and work activities. The wrist assumes a slightly dorsiflexed position.

Stage 3: Mild to moderate bilateral disease. Moderate disability involves a festinating gait. Retropulsion initially and propulsion later interfere with stopping, starting, turning, and stepping backward. Self-care activities are tediously performed and often require attendant help. Falls become a real threat to safety.

Stage 4: Severe disability. Marked rigidity, akinesis, and poor standing balance are severely disabling, as is fine motor incoordination. Thus, safe independent ambulation is confined to the home at best and self-care skills require assistance. Tremor is less pronounced.

Stage 5: Wheelchair bound or bedridden. This stage represents complete dependence and serious worsening of all preceding patterns of musculoskeletal disability. Aspiration, pneumonia, weight loss, malnutrition, dehydration, and fecal impaction often necessitate a feed tube.

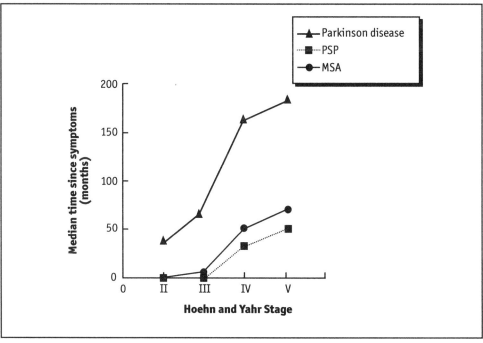

Figure 2.1. Rates of progression to various Hoehn and Yahr stages for individuals with Parkinson disease, progressive supranuclear palsy (PSP), and multiple system atrophy (MSA).

Perhaps the most comprehensive scale for recording information about an individual's functioning and symptoms is found in the Unified Parkinson Disease Rating Scale (UPDRS; Fahr, Elton, & UPDRS Development Committee, 1987; Stebbins & Goetz, 1998). This scale is based on interview and clinical examination, and uses a 5-point scale ranging from 0 (*no limitations*) to 4 (*severe problems*). The categories of dimensions rated are contained in Table 2.4. A number of the items on this scale, including the activities of daily living, are rated two times in the medication cycle, once during the "on" period and once during the "off" period.

The rate of progression of disease varies from patient to patient. Within individual patients, however, the progression of motor symptoms is fairly constant (Marttila & Rinne, 1991). Some of the interpatient variability may be explained by the existence of subgroups of patients (Zetusky, Jankovic, & Pirozzolo, 1985). One subgroup is characterized by a predominant bradykinesia and cognitive impairment, and another by predominant tremor and relatively intact intellectual function. The tremor-dominant group usually has a more favorable prognosis than the hypokinetic group. The tremor type is also associated with a family history of parkinsonism, earlier age at onset, less severe oropharyngeal involvement, and preservation of mental status. The poorest prognosis is associated with a "postural instability" subgroup (Zetusky et al., 1985). This group is characterized by more pronounced decline in functional and mental status, later age at onset, dysarthria, dysphagia, and more rapid progression. Risk factors for rapid progression include older age at onset, concomitant major depression, dementia, and akinetic symptom presentation (Poewe & Wenning, 1998).

TABLE 2.4

Categories Included in the Unified Parkinson Disease Rating Scale (UPDRS)

Mentation, Behavior, Mood	Activities of Daily Living	Motor Examination	Complications of Therapy
Intellectual impairment	Speech	Speech	Duration of dyskinesias
Thought disorder	Salivation	Facial expression	Disability related to dyskinesia
Depression	Swallowing	Tremor in face at rest	Painful dyskinesias
Motivation/ Initiation	Handwriting	Tremor in hands at rest	Early morning dystonia
	Cutting food, using utensils	Tremor in feet at rest	Predictable "off" periods
	Dressing	Action or postural tremor of hands	Sudden onset "off" periods
	Hygiene	Rigidity in neck	Percent of waking day as "off" period
	Turning in bed	Rigidity in upper extremity	
	Falling	Rigidity in lower extremity	Anorexia, nausea, vomiting
	Freezing when walking	Finger taps	Sleep disturbance
	Walking	Hand movement	Symptomatic orthostasis
	Tremor	Rapid alternative movements of hand	
	Sensory complaints	Foot agility	
		Rising from chair	
		Posture	
		Gait	
		Postural stability	
		Body bradykinesia and hypokinesia	

What Is the Medical Management
of Parkinson Disease?

Currently, there is no cure for Parkinson disease. In the absence of a cure, however, there are a number of general approaches to management. The following section reviews medication, surgery, and rehabilitative management of Parkinson disease.

MEDICATION

Pharmacologic intervention is a mainstay in management of Parkinson disease. Parkinson disease is the result of a reduction in dopamine, an important neurotransmitter in the brain. In simple terms, this reduction upsets the balance between two major neural transmitter systems, the dopamine system and the acetylcholine system. The primary goal of drug management is to reestablish this balance. Since the 1960s dramatic improvements have been made in the area of drug treatment, resulting in long-term relief from the symptoms of the disease. The pharmacologic management of Parkinson disease continues to change. Excellent review articles are available (Ahlskog, 2001; Munchau & Bhatia, 2000). Readers are also referred to Web sites such as that of the Mayo Clinic (www.mayoclinic.com/index.cfm) for general information about current drug and surgical management and the National Institute of Neurological Disorders and Stroke (www.ninds.nih.gov/parkinsonsweb/clinical_trials .htm) for the latest information about clinical trials. A number of different approaches may be used in the management of Parkinson disease.

Dopamine Replenishment

Dopamine replacement has become the gold standard of drug treatment in Parkinson's disease. Because dopamine does not cross the blood–brain barrier, it is not useful as a direct agent for intervention. The discovery of levodopa (L-dopa) in the late 1960s represented a major turning point. A small amount of levodopa crosses the blood–brain barrier and degrades readily into dopamine. Unfortunately, the dopamine that remains in the periphery causes side effects, including nausea and vomiting. Therefore, levodopa is usually given in combination with an enzyme inhibitor such as carbidopa that prevents breakdown before the levodopa crosses the blood–brain barrier, thus reducing nausea. Sinemet (which literally translates to "without vomit") is a common brand name for the levodopa/carbidopa combination (Duvoisin, 1991). Unfortunately as time passes, side effects may occur, including dyskinesia, motor fluctuations, and hallucinations (Jankovic, 2000a).

A number of characteristics of levodopa treatment are noteworthy. Marked drug cycle effects may be present. The medication is taken orally and, therefore, must be absorbed into the bloodstream before crossing the blood–brain barrier into the substantia nigra. Blood levels of levodopa reach their peak from $\frac{1}{2}$ to 2 hours after ingestion and gradually fall back to zero in 4 to 6 hours. The rate of absorption varies, depending on factors such as the type and amount of food in the stomach. Peak-dose dyskinesia is a common side effect of levodopa treatment and is characterized by chorea-like movements. These movements may include twitches, jerks, writhing movements, or restlessness. They are thought to be the result of overcorrection. Instead of a lack of spontaneous movement, there are constant involuntary movements induced by excessive amounts of dopamine. On–off effects may also be seen in patients after a few years of stable response to levodopa. On–off effects are end-of-dose periods of deterioration with severe and rapid fluctuations in mobility and dyskinesia. Patients compare the experience to an electric switch being turned off and on. Drug cycle effects may be managed by more continuous dopaminergic stimulation, such as that provided by controlled-release compounds; for example, Sinemet CR may be used, or Sinemet may be combined with other medications that reduce the fluctuations in the drug cycle.

Dopamine Imitators

A group of drugs known as dopamine receptor agonists mimic the action of dopamine. These drugs activate receptors in the brain in the same way dopamine does. Bromocriptine (Parlodel) is a common dopamine agonist used in combination with levodopa. Other drugs in this category include pergolide (Permax), pramipexole (Mirapex), and ropinirole (Requip). Bromocriptine is useful in reducing the drug cycle fluctuations that occur with levodopa alone because it lasts longer than levodopa, with peak concentrations reached in $\frac{1}{2}$ to 3 hours. Side effects include hallucinations, vivid dreams, and other symptoms similar to those of levodopa.

Dopamine Breakdown Inhibition

Dopamine in the brain is inactivated and metabolically broken down by monoamine oxidase (MAO). A group of drugs including selegiline (Deprenyl or Eldepryl) selectively inhibit an enzyme called monoamine oxidase-B (MAO-B), thereby slowing the breakdown of dopamine. Selegiline is now used as a routine adjunct to levodopa. It was thought that this drug might slow the progression of symptoms, but currently this is not thought to be the case. A new class of drugs, catechol-o-methyl transferase (COMT) inhibitors, prolong the effect of levodopa by blocking an enzyme that breaks down dopamine in the liver and other organs. Tolcapone (Tasmar) and entacapone are included in this class of drugs.

Anticholinergic Drugs

The earliest drug interventions to relieve parkinsonian symptoms involved a group of anticholinergic drugs that block the action of acetylcholine, thus restoring the balance between the dopamine and acetylcholine systems. One such anticholinergic drug, Artane, was first introduced around 1950. Anticholinergic drugs do not provide complete relief of symptoms and have a number of troubling side effects, including dry mouth, blurring of near vision, constipation, and weakening of the bladder.

The physician and patient face a number of issues in developing the most appropriate drug regime to manage the symptoms of Parkinson disease. The first is the timing of the introduction of levodopa. Because there are side effects of long-term use and because young patients are more prone to develop motor complications, it has been suggested that levodopa therapy be delayed for as long as other drugs such as dopamine agonists adequately relieve symptoms (Hristova & Koller, 2000; Jankovic, 2000b; Munchau & Bhatia, 2000). Deferring levodopa treatment is controversial, however, and is typically only suggested for the very young (less than 40–50 years of age). Another issue is the compromise between the benefits of symptom relief and tolerance for side effects. Both relief of symptoms and occurrence of unwanted side effects vary from patient to patient and must be considered carefully when developing an individualized management plan. Finally, symptoms are not equally responsive to drugs. Adequate management of one symptom such as rigidity may leave other symptoms untouched. An individual's sensitivity to a drug may also shift over time.

SURGERY

Before the advent of drug treatment, surgical management was the most common treatment for Parkinson disease. Recent surgical procedures have come back into favor for selected individuals with Parkinson disease (Hallett, Litvan, & Task Force on Surgery for Parkinson's Disease, 1999). Surgeries can be categorized into three types: (a) albative procedures such a thalamotomy and pallidotomy, (b) augmentative or nondestructive techniques such as deep brain stimulation, and (c) restorative techniques such as tissue transplantation or gene therapy. In ablative surgeries, an electric current is used to destroy a small amount of tissue. Current surgical techniques benefit from advances in neural imaging that allow for greater precision than earlier methods. Pallidotomy may improve the motor aspects of the disease (tremors, rigidity, and slow movements) by interrupting the neural pathway between the globus pallidus and the thalamus (Lacritz, Cullum, Frol, Dewey, & Giller, 2000; Laitnen, 2000; York, Levin, Grossman, & Hamilton, 1999). About 5% of patients experience some mild postoperative deterioration.

Deep brain stimulation, a nondestructive surgical technique, came into use in the late 1990s. A unit similar to a pacemaker is implanted in the chest and sends impulses through a wire to the thalamus or subthalamic nuclei, thus interrupting signals from the thalamus. Studies suggest that this procedure results in motor improvement and is relatively safe from the perspective of cognitive function (Fields & Troster, 2000). At this time, restorative surgeries such as tissue transplantation are considered experimental.

REHABILITATION

Rehabilitation efforts, including physical and occupational therapy programs, are adjuncts to appropriate drug management. The goal of all of these programs is to enhance and maintain the level of function of individuals with Parkinson disease. They have a role in management at any stage of progression of the disorder. In early stages of the disease, rehabilitation may take the form of informal fitness or home exercise programs (Lavigne & Roberts, 1982; Weiner & Singer, 1989). Individuals who were physically active before the onset of their disease are commonly encouraged to maintain the activities that they enjoy. For example, they are encouraged to continue participating in such activities as tennis, swimming, walking, or light exercise workouts. On the other hand, individuals who have always been sedentary probably will not start to participate in sports or vigorous physical activities. As the disease progresses, more traditional rehabilitative efforts designed to compensate for motor impairments and prevent secondary complications may be put into place. Table 2.5 contains a brief listing of some of the areas of focus for each of the rehabilitation disciplines.

What Other Problems Are Associated with Parkinson Disease?

Many individuals with Parkinson disease experience difficulties in addition to their motor problems. Primary among these difficulties are depression, cognitive changes, and subtle changes in language. A growing body of evidence supports the nonmotor functions of the basal ganglia (Middleton & Strick, 2000). This evidence includes the presence of multiple circuits or loops connecting the basal ganglia with the cortex, physiologic studies of the activity of neurons in the basal ganglia related to cognitive and sensory operations, and lesions in the basal ganglia resulting in primarily cognitive or sensory disturbances.

DEPRESSION

Depression, characterized by pessimism and hopelessness, decreased motivation and drive, and increased concern with health, is common in Parkinson disease (Gotham, Brown, & Marsden, 1986). Estimates of the occurrence of significant depression range considerably from study to study. Slaughter, Slaughter, Nichols, Holmes, and Martens (2001), in an analysis of 45 studies of depression in Parkinson disease, estimated a 31% prevalence. The specific origin of the depression is unclear. It may be a reactive depression, caused by the person's response to fears of coping with a potentially disabling disease. A mild to moderate depression can be expected in anyone who has a chronic disabling condition. On the other hand, the depression may be endogenous, reflecting some neurochemical aspects of the disease. It may also be the result of other factors such as aging. Because depression is common in old age, its occurrence in Parkinson disease may be coincidental. Diagnosis of depression, especially in early stages, is made somewhat difficult because of parkinsonian symptoms such as a masklike, expressionless face and changes in cognition. Depression is positively correlated with stage of the disease, global cognitive function, and functional capacity (Gupta & Bhatia, 2000). Fortunately, depression can be successfully treated with a variety of antidepressant drugs.

TABLE 2.5	Rehabilitation Therapeutics by Discipline in Parkinson Disease
Medical and Nursing	**Physical Therapy**
Monitoring for othostasis, postural hypotension	Relaxation techniques to decrease rigidity
Nutritional consultation	Range of motion and stretching exercises
Monitoring respiratory status including vital capacity	Functional mobility training
Bowel and bladder management	Progressive ambulation training
Artificial tears for lack of blinking	Use of assistive devices such as walkers
Sexual dysfunction evaluation	General cardiovascular fitness exercises
Anticholinergic medications for drooling	Family training and home exercise programs
Timing of medications and meals	**Speech–Language Pathology**
Occupational Therapy	Language assessment
Activities of daily living (ADLs) evaluation and training	Speech evaluation and treatment
Adaptive equipment for ADLs	Swallowing evaluation and treatment
Range of motion activities of upper extremities	**Psychology**
Fine motor coordination skills	Psychological support
Transfer training	Family counseling
Safety skills	Evaluation and management of depression
Handwriting skill	Cognitive evaluation
Position and posture training	
Family training and home exercises	

Note. Adapted from "Movement Disorders, Including Tremors," by S. S. Jain and S. C. Kirshblum, 1993, in *Rehabilitation Medicine: Principles and Practices*, edited by J. A. DeLisa and B. M. Gans, Philadelphia, PA: Lippincott.

COGNITIVE DEFICITS

Information about the presence, type, and extent of cognitive changes is critical in planning appropriate management programs. The risk of dementia is 6 times higher in individuals with Parkinson disease than in a nonimpaired population (Aarsland et al., 2001). Although the primary impairment associated with Parkinson disease is a motor deficit, a substantial number of individuals with the disease experience changes in cognition. Conservative estimates suggest that about 15% of individuals with Parkinson disease meet the *Diagnostic and Statistical Manual of Mental Disorders–Third Edition* (American Psychiatric Association, 1980) criteria for dementia (Levin, Tomer, & Rey, 1992). A higher proportion, as high as 90% of patients, exhibit milder or highly focal cognitive deficits (Stocchi & Brusa, 2000).

Estimates of the cognitive changes in Parkinson disease are complicated by a number of factors. The published studies in this area are difficult to compare because definitions of cognitive changes and dementia vary, as do techniques for measurement of cognition. The picture is also clouded by other characteristics of Parkinson disease, such as generalized slowness of movement, which limits performance on some measures of cognition. Occurrence of depression also complicates measurement of cognition.

The most frequently reported cognitive disturbances in Parkinson disease are visuospatial deficits, including visual analysis and synthesis; facial recognition; judgment of direction, orientation, and distance; constructional praxis; and spatial attention (Levin et al., 1991; Levin et al., 1992). Deficits in executive functioning are also reported in Parkinson disease resulting in a dementia of mild to moderate severity. Affected skills include anticipation, planning, initiation, and monitoring of goal-directed behaviors. These behaviors have been incorporated in the Frontal Assessment Battery (FAB) that can be administered clinically and is sensitive to frontal lobe dysfunction (Dubois, Slachevsky, Litvan, & Pillon, 2000). The following specific deficits have been identified in Parkinson disease (Levin et al., 1992):

- Failure to initiate activities spontaneously
- Inability to develop a successful approach to problem solving
- Impaired and slowed memory
- Impaired visuospatial perception
- Impaired concept formation
- Poor word-list generation
- Impaired set shifting
- Reduced rate of information processing

There is a growing body of evidence for the existence of more than one type of dementia in Parkinson disease. Cummings and Bensen (1984) suggest two types of dementia. The first is a subcortical dementia characterized by slowing, forgetfulness, depression, and impaired cognition. The second is a cortical dementia with features more typical of Alzheimer's disease.

Dementia is correlated with the overall severity of Parkinson disease (Ebmeier et al., 1991). Features in early stages of the disease include reduced recent memory, impairment of cognition, and somatic features of depression. These symptoms worsen as the disease advances. In the later stages of the disease, deficits are also noted in visuospatial skills, remote memory, language, and mood (Huber, Freidenberg, Shuttleworth, Paulson, & Christy, 1989). There also appears to be a relationship between the motor signs in Parkinson disease and dementia (Levin et al., 1992). If tremor is the predominant motor deficit, cognition is usually normal or near normal. On the other hand, if bradykinesia and rigidity predominate, cognition is more likely to be impaired.

LANGUAGE DEFICITS

Language abilities of individuals with Parkinson disease have received considerable attention (Bayles, 1990; Beatty & Monson, 1989; Cooper, Sagar, Jordan, Harvey, & Sullivan, 1991; Grossman et al., 1991; P. Lieberman, Friedman, & Feldman, 1990). These changes have been attributed to the disruption of the fronto-striatal network (Grossman, 1999). Understanding of potential language deficits in Parkinson disease is complicated by cognitive deficits and by the motor aspects of speech production, including altered speech prosody. Evidence exists that subjects with Parkinson disease differ from nondisabled peers on a number of language-related measures, including comprehension of complex commands (Cummings, 1988), sentence processing (Grossman et al., 1991), comprehension of prosody and lexical stress (Lloyd, 1999), generative naming (Bayles et al., 1997), and syntactic complexity in spontaneous speech (Illes, Metter, Hanson, & Iritani, 1988). There is a strong relationship between cognitive decline and language abilities such as discourse comprehension (Murray & Stout, 1999).

A number of studies of language and cognition highlight the differences between people with Parkinson disease and those with Alzheimer's disease (Cummings, 1988; Huber et al., 1989). In patients matched for degree of dementia, the patients with Alzheimer's disease showed far greater language deficits in naming, spontaneous verbalizations, and word-generation capacity than those with Parkinson disease. Other studies suggest that patients with Alzheimer's disease and those with Parkinson disease share some common language problems. McNamara, Obler, Au, Durso, and Albert (1992) found that both parkinsonian and Alzheimer's disease subjects corrected errors made during a verbal picture description task much less often than did nondisabled peers. They suggest that this impairment may be related to attentional and frontal lobe dysfunction in the two disease groups.

Speech Disorders

This section describes the common features of hypokinetic dysarthria associated with Parkinson disease and treatment approaches that target these features for speakers with mild, moderate, and severe dysarthria. The speech and swallowing evaluation protocol described in Chapter 1 is generally applicable to Parkinson disease.

What Speech Characteristics Are Associated with Parkinson Disease?

Dysarthria is common in Parkinson disease. Hartelius and Svensson (1994) surveyed 230 people with Parkinson disease. Seventy percent reported that speech and voice were worse than prior to disease onset. Table 2.6 lists the most frequently reported voice and speech problems in this population. Note that weak voice was the most frequent complaint. Results of self-reports of speech changes must be interpreted with caution because a sizable proportion of individuals with Parkinson disease are aware of their speech problems (Coates & Bakheit, 1997b).

Personal accounts of living with Parkinson disease also give insight into speech characteristics. Dr. Anthony Caruso, a professor in the School of Speech Pathology and Audiology at Kent State University, describes the experience of maintaining his role as a teacher and lecturer despite onset of Parkinson disease at an early age (Caruso, 2001). He describes the stiffness associated with the disease as feeling "more like the Tin Woodsman

TABLE 2.6   Most Frequently Reported Voice and Speech Problems in Parkinson Disease

Voice or Speech Problem	Percentage of Patients Reporting
Weak voice	61
Imprecise articulation	36
Hoarse voice	32
Difficulties getting started	27
Monotonous voice	17
Speech too slow	11
Tremor	10
Stuttering	9
Speech too fast	6
Impaired stress or rhythm	5
Voice too nasal	4

Note. Adapted from "Speech and Swallowing Symptoms Associated with Parkinson's Disease and Multiple Sclerosis," by L. Hartelius and P. Svensson, 1994, *Folia Phoniatrica et Logopaedica, 46,* pp. 9–17.

than the Scarecrow from 'The Wizard of Oz.'" Medications are analogous to Dorothy's oil in allowing him fluid and wide-ranging speech movements.

The perceptual features of the speech of individuals with hypokinetic dysarthria and Parkinson disease are distinctive. The following classic description of moderately severe hypokinetic dysarthria was provided by Darley, Aronson, and Brown (1975):

> . . . significantly reduced variability in pitch and loudness, reduced loudness level overall, and decreased use of all vocal parameters for achieving stress and emphasis. Markedly imprecise articulation is generated at variable rates in short bursts of speech punctuated by illogical pauses and often by inappropriate silences. Voice quality is sometimes harsh, sometimes breathy. (p. 195)

Dysarthria associated with Parkinson disease is distinct from other types of dysarthria. The following 10 speech dimensions are rated more deviant in speakers who have Parkinson disease than in any other group studied by Darley and his colleagues (1975):

* Monopitch
* Monoloudness
* Loudness decay
* Loudness level (overall)
* Increase of rate in segments
* Increase of rate overall
* Reduced stress
* Inappropriate silences
* Short rushes of speech
* Repeated phonemes

Note that the features that distinguish parkinsonism from other dysarthrias are related to altered prosody and rate. Hypokinetic dysarthria is the only type of dysarthria in which faster than normal rate is noted in some speakers.

The clinical picture that emerges from studies of the perceptual features of dysarthria in Parkinson disease is consistent with the underlying pathophysiology. For example, reduced ranges of movement may be reflected in the features of monopitch, monoloudness, reduced stress, and short phrases. Variable rate, short rushes of speech, and imprecise consonants may also be reflective of the reduced range of speech movements. Inappropriate silences may be related to bradykinesia, with its feature of difficulty in initiating movements. The deviant voice dimensions (breathiness, voice harshness, and low pitch) may be the result of rigidity of the laryngeal musculature.

The perceptual information related to dysarthria in Parkinson disease is consistent with a growing body of acoustic evidence (Illes et al., 1988; Ludlow, Connor, & Bassich, 1987; Metter & Hanson, 1986; Weismer, Jeng, Laures, Kent, & Kent, 2001). Acoustic features of parkinsonian dysarthria include reduced durations of vocalic segments, reduced formant transitions, and increased voice onset time compared with typically aging individuals (Forrest, Weismer, & Turner, 1989). In an acoustic analysis of the articulatory deficits of individuals with Parkinson disease, Ackermann and Ziegler (1991) suggested that these speakers have difficulties in running a sequence of motor programs linked together within a complex motor plan. In other words, parkinsonian speakers may have difficulty switching from one motor program to another, just as they appear to have a similar difficulty with limb motor control.

What Are the Characteristics of the Dysarthria Accompanying the Parkinson Plus Syndromes?

Parkinson disease usually presents with a single type of dysarthria—hypokinetic. If one sees a mixed dysarthria, especially early in the disease process, there is the likelihood that the dysarthria is associated with MSA or PSP more than Parkinson disease. The dysarthria accompanying MSA is often of mixed type and is variable from patient to patient. There are some variations one would expect in the dysarthria among the subtypes of MSA. The dysarthria associated with OPCA is primarily described as a mixed spastic–ataxic dysarthria, although there are few reports in the literature (Duffy, 1995). Although the dysarthrias accompanying SND have not been investigated, hypokinetic dysarthria would be expected, as would hyperkinetic or spastic dysarthria types. Dysarthria occurs frequently in SDS and may be a single dysarthria (ataxic or hypokinetic), but mixed types (hypokinetic–ataxic, ataxic–spastic, aspastic–ataxic–hypokinetic) also occur. The dysarthrias associated with MSA change over time, both in terms of severity and type(s). Unlike the dysarthria in Parkinson disease that usually occurs later in the disease process, dysarthria is often an early and salient symptom in PSP (Muller et al., 2001). The most common type of dysarthria associated with PSP is mixed. One should predict the possibility of several types of dysarthria (especially hypokinetic, ataxic, and spastic). Management of the dysarthria of the Parkinson plus syndromes requires changing intervention strategies as the disease progresses.

How Are the Components of the Speech Production Mechanism Altered in Parkinson Disease?

Table 2.7 contains a summary of the physiologic and perceptual characteristics of dysarthria associated with Parkinson disease. Included in the table is a brief description of the respiratory, phonatory, velopharyngeal, and articulatory aspects of speech production.

RESPIRATION

The perceptual features of hypokinetic dysarthria, including reduced loudness level, lead one to suspect that the respiratory system is involved. The literature in Parkinson disease paints a somewhat mixed picture, however. For example, some studies (Boshes, 1966; Canter, 1965) report a reduced ability to sustain phonation, whereas others (Kreul, 1972) report no differences between subjects with no neurological involvement and parkinsonian subjects. See Murdoch, Chenery, Bowler, and Ingram (1989) and Solomon and Hixon (1993) for reviews in this area. The differences in findings may be the result of the experimental tasks (speech vs. nonspeech tasks) and the relative severity of the disease. Differences may also reflect a problem in adjusting the "gain" when regulating speech loudness (Ho, Iansek, & Bradshaw, 1999). Individuals with hypokinetic dysarthria have been described as having an "inflexible" respiratory pattern for speech (Kim, 1968). This inflexibility may be the result of reduced compliance of the rib cage (Solomon & Hixon, 1993).

TABLE 2.7

Characteristics of Dysarthria in Parkinson Disease

	Physiologic Impairment	Speech Characteristics	Treatment Options
Respiration	Muscular rigidity, tremor, reduced amplitude of chest wall movement	Decreased loudness, decay of loudness, short phrases	Erect posture; deep breath before speaking; increasing respiratory effort during speech
Phonation	Muscular rigidity, incomplete closure of vocal folds, bowing, tremor, asymmetrical vocal folds; reduced laryngeal efficiency and flexibility	Breathy, hoarse, or tremulous voice quality; reduced prosody	Techniques to increase vocal fold adduction; high respiratory-phonatory effect during speech
Velopharyngeal Function	May be normal or rigid with reduced closure	Nasalization extending over several phonetic segments associated with reduced movements	VP typically not targeted for treatment other than by slowing rate
Articulation	Weakness in control signals, rigidity, acceleration, tremor	Imprecise articulation associated with reduced movements or fast rate, short rushes of speech, repeated phonemes, blurred syllables	Slow rate; overarticulation; increase emphatic stress patterning

Note. Adapted from "Speech Characteristics in Parkinson's Disease," by L. A. Ramig and W. J. Gould, 1986, *Neurological Consultant, 4,* pp. 1–6. Copyrigt 1986 by Lawrence DellaCorte Publications. Adapted with permission.

PHONATION

Voice disorders are common in Parkinson disease. Many of the perceptually deviant speech features studied by Darley et al. (1975) are associated with pitch, loudness, or changes in voice quality. Physically, the vocal folds appear normal in structure. Adductor and abductor movements are bilaterally symmetrical, but there may be incomplete closure of the vocal folds (Perez, Ramig, Smith, & Dromey, 1996), which accounts for the breathy voice quality (Aronson, 1985). Recent advances in instrumentation have allowed for better understanding of the voice changes in Parkinson disease. Electromyographic (EMG) measures show reduced levels of thyroarytenoid muscle activity in speakers with hypophonic voice disorders (Baker, Ramig, Luschei, & Smith, 1998). Cinegraphic observation of laryngeal function (Hanson, Gerratt, & Ward, 1984) suggests a direct relationship between symptoms of breathiness and reduced loudness and increasing amounts of glottic gap and bowing of the vocal folds. Aerodynamic measures of phonatory function suggest lower subglottal pressure and phonatory low rates in Parkinson disease (Murdoch, Manning, Theodoros, & Thompson, 1997). Acoustic analysis of sustained phonation has shown cycle-to-cycle shifts in intensity and frequency and increased spectral noise. These may be related to the listener's perception of hoarseness, breathiness, and roughness (Ramig & Gould, 1986). Long-term fluctuation in intensity (in the 5–10 Hz range) may be seen in the "tremulous" voice. Breakdowns in the coordination of voicing with other aspects of speech may account for some of the other features described by Ramig and Gould, including difficulty initiating voicing, voiceless transitions, abnormal control of fundamental frequency contours, and voice timing deficits.

VELOPHARYNGEAL FUNCTION

Velopharyngeal dysfunction is not a major aspect of parkinsonian dysarthria. Studies (Hoodin & Gilbert, 1989) suggest some abnormal airflow as the disease progresses.

The velopharyngeal port may not close completely because of the underlying motor problems.

ORAL ARTICULATION

Perceptually, imprecise consonant production is a common feature of dysarthria associated with Parkinson disease. Oral articulatory disorders may be associated with consonants that require the most constriction (Logemann & Fischer, 1981). For example, spirantization (friction segments of low intensity in place of stopgaps) is a common articulatory characteristic of parkinsonian speech. This feature suggests a lack of complete oral closure. Physiologic measures of the lip and tongue suggest slower rates of force development and difficulty maintaining a given contraction (Gentil, Perrin, Tournier, & Pollak, 1999). In addition, individuals with Parkinson disease have slight decreases in tongue strength and endurance (Solomon, Lorell, Robin, Rodnitzky, & Luschei, 1995; Solomon, Robin, & Luschei, 2000). However, these changes are not correlated with measures such as articulatory precision or overall speech defectiveness. Rigidity of the oral muscles has been associated with articulatory undershoot, the failure of articulators to achieve the intended target.

SPEECH RATE

The relationship between articulatory precision and speech rates has been the focus of considerable attention in the study of hypokinetic dysarthria. There is considerable variability in speaking rates across parkinsonian speakers, with some exhibiting a slower than normal rate and others exhibiting articulatory rates much more rapid than normal. The underlying mechanism for these rate alterations is a topic for speculation. Netsell, Daniel, and Celesia (1975) studied the "rushes of speech" in parkinsonian dysarthria. They found syllable production rates in excess of 13 syllables per second. Because these rates are at the limits of voluntary control, these investigators suggest that "the subject is in some neuromuscular mode over which he [the speaker] has no immediate control" (p. 173). The palilalia (involuntary repetition of syllables or phrases) also resembles the festinating gait pattern seen in some individuals with Parkinson disease.

What Is the Typical Progression of Dysarthria in Parkinson Disease?

Dysarthria severe enough to impose functional limitations usually comes relatively late in the course of Parkinson disease. It typically begins with voice changes and progresses to other speech systems. Mild speech changes have been documented in speakers with early Parkinson disease (Stewart et al., 1995). Logemann, Fisher, Boshes, and Blonsky (1978) reported a large-scale study of speech features in the parkinsonian population. By far the most common features were associated with laryngeal dysfunction (89% of subjects), including breathiness, roughness, hoarseness, and tremulousness. The second most common disorder was articulation, in 45% of subjects. This was followed by rate disorders (repetition of syllables, shortened syllables, or prolonged pauses) in 20% and hypernasality in 10% of the 200 subjects studied. Logemann and her colleagues also studied the co-occurrence of various speech features and found five groups of patients. These data are summarized in Table 2.8. Note that laryngeal dysfunction was the only symptom in a group comprising 45% of the population. With each group, a new speech feature was added until a group comprising 9% of the population exhibited all features listed, including dysfunction in the larynx, posterior tongue, tongue blade, lips, and tongue tip.

The perceptual and acoustic measures of voice have been examined in groups of individuals in the early and late stages of Parkinson disease (Holmes, Oates, Phyland, & Hughes, 2000). The results are summarized in Table 2.9 and suggest that some changes such as breathiness are observed at both stages. Some of these features worsen over time, whereas others do not. Tremor was observed only in late stages of the disease. Early changes in voice were also confirmed by Sapir and colleagues (2001), when they found abnormal voice characteristics in individuals with short duration of Parkinson disease and with low UPDRS scores. Further, individuals with longer duration and higher UPDRS scores also had more voice and speech abnormalities. Voice and speech changes did not correlate with depression, age, or gender.

Rating scales that describe in detail the progression of speech dysfunction are available. Table 2.10 contains one such scale, which ranges from 0 (*does not vocalize at all*) through 10 (*normal speech*). A scaled score may be assigned through an interview, and results may be used to compare level of function from one visit to another.

What Is the Impact of Treatment on Speech in Parkinson Disease?

There is consensus that intervention does not bring about the same changes in all motor systems. Therefore, the following section reviews the impact on speech of pharmacologic, surgical, and behavioral interventions. For a more detailed discussion of this topic, see Schulz and Grant (2000).

PHARMACOLOGIC INTERVENTION

Drug intervention does not eliminate dysarthria associated with Parkinson disease. Early studies of the consequences of levodopa on speech found some changes in speech, but these were not as dramatic as changes in limb function (Rigrodsky & Morrison, 1970). Many of these studies rated only subjective impression. More recent studies using physiologic or acoustic measures are inconsistent. On one hand,

TABLE 2.8	Percentage of Co-occurrence of Speech Features in Parkinson Disease				
Speech Feature					
Laryngeal dysfunction	+	+	+	+	+
Posterior lingual dysfunction		+	+	+	+
Tongue blade dysfunction			+	+	+
Labial dysfunction				+	+
Tongue-tip dysfunction					+
Percentage of Population	45	13.5	17	5.5	9

Note. Adapted from "Frequency and Co-occurrence of Vocal Tract Dysfunction in the Speech of a Large Sample of Parkinson Patients," by J. A. Logemann, H. B. Fisher, B. Boshes, and E. Blonsky, 1978, *Journal of Speech and Hearing Disorders, 43,* pp. 47–57.

TABLE 2.9   Progression of Voice Changes in Parkinson Disease

Changes found in both early and late stages
Limited pitch
Limited loudness variability
Breathiness
Harshness
Reduced loudness

Features not deteriorating over time
Harshness
High modal pitch and speaking fundamental frequency (in men)
Fundamental frequency variability (in women)
Low intensity
Jitter

Feature deteriorating over time
Breathiness
Monopitch
Monoloudness
Low loudness
Reduced maximum phonation frequency range

Only in late stages
Tremor

Note. Adapted from "Voice Characteristics of the Progression of Parkinson's Disease," by R. J. Holmes, J. M. Oates, D. J. Phyland, and A. J. Hughes, 2000, *International Journal of Language and Communication Disorders, 35*(3), pp. 407–418.

changes in lip function (Cahill et al., 1998), selected acoustic measures (Sanabria et al., 2001), and laryngeal muscle activity (Gallena, Smith, Zeffiro, & Ludlow, 2001) have been reported. On the other hand, studies of speech breathing (Solomon & Hixon, 1993), vocal stability (Larson, Ramig, & Scherer, 1994), and selected acoustic aspects of vowel production (Poluha, Teulings, & Brookshire, 1998) have reported no differences. Inconsistencies may reflect methodological differences such as variation in dysarthria severity.

SURGERY

The surgical procedure, thalamotomy, has been used to treat severe drug-resistant tremor in Parkinson disease. In their review of the impact of this surgery on speech, Schulz and Grant (2000) suggest that speech is not improved; instead more speech symptoms may occur. These indicate a worsening of dysarthria that may be characterized by monotonous voice, slow speech, decreased vocal loudness, and articulation difficulties. More recently, the surgical procedure pallidotomy has been used to release inhibition in the thalamic and brain stem centers, thus improving all major parkinsonian symptoms. Studies of the impact of such intervention on speech have begun to appear (Barlow, Iacono, Paseman, Biswas, & D'Antonio, 1998; Schulz, Peterson, Sapienza, Greer, & Friedman, 1999). Results suggest some positive changes in phonatory and articulatory measures, especially in speakers with mild hypokinetic dysarthria prior to the surgery. The impact of deep brain stimulation on speech production has not been studied extensively. Reports of side effects indicate that dysarthria occurs less frequently with deep brain stimulation than with thalamotomy (Tasker, 1998) and that symptoms can be reversed with a change in stimulation parameters (Taha, Janszen, & Favre, 1999). Results of studies of various speech parameters such as pitch and speech intelligibility are inconsistent both within and across subjects (Maruska, Smit, Koller, & Garcia, 2000).

BEHAVIORAL INTERVENTION (SPEECH TREATMENT)

There is a long history of reports documenting the effectiveness of speech intervention for individuals with Parkinson disease. Table 2.11 contains a summary of selected studies of speech intervention. A review of this table suggests considerable variability across studies. Although many studies are case reports, there are a growing number of studies in which groups of individuals are compared with controls or in which two types of intervention are compared. The focus of treatment varies. Some treatments are broad-based speech improvement programs designed to improve voice loudness, intonation, and articulation. Others focus on a single aspect of speech production. For example, the program by Ramig, Bonitati, Lemke, and Horii (1994), described later in this chapter, focused largely on improvement of phonation. Intensity of treatment varies from concentrated but relatively brief periods of intervention (i.e., the four sessions per week for 4 weeks used by Ramig and colleagues) to extended periods of less intensive treatment. Current studies report a broad range of physiologic, acoustical, and perceptual measures.

A number of trends in the treatment of parkinsonian dysarthria are apparent when reports are viewed chronologically. In the late 1960s and early 1970s, broad-based speech improvement programs were viewed as bringing about changes during the treatment session, but these changes reportedly were not maintained outside treatment (Allan, 1970; Sarno, 1968). The studies that followed had a somewhat different focus, perhaps in response to the lack of carryover reported in the earlier literature. Accounts by Helm (1979) and Downie, Low, and Lindsay (1981), among others, reported the success of such devices as pacing boards and portable delayed auditory feedback (DAF) devices. These devices were to be used whenever the individual was communicating. The goal was to compensate for the dysarthria rather than to restore normal function. These therapies were marked by success when the appropriate candidates were selected. In the 1980s, prospective studies of speech

(text continues on p. 113)

TABLE 2.10	Speech Scale
10	Normal speech
9	Speech entirely adequate; minor voice disturbance present
8	Speech easily understood, but voice or speech rhythm may be disturbed
7	Communication accomplished with ease, although speech impairment detracts from content
6	Speech can always be understood if listener pays close attention; both articulation and voice may be defective
5	Speech always employed for communication, but articulation is very poor; usually uses complete sentences
4	Uses speech for most communication, but articulation is highly unintelligible; may have occasional difficulty in initiating speech; usually speaks in single words or short phrases
3	Attempts to use speech for communication, but has difficulty initiating vocalization; may stop speaking in middle of phrase and be unable to continue
2	Vocalizes to call attention to self
1	Vocalizes, but rarely for communicative purposes
0	Does not vocalize at all

Note. Adapted from *Parkinson's Disease Disability Rating Scale*. Copyright by Sandoz Pharmaceuticals Corporation/Novartis. Adapted with permission.

TABLE 2.11

Studies of Speech Treatment in Parkinson Disease

Reference	# of Subjects	Primary Focus	Medical Diagnosis	Rationale for Treatment	Outcomes Impairment	Outcomes Activity	Outcomes Participation	Study Conclusions
Hanson & Metter, 1980	1	Delayed auditory feedback	PSP	Previously failed behavioral intervention	Vocal intensity during reading and counting	Speaking rate, speech intelligibility during reading and counting	Family reported increased participation	Improved speech rate, vocal intensity, and intelligibility.
Hanson & Metter, 1983	2	Delayed auditory feedback	PD	Poor response to behavioral intervention	Voice intensity; fundamental frequency; phonation time for vowel /a/	Speaking rate during reading; speech intelligibility from connected speech samples		Marked reduction in speech rate, an increase in vocal intensity, and improved speech intelligibility under DAF.
Scott & Caird, 1983	26	Prosodic exercises with and without a visual reinforcement device	PD	Feedback allowed monitoring of prosody		Perceived abnormality of prosody	Reports of relatives	Improved prosody and intelligibility.
Robertson & Thomson, 1984	12	Group therapy	PD	Need to improve capacity/control of respiration and coordination/control of voice production	Dysarthria profile (respiration and phonation)	Dysarthria profile (intelligibility)	Questionnaires from patients, relatives/friends	Higher scores on the dysarthria profile; maintained their improvements 3 months.
Rubow & Swift, 1985	1	Portable biofeedback device	PD	Microcomputer was intended to facilitate generalization of improved respiratory control	Perceptual ratings of speech dimensions		Probes outside of clinic (vocal intensity)	Skills transferred to the outside environment while wearing the feedback device.
Johnson & Pring, 1990	12	Treatment targeting pitch and volume with visual feedback	PD	To determine if treatment benefits could be achieved from a less intensive program	Acoustic measures, severity of dysarthria			Improved in terms of dysarthria severity and on volume and pitch measures.

(continues)

TABLE **2.11** *Continued.*

Reference	# of Subjects	Primary Focus	Medical Diagnosis	Rationale for Treatment	Outcomes			Study Conclusions
					Impairment	Activity	Participation	
Adams & Lang, 1992	10	Masking noise	PD	Decreased vocal intensity	Speech intensity	Speech intelligibility		Marked increase in speech intensity with masking; effect on rate and intelligibility was inconsistent.
Countryman & Ramig, 1993	1	LSVT	PD (with bilateral thalamotomy)	An intensive therapy program to improve perceptual characteristics	Multiple acoustic measures	Patient's self-ratings of slurring in speech; SLPs ratings of overall quality of speech/voice	Self ratings in natural settings	Acoustic outcome measures were significantly improved immediately following treatment.
Countryman, Ramig, & Pawlas, 1994	3	LSVT	Parkinson Plus Syndrome (PSP, MSA, Shy-Drager syndrome)	LSVT has been seen to benefit subjects with PD	Multiple acoustic measures	Perceptual rating of word and overall intelligibility	Depression inventories, Sickness Impact Profile, and Profile of Mood States	Objective and perceptual data supported improvement of speech and voice. By 6 months posttreatment, the patients' objective and perceptual data had declined, but patients and families reported that overall functional communication skills remained above pretreatment status.
Ramig, Bonitati, Lemke, & Horii, 1994	40	LSVT	PD	To improve perceptual characteristics of voice by targeting the hypothesized underlying laryngeal physical pathology	Multiple acoustic measures	Perceptual ratings of speech intelligibility and intonation		Findings support the effectiveness of LSVT for patients with PD. Improvements were maintained at 6 and 12 months whether or not subjects received additional treatment.
Dromey, Ramig, & Johnson, 1995	1	LSVT	PD	Patient's livelihood was dependent upon his oral communication	Multiple acoustic measures			LSVT resulted in increased vocal intensity; this also led to changes in articulation that were not targeted in treatment.

Reference	# of Subjects	Primary Focus	Medical Diagnosis	Rationale for Treatment	Outcomes			Study Conclusions
					Impairment	Activity	Participation	
Ramig, Countryman, Thompson, & Horii, 1995	45	LSVT vs. respiratory treatment	PD	Comparison of 2 intensive treatment programs: (1) respiratory support or (2) increase vocal fold adduction and respiratory support	Multiple acoustic measures	Family and subject self-ratings of intelligibility and initiation of conversation	Beck Depression Inventory and Sickness Impact Profile	LSVT, focusing on increased vocal fold adduction, is more effective than respiration treatment alone for improving vocal intensity and decreasing the impact of PD on communication.
Smith, Ramig, Dromey, Perez, & Samandari, 1995	22	LSVT vs. respiratory treatment	PD	Comparison of 2 intensive treatment programs: (1) respiratory support or (2) increase vocal fold adduction and respiratory support	Laryngostroboscopic findings			LSVT improved laryngeal adduction which was correlated with increased vocal intensity. No differences with respiratory only treatment.
Ramig & Dromey, 1996	17	Vocal and respiratory therapy (LSVT) versus respiration only therapy	PD	Comparison of 2 intensive treatment programs: (1) respiratory support or (2) increase vocal fold adduction and respiratory support	Aerodynamic and EGG measures			LSVT associated with increases in SPL through improved vocal fold adduction and increase in subglottal pressure. Respiratory training alone was not.
Ramig, Countryman, O'Brien, Hoehn, & Thompson, 1996	35	LSVT vs. respiratory treatment	PD	To improve perceptual characteristics of voice by targeting the hypothesized underlying laryngeal physical pathology	Multiple acoustic measures		Beck Depression Inventory and Sickness Impact Profile	Findings support the short- and long-term effectiveness of intensive voice therapy (LSVT) for improving vocal intensity in patients with PD.

(continues)

TABLE 2.11 *Continued.*

Reference	# of Subjects	Primary Focus	Medical Diagnosis	Rationale for Treatment	Outcomes			Study Conclusions
					Impairment	Activity	Participation	
Sullivan, Brune, & Beukelman, 1996	6	Group therapy	PD	To improve speech intelligibility followed by practice of the techniques and social time to allow practice in a functional setting; goals included increased-breath support and increased voice projection	Perceptual judgments of vocal tone, appropriate pitch and loudness	Perceptual judgments of speech naturalness	Questionnaires on communication strategies and communicative effectiveness (Yorkston et al., 1992)	Group speech intervention was effective. Five of the 6 participants improved their speech performance and maintained improvements for up to 10 months after treatment.
Countryman, Hicks, Ramig, & Smith, 1997	1	LSVT	PD	To improve the primary deficit (true vocal fold hypoadduction), reduce the need for secondary compensatory behavior (supraglottic hyperadduction), and result in improved loudness, intonation, and overall vocal quality	Multiple acoustic measures	Perceptual ratings of speech during reading of "Rainbow Passage"		Increased vocal loudness, decreased supraglottic hyperadduction, and improved intonation and overall voice quality.
de Angelis, Mourao, Ferraz, Behlau, Pontes, & Andrade, 1997	20	Increasing vocal intensity through group therapy	PD	Reduced vocal intensity was the main factor leading to unintelligible speech: treatment focused on phonatory function with tasks that facilitate greater glottic closure	Maximum phonation times; s/z ratio; air flow; vocal intensity	Self evaluation of oral communication (interview)		Voice rehabilitation resulted in a greater glottic efficiency, increased vocal intensity, decreased complaints of weak and strained-strangled voice, and monotonous, unintelligible speech.

Reference	# of Subjects	Primary Focus	Medical Diagnosis	Rationale for Treatment	Outcomes				Study Conclusions
					Impairment	Activity	Participation		
Cariski & Rosenbek, 1999	1	Speech Enhancer with and without behavioral therapy	PD	Subjects failed with traditional voice amplification in the past		Live transcription of orally read sentences for % speech intelligibility			The Speech Enhancer effectively improved speech intelligibility. Superior treatment results may be obtained when a patient receives speech therapy in conjunction with using an amplification device.
Theodoros, Thompson-Ward, Murdoch, Lethlean, & Silburn, 1999	1	LSVT	PD	To improve voice/speech deficits and to document the immediate and long-term effectiveness following thalamotomy and pallidotomy procedures	Multiple acoustic measures	Perceptual measures of word and sentence intelligibility, number of intelligible words per minute, and communication efficiency			Marked improvement in the subject's speech intelligibility immediately post-LSVT (increases in vocal volume, phonatory stability, respiratory—phonatory control, and a decrease in rate of speech). At 6 months posttreatment, initial gains in speech intelligibility and respiratory phonatory control were not maintained.
E. C. Ward, Theodoros, Murdoch, & Silburn, 2000	30	LSVT	PD with or without pallidotomy and/or thalamotomy	To determine whether surgical PD patients and nonsurgical PD patients responded similarly to LSVT	Multiple acoustic measures	Sentence intelligibility from the *Assessment of Intelligibility of Dysarthric Speech*			Both subject groups demonstrated significant improvements following LSVT across the measures of intelligibility and SPL in sustained phonation and reading. Assessment of tongue function, however, revealed that only the nonsurgical PD patients had an increased capacity to generate maximal effort tongue pressures following intervention.

(continues)

TABLE 2.11 *Continued.*

Reference	# of Subjects	Primary Focus	Medical Diagnosis	Rationale for Treatment	Outcomes			Study Conclusions
					Impairment	Activity	Participation	
Ramig, Sapir, Fox, & Countryman, 2001	14	LSVT	PD	To maximize phonatory efficiency through intensive, high-effort treatment. The respiratory system is "indirectly" stimulated during the speech tasks	SPL during four speaking tasks			Significant increase in voice SPL from baseline to post-treatment and from baseline to the 6-month follow-up. Subjects with PD who did not receive treatment, as well as control subjects without brain injury, did not demonstrate a significant increase in SPL.
Ramig, Sapir, Countryman, Pawlas, O'Brien, Hoehn, & Thompson, 2001	33	LSVT vs. respiratory treatment	PD	To assess the effectiveness of a respiratory–phonatory treatment (LSVT) versus a respiratory-only treatment, and measure the long-term (2-year) outcomes of treatment	Multiple acoustic measures			LSVT was significantly more effective than the respiratory-only therapy in improving SPL and pitch variability immediately posttreatment and maintaining those improvements at the 2-year follow-up.
Baumgartner, Sapir, & Ramig, 2001	20	LSVT vs. respiratory treatment	PD	To compare the effects of treatment emphasizing phonatory–respiratory effort with treatment emphasizing respiratory effort alone on perceived voice quality	Perceptual ratings of voice			Statistically significant pre- and posttreatment improvement in hoarseness and breathiness was observed in the LSVT group but not in the group that received respiratory therapy alone.

Note. PSP = Progressive supranuclear palsy; PD = Parkinson disease; DAF = delayed auditory feedback; LSVT = Lee Silverman Voice Treatment; SLP = speech–language pathologist; MSA = multiple system atrophy; EGG = electroglottography; SPL = sound pressure level.

treatment reported both immediate improvement and some maintenance of progress (Robertson & Thomson, 1984; Scott & Caird, 1983). The trend toward reporting positive speech treatment results continued into the 1990s (Le Dorze, Dioone, Ryalls, Julien, & Ouellet, 1992). Perhaps the most encouraging results have come from the Ramig group (Ramig, Countryman, O'Brien, Hoehn, & Thompson, 1996). They report the success of intensive treatment called Lee Silverman Voice Treatment (LSVT), focusing on phonation. This treatment is described in detail later. A more detailed description of evidence-based practice guidelines for dysarthria can be found elsewhere (Yorkston et al., 2002).

What Issues Are Particularly Important in Assessment of Parkinsonian Dysarthria?

INTERVIEW

A number of principles of assessment are important when evaluating the speech of individuals with Parkinson disease. An interview with both the patient and the spouse is critical in understanding their perspectives regarding the severity of the problem. This is especially important in Parkinson disease because many patients are not aware of the extent of their difficulties. Our clinical experience suggests that people with Parkinson disease underestimate their problems whereas spouses do not. A detailed interview is also necessary to understand the communication needs of the patient. Communication needs in this population vary considerably. Some individuals with Parkinson disease wish to play the highly demanding role of a public speaker. Others communicate only with a small network of familiar people. Patients and their spouses should also be questioned carefully about the patient's medication regime. What medications is the person currently taking? What side effects are being experienced? How does speech change as a function of the drug cycle?

EXAMINATION

In addition to a complete oral examination (details of which can be found in Chapter 1), it is particularly important to listen to the connected speech of individuals with Parkinson disease. Many of the movement problems associated with the disease involve difficulty initiating and carrying out complex sequences of movements. The extent of these problems cannot be fully appreciated by examining isolated speech movements or production of words in isolation. The speaker should be asked to perform a variety of speech activities, including reading long sentences or a paragraph, and spontaneous speech activities, such as picture description, monologue, or conversation. Some individuals with Parkinson disease perform noticeably better on relatively structured tasks such as reading than they do on more spontaneous tasks. The final issue we address in the assessment of parkinsonian dysarthria is stimulability. Knowing whether the speaker can modify his or her productions is critical in developing a treatment plan. Some of the approaches described in the next section are dependent on learning to modify speech production, whereas others are much less dependent on this ability.

What Approaches to Speech Treatment Are Available to Individuals with Parkinson Disease?

The following sections will describe a series of speech intervention approaches for individuals with Parkinson disease. Because the severity of dysarthria is a critical factor in developing intervention approaches, this section will be organized according to severity levels, with management suggestions for mild, moderate, and severe dysarthrias. See Table 2.12 for a summary of the speech features and treatment approaches for each severity group. Each treatment approach will be described in detail for the group of patients with whom the technique is most frequently applied. Of course, each of the treatment techniques can be modified for use with speakers with differing levels of involvement.

MILD DYSARTHRIA

Possibly because of the mixed findings of early studies of treatment efficacy, people with Parkinson disease and mild dysarthria are not consistently referred for speech intervention. Results of a large-scale survey of individuals with Parkinson disease indicated that 65% reported difficulty with speech, but only 4.4% had been seen by a speech–language pathologist (Mutch, Strudwick, Roy, & Downie, 1986). It has been our clinical experience that referrals typically come late in the progression of the disease after dysarthria has become moderate or even severe.

Despite the relatively low referral rates for mild dysarthria, early intervention may be appropriate for a number of reasons. First, even mild dysarthria may be a functional limitation in people for whom quality of speech is critical—for example, those with heavy communication demands in their work. Second, mild dysarthria in Parkinson disease is usually associated with phonation changes. The work of Ramig

TABLE 2.12 Summary of Speech Intervention Approaches in Parkinson Disease

Severity	Speech Features	Treatment Approaches
Mild	Mild or no reduction in speech intelligibility Symptoms include reduced loudness, monotony, and breathiness Speech scale rating of 9, 8, or 7	Increased vocal fold adduction Increased maximum duration of phonation Increased respiratory support Patient and family education Home practice drills
Moderate	Some reduction in speech intelligibility Symptoms include reduced loudness, monotony, breathiness, consonant imprecision Speech scale rating of 6 or 5	Rate control drills Delay auditory feedback Voice amplification Patient and family education
Severe	Natural speech is no longer functional Symptoms include severe difficulty initiating voice, and short rushes of poorly articulated speech Speech scale rating of 4 or less	Pacing boards Alphabet supplementation Portable typing devices Development of partner-supported communication techniques Patient and family education

and her colleagues (2001) has suggested that phonatory function is amenable to change in the parkinsonian population. People may be better able to learn good speaking habits early than if they wait until the underlying problems are so severe that new learning is difficult. Finally, belief in one's ability to change and to maintain good communication skills may be a tremendously motivating factor. Good communication skills may prevent some of the depression so often noted as the disorder advances.

Speech Features

Typically, change in phonation is the first speech feature to become apparent in Parkinson disease. Although changes in voicing may be accompanied by other features of dysarthria, voicing changes occur as the only feature of dysarthria in nearly half of individuals studied (Logemann, Fisher, Boshes, & Blonsky, 1978). Table 2.13 contains a framework and rationale for the speech treatment. Note that the program is driven by a number of perceptual features of phonation in Parkinson disease. These include reduced loudness; breathy or weak voice; reduced pitch variability; and an unsteady, hoarse, or rough voice. For individuals in the mild range of severity, these vocal features, although noticeable, do not disrupt speech intelligibility.

The ideal candidate for an intervention such as LSVT is someone with idiopathic Parkinson disease and hypoadduction of the vocal folds (Ramig, 1993). The following treatment tasks encourage maximum phonatory effort in order to bring the vocal folds together and improve voice quality. The most successful candidates are those who are highly motivated and for whom oral communication is an important aspect of daily living. As with many behavioral therapy approaches, the best candidates are stimulable, in that they are able to produce louder phonation when asked to do so. They also exhibit an adequate appreciation of the quality of their speech production. Finally, because this treatment approach is dependent on learning to modify speech production, normal cognition enhances the likelihood of success.

In contrast, Ramig, Pawlas, and colleagues (1995) suggest a number of features that characterize individuals who are less likely to succeed. Negative prognostic indicators include severe dementia with difficulty following directions, severe depression, symptoms in addition to those typical of Parkinson disease (i.e., those seen in progressive supranuclear palsy or Parkinson plus), severe drug-related dyskinesia, and strong vocal tremor.

Treatment Approaches

The main goal of the LSVT is to increase phonatory effort (Ramig, Pawlas, et al., 1995). This is translated into the instruction, **"Think Loud!"** Increased phonatory effort is accomplished in a series of graded therapy tasks that focus on increasing loudness, increasing intonation, and reducing hoarse voice quality. Sessions typically include both practice on simple phonatory tasks (such as sustaining phonation as long as possible) and practice in maintaining that phonatory effort in speech activities, beginning with short phrases and progressing to longer utterances. The role of the speech–language pathologist is to give patients objective feedback about their performance: Examples are length of maximum phonation or fundamental frequency range. Clinicians strongly encourage maximum performance throughout the session, provide home practice drills, and serve as energetic motivators to elicit maximal levels of performance.

Another integral component of the program is speaker "calibration." Individuals with Parkinson disease appear to have difficulty gauging what is an appropriate level of effort. In the early phases of treatment, many will comment that they feel as if they are "shouting" during the practice sessions. With continuous feedback and

TABLE 2.13

Framework and Rationale for Speech Therapy in Parkinson Disease

Perceptual Characteristics	Hypothesized Laryngeal and/or Respiratory Pathophysiology	Therapy Goals and Tasks	Acoustic, Physiology Variables Measured	Perceptual Variables Measured
Reduced loudness, breathy, weak voice (Logemann et al., 1978; Aronson, 1985)	Bowed vocal folds (Hanson et al., 1984), rigidity, hypokinesia in laryngeal and/or respiratory muscle; reduced adduction; reduced inspiratory, expiratory volume (Critchley, 1981)	1. Increase voice fold adduction - pushing, lifting with phonation Increase maximum duration vowel phonation at increased intensity • think "shout" • speak over background noise	Maximum duration of sustained vowel phonation	Loudness Breathiness Intelligibility
		2. Increase respiratory support • posture • deep breath before speak • frequent breaths • phrasing of sentences	Vital capacity	
Reduced pitch variability monopitch (Logemann et al., 1978)	Rigidity cricothyroid muscle (Aronson, 1985)	1. Increase maximum fundamental frequency range • high and low pitch scales • sustain phonation at highest and lowest pitches	Maximum range of fundamental frequency	
		2. Increase fundamental frequency variation in connected speech • word emphasis • intonation in questions	Variability of fundamental frequency in connected speech	Monotone Intelligibility
Unsteady, hoarse, rough voice (Logemann et al., 1978)	Rigidity, hypokinesia tremor in laryngeal and respiratory muscles (Hanson et al., 1984)	1. Increase steadiness of phonation • maximum duration tasks with constant intensity • consistent, firm voice throughout sentence	Improved measure of phonatory stability	Steadiness of voice, hoarse, tremorous intelligibility

Note. Adapted from "The Role of Phonation in Speech Intelligibility" (pp. 119–156), by L. Ramig, 1992, in *Intelligibility in Speech Disorders,* edited by R. D. Kent, Philadelphia: John Benjamins.

other techniques such as review of audiotape recordings, speakers are taught to become comfortable with the new loudness level.

The subjects who participated in Ramig's (1992) treatment efficacy study received four treatment sessions per week for 4 weeks. Outcome measures included a comprehensive range of aerodynamic, acoustic, and perceptual measures. Table 2.14 contains the visual analogue perceptual rating scale used in the study. Preliminary results suggested a positive treatment outcome, with reduction in monotony and shakiness of voice most closely associated with improvements in intelligibility. These changes were maintained at a 6-month follow-up. Because of the degenerative nature

TABLE 2.14

Rating Scale for Speech Characteristics in Parkinson Disease

Always loud enough	├————————————┤	Never loud enough
Never a shaky voice	├————————————┤	Always a shaky voice
Never a hoarse, scratchy voice	├————————————┤	Always a hoarse, scratchy voice
Never monotone	├————————————┤	Always monotone
Never slurs speech	├————————————┤	Always slurs speech
Never mumbles	├————————————┤	Always mumbles
Always speaks so others can understand	├————————————┤	Never speaks so others can understand
Always participates in a conversation	├————————————┤	Never participates in a conversation
Always starts a conversation	├————————————┤	Never starts a conversation

Note. From "The Role of Phonation in Speech Intelligibility" (pp. 119–156), by L. Ramig, 1992, in *Intelligibility in Speech Disorders,* edited by R. D. Kent, Philadelphia: John Benjamins. Copyright 1992 by John Benjamins North America, Inc. Reprinted with permission.

of the disorder, Ramig recommends 6-month checkups. If the patient's speech has deteriorated or has "fallen out of calibration," a small number of sessions may be needed to reinstate the gains made during earlier, more intensive work. In some cases, the treatment targets must be modified because of progression of the disease.

Ramig and her colleagues suggest that there are a number of keys to the success of this type of treatment:

- *Treatment should be simple.* The therapy is simple, focusing only on the phonatory aspects of speech production. Because people with Parkinson disease are known to have difficulty simultaneously executing two movements, simplifying the focus and instructions may increase the probability of successful learning. It should be noted that positive changes have also been noted in "nonphonatory" aspects of speech production. Speaking rates may be slowed, oral articulatory gestures may be extended, and overall speech intelligibility may be improved. This may be related to an overall increase in physiologic effort.
- *Intensive treatment is motivating.* The intensive treatment with immediate transfer of skills to speech is highly motivating. Speakers and their spouses report immediate improvements, thus encouraging them to work even harder to bring about more changes.
- *Level of effort must be recalibrated.* Finally, patient testimonies also suggest that their perceived level of effort must be "recalibrated" to ensure successful carryover (Ramig, 1993). Speakers often report that they had not realized their voices were soft or weak prior to treatment. Early in treatment many report feeling as if they are shouting in order to produce "normal" voicing. Therefore, a focus on self-awareness and accurate calibration of the amount of effort needed to produce acceptable voice also appear to be critical treatment features.

MODERATE DYSARTHRIA

Reduction in speech intelligibility in certain situations is a key feature distinguishing mild from moderate dysarthria. Patients and their spouses will report that requests for repetitions are more frequent and that communication is difficult in adverse environments such as noisy situations. Speaking in groups is difficult, and many individuals with moderate dysarthria tend to listen rather than speak at social gatherings.

Speech Features

The speech patterns of individuals with moderate dysarthria are characterized by the same changes in voice that were described for mild dysarthria. Vocal loudness is reduced, intonation is monotonous, and vocal quality may be breathy. In addition to these vocal features, moderate dysarthria is typically characterized by oral articulatory imprecision. The range of oral movements is limited. The speaker may fail to reach articulatory targets, thus blurring consonant contrasts. Some speakers with moderate dysarthria pause inappropriately; that is, their pauses may be longer than normal or may occur at inappropriate locations. These inappropriate pauses may be caused by difficulty initiating speech movements. Some individuals with moderate dysarthria may also speak at excessively rapid rates.

Treatment Approaches

People with moderate dysarthria are more commonly referred for speech intervention than are people with mild dysarthria. This may be due in part to the fact that the reduction in speech intelligibility associated with moderate dysarthria poses important functional limitations for the speaker. Because articulatory undershooting and excessive articulatory rates are characteristic of moderate dysarthria in Parkinson disease, many treatment approaches involve slowing the rate of speech. Some of these techniques rely on a behavioral intervention in which the speaker is taught to modify productions. Other techniques impose a slow rate on the speaker through the use of devices such as delayed auditory feedback (DAF).

Creating a "Theater Voice." The analogue of speaking like a stage performer is a useful one for individuals with Parkinson disease (Sullivan, Brune, & Beukelman, 1996). A "theater voice" is different from conversational speech in a number of ways. It is characterized by exaggeration in loudness, a slowed rate, and emphatic stress. Although performers modify their speech in complex ways, the behaviors can be called up by a single trigger—to use a "stage voice." Many speakers with moderate dysarthria associated with Parkinson disease can learn to call upon a stage voice in conversation.

Behavioral Rate-Control Techniques. For many speakers with moderate dysarthria, behavioral interventions such as those described for mild dysarthria may be appropriate. There are advantages and disadvantages to behavioral interventions. On the positive side, these techniques preserve or enhance the natural prosody of speech. On the negative side, they require an investment of time and training. Therefore, potential candidates must be motivated to practice and able to learn new approaches to speech.

Behavioral techniques for rate reduction take a variety of forms. Increasing overall loudness level has the effect of increasing overall level of effort and thus slowing production rates. Drills that encourage exaggerated stress patterns also have the effect of slowing overall speaking rate and thus improving speech intelligibility.

Other techniques target rate reduction more directly. Visual feedback in the form of intensity-by-time tracings on oscilloscopic screens (such as the "Visipitch") (Berry, 1983) or software programs has been used to teach speakers to prolong utterances. A computerized pacing program (Beukelman, Yorkston, & Tice, 1997) has also been used to prompt individuals to speak at selected rates. Passages are entered into computer files along with timing information that approximates the rhythmic durational relationships of words in normal connected speech. As the speaker reads a passage aloud, a cursor moves along the passage to cue the target rate.

Pauses may be inserted at phrasal boundaries or at punctuation marks. Once the speaker can produce speech at the target rate, the computer cues are systematically faded. The typical stages of a training program are as follows:

1. *Select an optimal rate.* Normal reading rates range from 170 to 190 words per minute, depending on the task. A subgroup of people with Parkinson disease exhibit speaking rates far in excess of these normal rates. The general goal in rate selection for individuals with Parkinson disease is to choose a speaking rate that is consistent with intelligibility and natural-sounding speech. The specific rate may vary from one individual to another. The rate-selection process may involve the recording of trials at various rates so that the clinician and speaker can come to a consensus about the "best-sounding" rate.

2. *Practice optimal rate with computer cueing of reading passages.* Once an optimal rate has been selected, that rate is practiced in various passages until the speaker is comfortable with the new rate. At this point each patient may create an audiotape for home practice. We encourage speakers to "calibrate" themselves every day by reading along with the audiotape recorded during the therapy session.

3. *Practice maintaining the rate on the same reading passages without computer cueing.* Once the speaker is comfortable with the optimal rate, the computer cues are faded. During this stage, the speaker reads a passage without cues and is given feedback regarding speaking rate. Reading rates can be monitored "online" using the "Pacer/Tally" computer software (Beukelman et al., 1997).

4. *Practice maintaining the rate in conversation.* Once the speaker can comfortably maintain the optimal speaking rate during reading, tasks such as monologues or conversations are practiced. Speaking rates on these tasks can also be monitored using the "Pacer/Tally" software program.

Delayed Auditory Feedback (DAF). DAF may serve as an intermediary technique between behavioral intervention and the more rigid rate-control devices that are typically employed with severely dysarthric speakers. The speaker wears a portable device consisting of a microphone, a pocket-sized delay unit/battery, and earphones. This unit delays speech for a fraction of a second (from 50 to 200 msec.). The overall effect is to slow the individual's speaking rate. A number of independent investigators have reported successful use of the device in hypokinetic dysarthria (Adams, 1994, 1997; Downie et al., 1981; Hanson & Metter, 1983). With DAF treatment, a number of speech features reportedly become less deviant in these individuals, including duration, articulation time, fundamental frequency variability, mean intensity, and intensity variability. Because speakers typically do not adapt to the delay, the device can be used for extended periods of time.

The best candidates for DAF intervention share a number of features:

1. They tend to exhibit speech that is more rapid than normal. This is the only type of dysarthria in which speech is excessively rapid rather than slowed.

2. The speaker's voice must be sufficiently loud that the device can receive it, impose a timing delay, and present it to the speaker through

earphones. Therefore, individuals with severely reduced loudness levels or severe vocal initiation problems are not ideal candidates for the device.

3. No carryover can be expected with the device. In other words, once the device is removed, speakers with hypokinetic dysarthria will revert to habitual patterns. Therefore, individuals with the motivation, time, and ability to learn behavioral techniques may not be appropriate candidates for DAF.

Voice Amplifiers. Portable vocal amplifiers may also be of assistance for some individuals with Parkinson disease (Beukelman & Mirenda, 1998). The best candidates for such devices are speakers who have consistent voicing but at reduced loudness levels. Voice amplifiers are typically not a satisfactory solution for individuals with severe vocal initiation problems. New technology that suppresses background noise as well as enhancing the speech signal is also available (Cariski & Rosenbek, 1999).

SEVERE DYSARTHRIA

In severe hypokinetic dysarthria, natural speech is no longer a functional means of communication. Speakers will require some degree of support from their communication partners and may rely entirely or in part on augmentative communication.

Speech Features

Speech may be characterized by severe difficulty initiating voicing and short rushes of poorly articulated speech. Once speech is initiated, the speaker may freeze in mid-utterance and be unable to continue. Perhaps because of associated cognitive problems, language production may be sparse. Responses may be limited to single words or short phrases. Individuals at this level of severity may also experience "on/off periods" in which performance is notably worse during the "off" periods than during the "on" periods.

Treatment Approaches

The following treatment approaches typically require some level of partner support. Therefore, it is critical that frequent communication partners are trained in techniques for managing communicative interactions. The following rate-control techniques are considered rigid in that they impose a reduced rate upon the speaker. The chief advantage of rigidly imposed rate-control techniques is that they may be effective when other techniques have failed. On the negative side, however, these techniques may impair the naturalness of speech, require artificial devices, and demand a supportive and knowledgeable communication partner for successful implementation.

Pacing Board. The pacing board is a simple device consisting of a series of colored squares separated by ridges. The speaker touches one square while saying each word, thus separating the words and metering speech production. The device is recommended for individuals with severe palilalia, that is, repetitive production of syllables or words (Helm, 1979). Its use is felt to bring an automatic act under voluntary control. Our clinical experience suggests that pacing boards are somewhat limited by the fact that the hand movement that initially meters output may become overlearned. As the hand movement becomes automatic, it no longer imposes control over excessively rapid speech. After extended use, many people will develop a festinating pattern of progressively more rapid tapping on the squares of the board. Because this pattern mirrors the festinating speech, it no longer serves to slow rate.

Alphabet Supplementation. In alphabet supplementation, the speaker uses an alphabet board to identify the first letter of each word as it is spoken. This approach slows speaking rate and provides the communication partner with the first letter of each word. For individuals with Parkinson disease, this technique has the advantage of not relying on a simple, repeated movement that can be overlearned. Instead, the speaker must locate a different letter for each word. The technique may be helpful for individuals with vocal initiation problems. When a communication breakdown occurs, the speaker can use the alphabet board to spell the entire message.

Portable Typing Devices. For most individuals with Parkinson disease, even those with severe dysarthria, natural speech is a component of their communication systems. For some individuals, communication must be supplemented with a portable typing system. With such a device, the user can type messages in a letter-by-letter fashion. Because reduced range of movement is often a problem, small keyboards are usually preferred. Individuals with prominent tremor may need to stabilize the typing hand on the device in order to dampen the tremor. A keyguard may also be used to compensate for tremor.

Swallowing Disorders

This section reviews swallowing symptoms associated with Parkinson disease. Approaches to assessment and intervention are also described.

Why Do Individuals with Parkinson Disease Experience Swallowing Problems?

Dysphagia in Parkinson disease appears to be related to changes in both striated musculature under dopaminergic control and smooth musculature under autonomic control (Morrell, 1992). All three stages of swallowing may be affected. Dysphagia may be manifested at any stage of disease and its presence predicted by the severity of tremor and speech disturbance (Coates & Bakheit, 1997a). In the oral stage (much of which is under voluntary control), dysfunction appears to result largely from rigidity of the lingual musculature, rather than weakness (Athlin, Norberg, Axelsson, Moller, & Nordstrom, 1989; A. N. Lieberman et al., 1980; Morrell, 1992). Jaw rigidity has also been implicated (Leopold & Kagel, 1996). The contractions of the striated muscles of the pharynx, which are under the control of the lower brain stem, are often delayed during swallowing (Robbins, Logemann, & Kirschner, 1986). Complex interactions between the lower motor neurons and cortical control systems may be involved in the disease (Blonsky, Logemann, Boshes, & Fisher, 1975; A. J. Miller, 1982). In addition, the basal ganglia have an influence on sensory components in the trigeminal system and may contribute to abnormalities in sensorimotor responses during the oropharyngeal stage of swallowing (Labuszewski & Lidsky, 1979). Pathology in the dorsal motor nucleus of the vagus nerve and in the medullary reticular formation has also been associated with Parkinson disease, possibly accounting for additional pharyngeal stage abnormality (Forno, 1981). Eadie and Tyrer (1965), who reported a higher incidence of esophageal spasm, hiatal hernia, and gastroesophageal reflux in patients with Parkinson disease as compared to matched controls, speculated involvement of the dorsal vagal nucleus. Autonomic dysfunction may partially account for the observations of reduced esophageal motility (Bramble, Cunliffe, & Dellipiani, 1978). Logemann, Boshes, Blonsky, and Fisher (1977) also presented evidence of slowed esophageal transit times for patients with Parkinson disease, regardless of disease stage.

Studies have failed to demonstrate that levodopa has a positive effect on swallowing in Parkinson disease (Bushman, Bomeyer, Leeker, & Perlmutter, 1989; Hunter, Crameri, Austin, Woodward, & Hughes, 1997). Because levodopa has a positive effect on the basal ganglia, other nondopamine structures must also be impaired. The central pattern generator for swallowing, which lies in the medulla, appears to be implicated. In Parkinson disease, this neural network fails to smoothly control the series of muscle actions needed to produce a coordinated swallow.

It appears, then, that swallowing disorders in individuals with Parkinson disease may be only partially accounted for by the primary pathology in the basal ganglia and the resulting muscular rigidity and bradykinesia. Impairment may also be present in the interactions among the cortical and bulbar motor tracts, the basal ganglia, and the trigeminal sensorimotor systems, and in the medullary structures of the dorsal motor nucleus of the vagus nerve and the reticular formation. The pathology is manifested as a disruption to the normal sequencing of a swallow and fits with other disruptions in motor sequencing found in Parkinson disease (Hunter et al., 1997). The specific nature and severity of the resulting swallowing symptoms appear to be independent of the overall disease stage.

What Swallowing Characteristics Are Associated with Parkinson Disease?

The incidence of dysphagia in people with Parkinson disease has been reported to be as high as 95% (Blonsky et al., 1975). It is evident, however, that the percentage of individuals who complain of or even recognize that a problem exists is much smaller (Bushman et al., 1989; Robbins et al., 1986). In a questionnaire completed by 230 people with Parkinson disease in Sweden, 41% reported that their ability to chew and swallow was worse than prior to disease onset (Hartelius & Svensson, 1994).

Table 2.15 lists common symptoms of swallowing difficulties in Parkinson disease. Note that symptoms may occur in the oral, pharyngeal, or esophageal stage. The oral stage of swallowing has been variously described as delayed, inefficient, and piecemeal. Increased mastication time and limited mandibular excursion are frequent symptoms (Calne, Shaw, Spiers, & Stern, 1970; Leopold & Kagel, 1996b). The oral stage is further characterized by repetitive tongue pumping, difficulty with bolus formation, and hesitancy in initiating the swallow (Wintzen et al., 1994). Patients often fail to lower the posterior tongue during this voluntary phase of swallowing, thus forcing the bolus to return to a more anterior position. They may repeat this backward-forward-backward movement several times before generating enough force to propel the bolus into the pharynx (Logemann, 1983). Logemann describes this repetitive action as a type of "festination" in lingual movement and suggests that it may reflect a form of muscle rigidity. The frequency with which individuals with Parkinson disease swallow is also reduced. Pehlivan and colleagues (1996) describe Parkinson patients as having less frequent spontaneous swallows and taking more time to swallow a volume of water than unimpaired individuals. This difficulty may be made worse by adding the stress of forcing repetitive swallows (Nilsson, Ekberg, Olsson, & Hindfelt, 1996).

Once a bolus is propelled into the pharyngeal cavity, there may be a delay in triggering pharyngeal contractions. Some people report little or no problem with the pharyngeal stage of swallowing (Calne et al., 1970). Others, while describing a variety of abnormalities, report that the durational changes in the pharyngeal phase are similar to elderly control subjects (Nagaya, Kachi, Yamada, & Igata, 1998). Most investigators, however, report reduced force of contractions, excessive residue in the valleculae and pyriform sinuses, and a prevalence of silent aspiration (Bird, Woodward, Gibson, Phyland, & Fonda, 1994; Bushman et al., 1989; Robbins et al., 1986). In some cases, pharyngeal contractions are not elicited until the bolus reaches the valleculae. Over successive swallows, patients may accumulate residue in the valleculae and pyriform sinuses, causing the potential for aspiration if this residual material

TABLE 2.15

Symptoms of Swallowing Difficulties in Parkinson Disease

124

Oral Stage	Pharyngeal Stage	Esophageal Stage
Drooling	Moderate delay in swallow	Cinefluorography may reveal reduced esophageal peristalsis
Tongue tremor	Response triggered from the valleculae	
Disturbed lingual peristalsis	Reduced pharyngeal peristalsis	
Difficulty initiating lingual movement	Coating of the pharyngeal walls	
Slowed oral transit time	Decreased relaxation of the pharynx after swallow	
Tongue pumping action; the posterior tongue remains elevated, preventing food from leaving the oral cavity	Pooling in the valleculae and pyriform sinuses	
Repetitive anterior-to-posterior rolling pattern	Increased risk of aspiration after swallow	
Prolonged ramp-like posture	Incomplete laryngeal closure	
Piecemeal deglutition	Aspiration during swallow	
Bolus falling over the base of the tongue	Aspiration after swallow	
Reflux from base of tongue into mouth	Vestibular aspiration	
	Tracheal aspiration	
	Decreased laryngeal elevation	
	Cricopharyngeal spasm	

Note. Adapted from Bushman et al. (1989); Kirschner (1986); Logemann (1983); Robbins, Logemann, and Kirschner (1986); and Serradura and Hill (1989).

spills into the open airway after a swallow is complete. Problems specific to the cricopharyngeus generally have not been recognized (Eadie & Tyrer, 1965; Logemann, 1983; Penner & Drukerman, 1942), although Palmer (1974) believed that dysphagia in parkinsonism is almost always caused by cricopharyngeal achalasia (failure to relax of the smooth muscle fibers of the gastrointestinal tract) and can be treated by cricopharyngeal myotomy. It appears that although there may be a higher incidence of cricopharyngeal dysfunction in this population (Ali et al., 1996; Donner & Silbiger, 1966), the problem stems from impaired pharyngeal and esophageal contractions rather than from an isolated pharyngeal–esophageal sphincteric achalasia. Some reports indicate improved swallowing in a small number of patients who demonstrate evidence of cricopharyngeal dysfunction and undergo myotomy (Born, Harned, Rikkers, Pfeiffer, & Quigley, 1996).

Once the bolus passes through the upper esophageal sphincter, the transit continues at a slow pace through the body of the esophagus. It is not uncommon for individuals with Parkinson disease to complain of symptoms such as esophageal obstruction, acid regurgitation, heartburn, and noncardiac chest pain (Bassotti et al., 1998). Primary esophageal peristalsis tends to be inefficient or even absent, and tertiary waves are frequently elicited. These abnormalities may be found in any patient, regardless of duration or severity of Parkinson disease (Bassotti et al., 1998; Castell et al., 2001). Hesitation at the lower esophageal sphincter is common, and esophageal reflux may be evident (Leopold & Kagel, 1997b). There is even some evidence that patients with Parkinson disease are prone to gastrointestinal dysfunction. This may be related to delayed colon transit and impaired anorectal muscle coordination (Pfeiffer, 1998).

In summary, specific characteristics of dysphagia in parkinsonism vary from patient to patient. Oral, pharyngeal, and esophageal stages, in various degrees, are all susceptible to dysfunction. Problems can be experienced in any of these phases of swallowing at any time during the course of the disease. Impairments, including aspiration, are frequently demonstrated in patients who have no swallowing complaints.

What Is Progressive Supranuclear Palsy and How Does It Differ from Parkinson Disease?

Progressive supranuclear palsy (PSP) is a degenerative disease of the extrapyramidal system that may appear very similar to Parkinson disease. Patients with PSP have many of the same symptoms as those with Parkinson disease, including rigidity and bradykinesia. Both speech and swallowing may be affected and show characteristics similar to those described for Parkinson disease. Individuals with PSP do not tend to improve in symptoms or function with levodopa. Difficulty with voluntary eye movements is often a feature of PSP. Dementia, while present in some individuals with Parkinson disease, is more common in PSP.

Oral stage swallowing abnormalities in PSP have been reported to include uncoordinated tongue movements, impaired elevation of the soft palate, and premature leakage of the bolus into the pharynx. Compared to Parkinson disease, oral stage difficulties are more common in PSP patients (Johnston et al., 1997). During the pharyngeal stage, the epiglottis does not fully deflect down and vallecular pooling is evident (Leopold & Kagel, 1997a). However, pharyngeal abnormalities for individuals with PSP do not appear to differ from those with Parkinson disease (Johnston et al., 1997). Litvan, Sastry, and Sonies (1997) note that generally, as cognitive deficits become more severe, swallowing complaints increase. Further, in their report, swallowing abnormalities were detected in all patients with PSP, whereas only 75% had abnormal speech.

How Is Swallowing Evaluated in Parkinson Disease?

Individuals with Parkinson disease may not complain of dysphagia in spite of having symptoms of weight loss, dehydration, and even pneumonia. When they do complain, their complaints are frequently associated with oral stage dysfunction—for example, difficulty chewing, food sticking on the roof of the mouth, slowness in the initiation of the swallow, and drink or saliva escaping through the lips. Complaints associated with the pharyngeal stage relate to coughing or choking and to solid food or pills sticking in the throat. Problems related to the esophageal stage generally go unnoticed. Although patients may complain of acid regurgitation or heartburn, they often do not relate this to dysphagia. Table 2.16 lists the frequency of occurrence of a variety of swallowing symptoms. Note that liquids escaping through the lips is the most frequent complaint, followed by choking on food or drink.

INTERVIEW

The case history should be detailed and comprehensive. The duration of the problem and the frequency of difficulty should be specified. The relationship between symptoms, severity of symptoms, and the timing of medications should be identified. The relative influence of bolus texture (solid, semisolid, or liquid) on swallowing should be explored. Associated symptoms such as the sensation of obstruction; mouth, throat, or chest pain; choking; and the sensation of heartburn or reflux should be noted. Changes in weight, eating habits, and appetite must be documented. The patient should be questioned about other ancillary symptoms such as speech or voice abnormalities and drooling.

A general medical history should attempt to document family history, the results of neurologic examination, and all previous swallowing studies. Special note should be made of any pulmonary disorders and surgeries that might affect deglutition. All current and past medications taken, both prescription and over-the-counter, should be listed and scrutinized for their possible side effects on swallowing, including drying of the mouth, sedating, and dyskinesia.

EXAMINATION

Because of reports that there is no significant relationship between the patient's complaints of swallowing difficulty and radiographic or manometric evidence of abnormalities (Bassotti et al., 1998; Bushman et al., 1989; Castell et al., 2001), and because symptoms may occur even in the earliest stages of the disease and remain unrelated to the severity of disease, a thorough clinical and radiographic examination is usually warranted. Weight loss is not only an important index of swallowing difficulty, it may be an important characteristic symptom of Parkinson disease (Jankovic, Wooten, Van der Linden, & Jansson, 1992). Therefore, obtain a baseline weight and monitor weight regularly. Thoroughly examine the peripheral musculature for swallowing, including the laryngeal mechanism. Observations of the patient during a meal can be invaluable in documenting the problems and identifying the underlying mechanisms contributing to them.

In most instances, radiographic assessment of swallowing is warranted, because the problem is multifactorial and extends to stages of swallowing that cannot be adequately assessed by the clinical examination alone. Cricopharyngeal and esophageal functions deserve particular attention on the radiographic examination. In many cases, you will want to employ provocative measures to assess for esophageal reflux.

TABLE 2.16	Frequency of Swallowing Difficulties in Parkinson Disease	
	Symptom	**Percentage**[a]
	Liquid or saliva escaping through lips	26
	Choking on food or drink	21
	Difficulty swallowing solids	18
	Difficulty swallowing liquids	17
	Difficulty chewing	12

[a]Percentages indicate the proportion of the population reporting that problem occurs "fairly often" ($N = 230$).
Note. Adapted from "Speech and Swallowing Symptoms Associated with Parkinson's Disease and Multiple Sclerosis," by L. Hartelius and P. Svensson, 1994, *Folia Phoniatrica et Logopaedica, 46*, pp. 9–18.

TABLE 2.17	Dysphagia Severity Rating Scale for Parkinson Disease	
Rating	**Description**	
7	**Normal swallowing mechanism**	
6	**Minimal dysphagia:** Videofluoroscopy shows slight deviance from a normal swallow. Client may report a change in sensation during swallow. No change in diet is required.	
5	**Mild dysphagia:** Oropharyngeal dysphagia is present but can be managed by specific swallowing suggestions. Slight modification in consistency of diet may be indicated.	
4	**Mild–moderate dysphagia:** Potential for aspiration exists but is diminished by specific swallowing techniques and a modified diet. Time required for eating is significantly increased, and supplemental nutrition may be indicated.	
3	**Moderate dysphagia:** Significant potential for aspiration exists. Trace aspiration of one or more consistencies may be seen under videofluoroscopy. Patient may eat certain consistencies by using specific techniques to minimize potential for aspiration or to facilitate swallowing. Supervision at mealtimes is required. Patient may require supplemental nutrition orally or via tube feeding.	
2	**Moderate–severe dysphagia:** Patient aspirates 5% to 10% on one or more consistencies, with potential for aspiration of all consistencies. Potential for aspiration is minimized by use of specific swallowing instructions. Cough reflex is absent or nonprotective. Alternative mode of feeding is required to maintain patient's nutritional needs. If pulmonory status is compromised "nothing by mouth" may be indicated.	
1	**Severe dysphagia:** More than 10% aspiration for all consistencies. "Nothing by mouth" recommended.	

Note. Adapted from "Nutritional Aspects and Swallowing Function of Patients with Parkinson's Disease," by M. J. Waxman, D. Durfee, M. Moore, and R. A. Morantz, 1990, *Nutrition in Clinical Practice, 5*(5), pp. 196–199. Copyright 1990 by American Society for Parenteral & Enteral Nutrition. Adapted with permission.

Waxman, Durfee, Moore, and Morantz (1990) have proposed a Dysphagia Severity Rating Scale for staging purposes. The authors utilize a 7-point scale ranging from *normal swallowing mechanism* to *severe dysphagia* (see Table 2.17). Gradations in the rating of severity are based on the patient's report, observations of family members or caregivers, and the results of a radiographic examination.

What Approaches to Treatment Are Available for Swallowing Disorders in Parkinson Disease?

The problems associated with eating and swallowing are managed on a case-by-case basis, dictated by the findings of all examination procedures. Table 2.18 contains a summary of swallowing intervention approaches at various severity levels for individuals with Parkinson disease. The management techniques employed may be either of a general nature and designed to improve overall function or specific to a single dysfunctional element in the swallow sequence. Serradura and Hill (1989) provide a summary of management techniques. Throughout the course of the disease and at every swallowing evaluation, the patient and spouse should be counseled regarding the findings and likely prognosis for progression. To the extent possible, problems should be anticipated and supportive measures employed to obviate such complications as aspiration, inadequate nutrition, and dehydration. Referrals should be made to appropriate support agencies whenever possible.

TABLE 2.18

Summary of Swallowing Intervention in Parkinson Disease

	Normal Swallow	**Early Swallowing Problems**	**Moderate Swallow Disability**	**Severe Swallow Disability**
Presenting Features	• No observable changes	• Reduction in pharyngeal peristalsis • Repetitive rocking motion of the tongue	• Pharyngeal peristalsis worsens • Delay in swallowing reflex • Cricopharyngeal dysfunction • Laryngeal closure during swallowing may be inadequate	• Aspiration occurring both during and after swallow
Intervention	• Monitor weight • Answer questions	• Counseling to bring swallowing under voluntary control • Monitor weight • Coordinate eating with drug cycle	• Introduce aids and devices to promote independence • Increase sensory input • Teach double swallow • Small, frequent highly nutritious meals	• Chin tuck swallowing • Switch to soft diet

DYSPHAGIA AND MEDICATIONS

Although levodopa has not been shown to improve swallowing, some of the motor events related to eating and swallowing may be enhanced with the medication. Therefore, the timing of dopaminergic medication should be monitored to ensure that the maximum effect of the medications can be used to facilitate upper extremity, oral, and pharyngeal functions during meals. Some cautions should be noted with regard to the interaction between parenteral routes for intake and medications. Anticholinergics may not be as effective when taken parenterally as when taken orally (Bushman et al., 1989). Vallecular pooling of medications will lead to irregular absorption and subsequent lack of clinical response. Furthermore, esophageal motility problems may compromise absorption (R. Miller & Groher, 1992). When medications are discontinued to evaluate a clinical response to new drugs or to adjust dosage levels, patients may be placed at greater risk for aspiration. In these cases, the patients should be monitored closely for any signs of compromised swallowing.

FEEDING AND DIETARY MODIFICATIONS

Adaptive utensils and devices may be used to promote independence in eating by compensating for movement disorders. Independent self-feeding with supervision will allow the eater to control the timing of each swallow and the speed and duration of the meal. Frequently, patients report improved nutritional management when they take more frequent, small, nutritious meals. Alterations in diet texture to avoid dry and crumbly foods while emphasizing moist and cohesive food boluses may obviate potential problems. Increasing sensory input from the bolus by adding flavor, visual presentation, and smell may facilitate both chewing and swallowing.

COMPENSATORY SWALLOWING TECHNIQUES

For the most part, the compensations that assist the person with Parkinson disease with swallowing are techniques that bring swallowing under voluntary control. Therapies focusing on effort, such as LSVT, may be effective for both speech and swallowing. Posturing the person in an upright, neck-flexed position will assist in airway protection during swallows. Using conscious airway-protection techniques, such as a double swallow followed by a voluntary cough, has been found useful in some cases (Logemann, 1983; Serradura & Hill, 1989). Logemann also advocates using the "supraglottic swallow" technique for individuals who aspirate during the swallow, as opposed to those who aspirate residue pooled in the pharynx after the swallow. Aspiration as a result of ineffective laryngeal closure may be treated by having the person inhale, hold a breath, swallow, cough, and reswallow. When performed with the head tilted forward to divert the food away from the laryngeal inlet, this technique may be effective in minimizing aspiration risks. At some point, supervised feeding may be required. Since there is evidence that it takes patients longer to swallow and clear a bolus, individuals with Parkinson disease should be allowed a longer time to eat. Verbal prompting to reswallow and clear any pooled residue may facilitate their swallow (Pinnington, Muhiddin, Ellis, & Playford, 2000).

LATE STAGES OF THE DISEASE

Patients with severe dysphagia may be unable to masticate adequately or feed themselves, and trained feeders may be employed in some cases to assist in nutritional management. Soft foods, even blenderized diets, may be necessary to maintain adequate nutritional support. Enteral feeding with a percutaneous endoscopic gastrostomy (PEG) may be indicated to improve quality of life by providing the person with a convenient and efficient means of nutritional support. People with a PEG can, if capable, continue to take some nutrition by mouth for pleasure or to supplement their tube feedings.

References

Aarsland, D., Andersen, K., Larsen, J. P., Lolk, A., Nielsen, H., & Kragh-Sorensen, P. (2001). Risk of dementia in Parkinson's disease. *Neurology, 56,* 730–736.

Ackermann, H., & Ziegler, W. (1991). Articulatory deficits in parkinsonian dysarthria: An acoustic analysis. *Journal of Neurology, Neurosurgery, and Psychiatry, 54*(12), 1093–1198.

Adams, S., & Lang, A. (1992). Can the Lombard effect be used to improve low voice intensity in Parkinson's disease? *European Journal of Disorders of Communication, 27*(2), 121–127.

Adams, S. G. (1994). Accelerating speech in a case of hypokinetic dysarthria: Descriptions and treatment. In J. A. Till, K. M. Yorkston, & D. R. Beukelman (Eds.), *Motor speech disorders: Advances in assessment and treatment* (pp. 213–228). Baltimore: Brookes.

Adams, S. G. (1997). Hypokinetic dysarthria in Parkinson's disease. In M. R. McNeil (Ed.), *Clinical management of sensorimotor speech disorders* (pp. 261–286). New York: Thieme.

Ahlskog, J. E. (2001). Parkinson's disease: Medical and surgical treatment. *Neurologic Clinics, 19*(3), 579–605.

Ali, G. N., Wallace, K. L., Schwartz, R., DeCarle, D. J., Zagami, A. S., & Cook, I. J. (1996). Mechanism of oral-pharyngeal dysphagia in patients with Parkinson's disease. *Gastroenterology, 110,* 383–392.

Allan, C. M. (1970). Treatment of non-fluent speech resulting from neurological diseases: Treatment of dysarthria. *British Journal of Disorders of Communication, 5,* 3–5.

American Psychiatric Association. (1980). *Diagnostic and statistical manual of mental disorders* (3rd ed.). Washington, DC: Author.

Aronson, A. E. (1985). *Clinical voice disorder: An interdisciplinary approach* (2nd ed.). New York: Thieme.

Athlin, E., Norberg, A., Axelsson, K., Moller, A., & Nordstrom, G. (1989). Aberrant eating behavior in elderly parkinsonian patients with and without dementia. *Research in Nursing & Health, 12*, 41–51.

Baker, K. L., Ramig, L. O., Luschei, E. S., & Smith, M. E. (1998). Thyroarytenoid muscle activity associated with hypophonia in Parkinson disease and aging. *Neurology, 51*(6), 1592–1598.

Barlow, S. M., Iacono, R. P., Paseman, L. A., Biswas, A., & D'Antonio, L. (1998). The effects of posteroventral pallidotomy on force and speech aerodynamics in Parkinson's disease. In M. Cannito, K. M. Yorkston, & D. R. Beukelman (Eds.), *Neuromotor speech disorders: Nature, assessment, and management* (pp. 117–156). Baltimore: Brookes.

Bassotti, G., Germani, U., Pagliaricci, S., Plesa, A., Giulietti, O., Mannarino, E., & Morelli, A. (1998). Esophageal manometric abnormalities in Parkinson's disease. *Dysphagia, 13*, 28–31.

Baumgartner, C., Sapir, S., & Ramig, L. O. (2001). Voice quality changes following phonatory-respiratory effort treatment (LSVT) versus respiratory effort treatment for individuals with Parkinson disease. *Journal of Voice, 15*(1), 105–114.

Bayles, K. A. (1990). Language and Parkinson disease. *Alzheimer Disease and Associated Disorders, 4*(3), 171–180.

Bayles, K. A., Tomoeda, C. K., Wood, J. A., Montgomery, E. B., Cruz, R. F., & Azuma, T. (1997). The effect of Parkinson's disease on language. *Journal of Medical Speech–Language Pathology, 5*(3), 157–166.

Beatty, W. W., & Monson, N. (1989). Lexical processing in Parkinson's disease and multiple sclerosis. *Journal of Geriatric Psychiatry and Neurology, 2*, 145–152.

Berry, W. R. (1983). Treatment of hypokinetic dysarthria. In W. H. Perkins (Ed.), *Dysarthria and apraxia* (pp. 91–100). New York: Theime-Stratton.

Beukelman, D. R., & Mirenda, P. (1998). *Augmentative and alternative communication: Management of severe communication disorders in children and adults* (2nd ed.). Baltimore: Brookes.

Beukelman, D. R., Yorkston, K. M., & Tice, R. (1997). *Pacer/tally rate measurement software.* Lincoln, NE: Madonna Rehabilitation Hospital.

Beyer, M. K., Herlofson, F., Arsland, D., & Larsen, J. P. (2001). Causes of death in a community-based study of Parkinson's disease. *Acta Neurologica Scandinavica, 103*(1), 7–11.

Bird, M. R., Woodward, M. C., Gibson, E. M., Phyland, D. J., & Fonda, D. (1994). Asymptomatic swallowing disorders in elderly patients with Parkinson's disease: A description of findings on clinical examination and videofluoroscopy in sixteen patients. *Age and Aging, 23*, 251–254.

Blonsky, E. R., Logemann, J. A., Boshes, B., & Fisher, H. B. (1975). Comparison of speech and swallowing function in patients with tremor disorders and in normal geriatric patients: A cinefluorographic study. *Journal of Gerontology, 30*, 299–303.

Born, L. J., Harned, R. H., Rikkers, L. F., Pfeiffer, R. F., & Quigley, E. M. (1996). Cricopharyngeal dysfunction in Parkinson's disease: Role in dysphagia and response to myotomy. *Movement Disorders, 11*, 53–58.

Boshes, B. (1966). Voice changes in parkinsonism. *Journal of Neurosurgery, 24*, 286–288.

Bramble, M. G., Cunliffe, J., & Dellipiani, W. (1978). Evidence for a change in neurotransmitter affecting esophageal motility in Parkinson's disease. *Journal of Neurology, Neurosurgery and Psychiatry, 41*, 709–712.

Brown, P., & Marsden, C. D. (1998). What do the basal ganglia do? *Lancet, 351*, 1801–1804.

Bushman, M., Bomeyer, S. M., Leeker, L., & Perlmutter, J. S. (1989). Swallowing abnormalities and their response to treatment in Parkinson's disease. *Neurology, 39*(10), 1309–1314.

Cahill, L. M., Murdoch, B. E., Theodoros, D. G., Triggs, E. J., Charles, B. G., & Yao, A. A. (1998). Effect of oral levodopa treatment on articulatory function in Parkinson's disease: Preliminary results. *Motor Control, 2*(2), 161–172.

Calne, D. B., Shaw, D. G., Spiers, A. S. D., & Stern, G. M. (1970). Swallowing in parkinsonism. *British Journal of Radiology, 43*, 456–457.

Canter, G. C. (1965). Speech characteristics of patients with Parkinson's disease: II. Physiological support for speech. *Journal of Speech and Hearing Disorders, 30,* 44–49.

Cariski, D., & Rosenbek, J. (1999). Clinical note: The effectiveness of the speech enhancer. *Journal of Medical Speech–Language Pathology, 7*(4), 315–322.

Caruso, A. J. (2001, July 24). Parkinson's disease and me. *The ASHA Leader, 7.*

Castell, J. A., Johnston, B. T., Colcher, A., Li, Q., Gideon, R. M., & Castell, D. O. (2001). Manometric abnormalities of the oesophagus in patients with Parkinson's disease. *Neurogastroenterology and Motility, 13*(4), 361–364.

Coates, C., & Bakheit, A. M. (1997a). Dysphagia in Parkinson's disease. *European Neurology, 38*(1), 49–52.

Coates, C., & Bakheit, A. M. (1997b). The prevalence of verbal communication disability in patients with Parkinson's disease. *Disability and Rehabilitation, 19*(3), 104–107.

Cooper, J., Sagar, H., Jordan, N., Harvey, N., & Sullivan, E. (1991). Cognitive impairment in early, untreated Parkinson's disease and its relationship to motor disability. *Brain, 114,* 2095–2122.

Countryman, S., Hicks, J., Ramig, L. O., & Smith, M. E. (1997). Supraglottal hyperadduction in an individual with Parkinson disease: A clinical treatment note. *American Journal of Speech–Language Pathology, 6*(4), 74–84.

Countryman, S., & Ramig, L. O. (1993). The effects of intensive voice therapy on voice deficits associated with bilateral thalamotomy in Parkinson's disease: A case study. *Journal of Medical Speech–Language Pathology, 1,* 233–250.

Countryman, S., Ramig, L. O., & Pawlas, A. A. (1994). Speech and voice deficits in parkinsonism plus syndromes: Can they be treated? *Journal of Medical Speech–Language Pathology, 2*(3), 211–226.

Critchley, E. M. R. (1981). Speech disorders of parkinsonism: A review. *Journal of Neurology, Neuropsychiatry and Psychiatry, 44,* 751–758.

Cummings, J. (1988). Intellectual impairment in Parkinson's disease: Clinical pathologic, and biochemical correlates. *Journal of Geriatric Psychiatry and Neurology, 1,* 24–36.

Cummings, J. L., & Bensen, F. (1984). Subcortical dementia: Review of an emerging concept. *Archives of Neurology, 14,* 874–879.

Darley, F. L., Aronson, A. E., & Brown, J. R. (1975). *Motor speech disorders.* Philadelphia: Saunders.

de Angelis, E. C., Mourao, L. F., Ferraz, H. B., Behlau, M. S., Pontes, P. A., & Andrade, L. A. (1997). Effect of voice rehabilitation on oral communication of Parkinson's disease patients. *Acta Neurologica Scandinavica, 96*(4), 199–205.

Donner, M., & Silbiger, M. (1966). Cinefluorographic analysis of pharyngeal swallowing in neuromuscular disorders. *American Journal of Medical Sciences, 251,* 600–616.

Downie, A. W., Low, J. M., & Lindsay, D. D. (1981). Speech disorders in parkinsonism: Usefulness of delayed auditory feedback in selected cases. *British Journal of Disorders of Communication, 16,* 135–139.

Dromey, C., Ramig, L. O., & Johnson, A. B. (1995). Phonatory and articulatory changes associated with increased vocal intensity in parkinson disease: A case study. *Journal of Speech and Hearing Research, 38*(4), 751–764.

Dubois, B., Slachevsky, A., Litvan, I., & Pillon, B. (2000). The FAB: A frontal assessment battery at bedside. *Neurology, 55,* 1621–1626.

Duffy, J. R. (1995). *Motor speech disorders: Substrates, differential diagnosis, and management.* St. Louis, MO: Mosby.

Duvoisin, R. C. (1991). *Parkinson's disease: A guide for patient and family* (3rd ed.). New York: Raven Press.

Eadie, M. J., & Tyrer, J. H. (1965). Alimentary disorders in parkinsonism. *Australian Annals of Medicine, 14,* 13–22.

Ebmeier, K. P., Calder, S. A., Crawford, J. R., Stewart, L., Cochrane, R. H., & Besson, J. A. (1991). Dementia in idiopathic Parkinson's disease: Prevalence and relationship with symptoms and signs of parkinsonism. *Psychological Medicine, 21,* 69–76.

Fahr, S., Elton, R. I., & UPDRS Development Committee. (1987). Unified Parkinson's Disease Rating Scale. In S. Fahn, C. D. Marsden, D. B. Calne, & M. Goldstein (Eds.), *Recent developments in Parkinson's disease* (pp. 153–304). New York: Macmillan.

Fields, J. A., & Troster, A. I. (2000). Cognitive outcomes after deep brain stimulation for Parkinson's disease: A review of initial studies and recommendations for future research. *Brain and Cognition, 42*(2), 268–293.

Forno, L. S. (1981). Pathology of Parkinson's disease. In D. Marsden & S. Fahn (Eds.), *Neurology II: Movement disorders.* Stoneham, MA: Butterworth.

Forrest, K., Weismer, G., & Turner, G. S. (1989). Kinematic, acoustic, and perceptual analyses of connected speech produced by Parkinsonian and normal geriatric adults. *Journal of the Acoustical Society of America, 85*(6), 2608–2622.

Gallena, S., Smith, P. J., Zeffiro, T., & Ludlow, C. L. (2001). Effects of levodopa on laryngeal muscle activity for voice onset and offset in Parkinson disease. *Journal of Speech, Language, and Hearing Research, 44*(6), 1284–1299.

Gentil, M., Perrin, S., Tournier, C., & Pollak, P. (1999). Lip, tongue and forefinger force control in Parkinson's disease. *Clinical Linguistics & Phonetics, 13*(1), 45–54.

Gotham, A. M., Brown, R. G., & Marsden, C. D. (1986). Depression in Parkinson's disease: A quantitative and qualitative analysis. *Journal of Neurology, Neurosurgery and Psychiatry, 46,* 381–389.

Graybiel, A. M. (1998). The basal ganglia and chunking of action repertoires. *Neurobiology of Learning and Memory, 70*(1–2), 119–136.

Grossman, M. (1999). Sentence processing in Parkinson's disease. *Brain and Cognition, 40,* 387–413.

Grossman, M., Carvell, S., Gollomp, S., Stern, M. B., Vernon, G., & Hurtig, H. I. (1991). Sentence comprehension and praxia deficits in Parkinson's disease. *Neurology, 41,* 1620–1626.

Gupta, A., & Bhatia, S. (2000). Depression in Parkinson's disease. *Clinical Gerontologist, 22*(2), 59–70.

Hallett, M., Litvan, I., & Task Force on Surgery for Parkinson's Disease. (1999). Evaluation of surgery for Parkinson's disease. *Neurology, 53,* 1910–1921.

Hanson, D., Gerratt, B. R., & Ward, P. H. (1984). Cinegraphic observations of laryngeal function in Parkinson's disease. *Laryngoscope, 94,* 348–353.

Hanson, W., & Metter, E. J. (1980). DAF as instrumental treatment for dysarthria in progressive supranuclear palsy: A case report. *Journal of Speech and Hearing Disorders, 45,* 268–276.

Hanson, W., & Metter, E. (1983). DAF speech rate modification in Parkinson's disease: A report of two cases. In W. Berry (Ed.), *Clinical dysarthria* (pp. 231–254). Austin, TX: PRO-ED.

Hartelius, L., & Svensson, P. (1994). Speech and swallowing symptoms associated with Parkinson's disease and multiple sclerosis: A survey. *Folia Phoniatrica et Logopaedica, 46,* 9–17.

Helm, N. (1979). Management of palilallia with a pacing board. *Journal of Speech and Hearing Disorders, 44,* 350–353.

Ho, A. K., Iansek, R., & Bradshaw, J. L. (1999). Regulation of parkinsonian speech volume: The effect of interlocuter distance. *Journal of Neurology, Neurosurgery and Psychiatry, 67*(2), 199–202.

Hoehn, M. M., & Yahr, M. D. (1967). Parkinsonism: Onset, progression and mortality. *Neurology, 17,* 427–442.

Holmes, R. J., Oates, J. M., Phyland, D. J., & Hughes, A. J. (2000). Voice characteristics of the progression of Parkinson's disease. *International Journal of Language & Communication Disorders, 35*(3), 407–418.

Hoodin, R. B., & Gilbert, H. R. (1989). Nasal airflows in parkinsonian speakers. *Journal of Communication Disorders, 22,* 169–180.

Hristova, A. H., & Koller, W. C. (2000). Early Parkinson's disease: What is the best approach to treatment? *Drugs and Aging, 17*(3), 165–181.

Huber, S. J., Freidenberg, D. L., Shuttleworth, E. C., Paulson, G. W., & Christy, J. S. (1989). Neuropsychological impairments associated with severity of Parkinson's disease. *Journal of Neuropsychiatry and Clinical Neurosciences, 1*(2), 154–158.

Hunter, P. C., Crameri, J., Austin, S., Woodward, M. C., & Hughes, A. J. (1997). Response of parkinsonian swallowing dysfunction to dopaminergic stimulation. *Journal of Neurology, Neuropsychiatry, and Psychiatry, 63,* 579–583.

Illes, J., Metter, E. J., Hanson, W. R., & Iritani, S. (1988). Language production in Parkinson's disease: Acoustic and linguistic considerations. *Brain and Language, 33,* 146–160.

Jain, S. S., & Kirshblum, S. C. (1993). Movement disorders, including tremors. In J. A. DeLisa & B. M. Gans (Eds.), *Rehabilitation medicine: Principles and practices.* Philadelphia: Lippincott.

Jankovic, J. (2000a). Complications and limitations of drug therapy for Parkinson's disease. *Neurology, 55*(12 Suppl. 6), S2–6.

Jankovic, J. (2000b). Parkinson's disease therapy: Tailoring choices for early and later disease, young and old patients. *Clinical Neuropharmacology, 23*(5), 252–261.

Jankovic, J., Wooten, M., Van der Linden, C., & Jansson, B. (1992). Low body weight in Parkinson's disease. *Southern Medical Journal, 85*(4), 351–354.

Johnson, J. A., & Pring, T. R. (1990). Speech therapy and Parkinson's disease: A review and further data. *British Journal of Disorders of Communication, 25,* 183–194.

Johnston, B. T., Castell, J. A., Stumacher, S., Colcher, A., Gideon, R. M., Li, Q., & Castell, D. O. (1997). Comparison of swallowing function in Parkinson's disease and progressive supranuclear palsy. *Movement Disorders, 12*(3), 322–327.

Kim, R. (1968). The chronic residual respiratory disorder in post-encephalitic parkinsonism. *Journal of Neurology, Neurosurgery and Psychiatry, 31,* 393–398.

Kompoliti, K., Goetz, C. G., Litvan, I., Jellinger, K., & Verny, M. (1998). Pharmacological therapy in progressive supranuclear palsy. *Archives of Neurology, 55*(8), 1099–1102.

Kreul, E. (1972). Neuromuscular control examination (NMC) for Parkinsonism: Vocal prolongations and diadokokinetic and reading rates. *Journal of Speech and Hearing Research, 15,* 72–83.

Labuszewski, T., & Lidsky, T. I. (1979). Basal ganglia influence on brain stem trigeminal neurons. *Experimental Neurology, 65,* 471–477.

Lacritz, L. H., Cullum, C. M., Frol, A. B., Dewey, R. B., & Giller, C. A. (2000). Neuropsychological outcome following unilateral stereotactic pallidotomy in intractable Parkinson's disease. *Brain and Cognition, 42*(3), 364–378.

Laitnen, L. (2000). Behavioral complications of early pallidotomy. *Brain and Cognition, 42*(3), 313–323.

Larson, K. K., Ramig, L. O., & Scherer, R. C. (1994). Acoustic and glottographic voice analysis during drug-related fluctuations in Parkinson disease. *Journal of Medical Speech–Language Pathology, 2*(3), 227–239.

Lavigne, J., & Roberts, K. M. (1982). *Home exercises for patients with Parkinson's disease.* New York: American Parkinson Disease Association.

Le Dorze, G., Dioone, L., Ryalls, J., Julien, M., & Ouellet, L. (1992). The effects of speech and language therapy for a case of dysarthria associated with Parkinson's disease. *European Journal of Disorders of Communication, 27*(4), 313–324.

Leopold, N. A., & Kagel, M. C. (1996). Prepharyngeal dysphagia in Parkinson's disease. *Dysphagia, 11,* 14–22.

Leopold, N. A., & Kagel, M. C. (1997a). Dysphagia in progressive supranuclear palsy: Radiologic features. *Dysphagia, 12*(3), 140–143.

Leopold, N. A., & Kagel, M. C. (1997b). Pharyngo-esophageal dysphagia in Parkinson's disease. *Dysphagia, 12,* 11–18.

Levin, B. E., Llabre, M. M., Reisman, S., Weiner, W. J., Sanchez-Ramos, J., Singer, C., & Brown, M. C. (1991). Visuospatial impairment in Parkinson's disease. *Neurology, 41,* 365–369.

Levin, B. E., Tomer, R., & Rey, G. J. (1992). Cognitive impairments in Parkinson's disease. *Neurologic Clinics, 10*(2), 471–481.

Lieberman, A. N., Hirowitz, L., Redmond, P., Redmond, L., Lieberman, I., & Leibowitz, M. (1980). Dysphagia in Parkinson's disease. *American Journal of Gastroenterology, 74,* 157–160.

Lieberman, P., Friedman, J., & Feldman, L. (1990). Syntax comprehension deficits in Parkinson's disease. *Journal of Nervous and Mental Disorders, 178,* 360–365.

Litvan, I., Sastry, N., & Sonies, B. C. (1997). Characterizing swallowing abnormalities in progressive supranuclear palsy. *Neurology, 48*(6), 1654–1662.

Lloyd, A. J. (1999). Comprehension of prosody in Parkinson's disease. *Cortex, 35*(3), 389–402.

Logemann, J. (1983). *Evaluation and treatment of swallowing disorders.* Boston: College-Hill Press.

Logemann, J. A., Boshes, B., Blonsky, R. E., & Fisher, H. E. (1977). Speech and swallowing evaluation in the differential diagnosis of neurologic disease. *Neurologica Neurocirugia Psiquiatria, 18,* 71–78.

Logemann, J., & Fischer, H. (1981). Vocal tract control in Parkinson's disease: Phonetic feature analyses of misarticulations. *Journal of Speech and Hearing Disorders, 46,* 348.

Logemann, J. A., Fisher, H. B., Boshes, B., & Blonsky, E. (1978). Frequency and co-occurrence of vocal tract dysfunction in the speech of a large sample of Parkinson patients. *Journal of Speech and Hearing Disorders, 43,* 47–57.

Ludlow, C. L., Connor, N. P., & Bassich, C. J. (1987). Speech timing in Parkinson's and Huntington's disease. *Brain and Language, 32,* 195–214.

Marsden, C. D. (1984). The pathophysiology of movement disorders. *Neurologic Clinics, 2,* 435–459.

Marttila, R., & Rinne, U. (1991). Progression and survival in Parkinson's disease. *Acta Neurologica Scandinavica, 136,* 24–28.

Maruska, K. G., Smit, A. B., Koller, W. C., & Garcia, J. M. (2000). Sentence production in Parkinson disease treated with deep brain stimulation and medication. *Journal of Medical Speech–Language Pathology, 8*(4), 265–270.

Metter, E. J., & Hanson, W. R. (1986). Clinical and acoustical variability in hypokinetic dysarthria. *Journal of Communication Disorders, 19,* 347–366.

Middleton, F. A., & Strick, P. L. (2000). Basal ganglia output and cognition: Evidence from anatomical, behavorial, and clinical studies. *Brain and Cognition, 42*(2), 183–200.

Miller, A. J. (1982). Deglutition. *Physiological Reviews, 62,* 128–184.

Miller, R., & Groher, M. E. (1992). General treatment of neurologic swallowing disorders. In M. E. Groher (Ed.), *Dysphagia: Diagnosis and management* (pp. 111–132). Stoneham, MA: Butterworth-Heinemann.

Morrell, R. M. (1992). Neurologic disorders of swallowing. In M. E. Groher (Ed.), *Dysphagia: Diagnosis and management.* Stoneham, MA: Butterworth-Heinemann.

Muller, J., Wenning, G. K., Jellinger, K., McKee, A. S., Poewe, W., & Litvan, I. (2000). Progression of Hoehn and Yahr stages in parkinsonian disorders: A clinicopathologic study. *Neurology, 55,* 888–891.

Muller, J., Wenning, G. K., Verny, M., McKee, A. S., Chaudhuri, K. R., Jellinger, K., Poewe, W., & Litvan, I. (2001). Progression of dysarthria and dysphagia in postmortem-confirmed Parkinsonian disorders. *Archives of Neurology, 58*(2), 259–264.

Munchau, A., & Bhatia, K. P. (2000). Pharmacological treatment of Parkinson's disease. *Postgraduate Medical Journal, 76,* 602–610.

Murdoch, B. E., Chenery, H. J., Bowler, S., & Ingram, J. C. L. (1989). Respiratory function in Parkinson's subjects exhibiting a perceptible speech deficit: A kinematic and spirometric analysis. *Journal of Speech and Hearing Disorders, 54,* 610–626.

Murdoch, B. E., Manning, C. Y., Theodoros, D. G., & Thompson, E. C. (1997). Laryngeal and phonatory dysfunction in Parkinson's disease. *Clinical Linguistics & Phonetics, 11,* 245–266.

Murray, L. L., & Stout, J. C. (1999). Discourse comprehension in Huntington's and Parkinson's disease. *American Journal of Speech–Language Pathology, 8*(2), 137–148.

Mutch, W. J., Strudwick, A., Roy, S. K., & Downie, A. W. (1986). Parkinson's disease: Disability, review and management. *British Medical Journal, 293,* 675–677.

Nagaya, M., Kachi, T., Yamada, T., & Igata, A. (1998). Videofluorographic study of swallowing in Parkinson's disease. *Dysphagia, 13,* 95–100.

Nathan, U., Ben-Shlomo, Y., Thomson, R., Morris, H. L., Wood, N. W., Lees, A. J., & Burn, D. (2001). The prevalence of progressive supranuclear palsy (Steele-Richardson-Olszewski syndrome) in the UK. *Brain, 124,* 1438–1449.

Netsell, R., Daniel, B., & Celesia, G. G. (1975). Acceleration and weakness in parkinsonian dysarthria. *Journal of Speech and Hearing Disorders, 40,* 170–178.

Nilsson, H., Ekberg, O., Olsson, R., & Hindfelt, B. (1996). Quantitative assessment of oral and pharyngeal function in Parkinson's disease. *Dysphagia, 11,* 144–150.

Obeso, J. A., Rodriguez, M. C., Rodriguez, M., Lanciego, J. L., Artieda, J., Gonzalo, N., & Olanow, C. W. (2000). Pathophysiology of the basal ganglia in Parkinson's disease. *Trends in Neurosciences, 23*(Suppl. 10), S8–19.

Okamoto, G. A. (Ed.). (1984). *Physical medicine and rehabilitation.* Philadelphia: Saunders.

Palmer, E. D. (1974). Dysphagia in parkinsonism. *Journal of the American Medical Association, 229,* 1349.

Parkinson's Disease. (2001). Retrieved December 17, 2001, from http://www.mayoclinic.com

Pehlivan, M., Yuceyar, N., Ertekin, C., Celebi, G., Ertas, M., Kalayci, T., & Aydogdu, I. (1996). An electronic device measuring the frequency of spontaneous swallowing: Digital phagometer. *Dysphagia, 11,* 259–264.

Penner, A., & Drukerman, L. (1942). Segmental spasms of the esophagus and their relation to parkinsonism. *American Journal of Digestive Disease, 9,* 282–287.

Perez, K. S., Ramig, L. O., Smith, M. E., & Dromey, C. (1996). The Parkinson larynx: Tremor and videostroboscopic findings. *Journal of Voice, 10*(4), 354–361.

Pfeiffer, R. F. (1998). Gastrointestinal dysfunction in Parkinson's disease. *Clinical Neuroscience, 5*(2), 136–146.

Pinnington, L. L., Muhiddin, K. A., Ellis, R. E., & Playford, E. D. (2000). Non-invasive assessment of swallowing and respiration in Parkinson's disease. *Journal of Neurology 247*(10), 773–777.

Poewe, W. H., & Wenning, G. K. (1998). The natural history of Parkinson's disease. *Annual of Neurology, 44*(3 Suppl. 1), S1–9.

Poluha, P. C., Teulings, H. L., & Brookshire, R. H. (1998). Handwriting and speech changes across the levodopa cycle in Parkinson's disease. *Acta Psychologia, 100,* 71–84.

Ramig, L. (1992). The role of phonation in speech intelligibility: A review and preliminary data from patients with Parkinson's disease. In R. D. Kent (Ed.), *Intelligibility in speech disorders* (pp. 119–156). Philadelphia: John Benjamins.

Ramig, L. A., & Gould, W. J. (1986). Speech characteristics in Parkinson's disease. *Neurological Consultant, 4,* 1–6.

Ramig, L. O. (1993). *Voice therapy for patients with Parkinson's disease* [Videotape]. Tucson, AZ: National Center for Neurogenic Communication Disorders.

Ramig, L. O., Bonitati, C. M., Lemke, J. H., & Horii, Y. (1994). Voice treatment for patients with Parkinson disease: Development of an approach and preliminary efficacy data. *Journal of Medical Speech–Language Pathology, 2*(3), 191–210.

Ramig, L. O., Countryman, S., O'Brien, C., Hoehn, M., & Thompson, L. (1996). Intensive speech treatment for patients with Parkinson disease: Short- and long-term comparison of two techniques. *Neurology, 47,* 1496–1503.

Ramig, L. O., Countryman, S., Thompson, L. L., & Horii, Y. (1995). A comparison of two forms of intensive speech treatment in Parkinson disease. *Journal of Speech and Hearing Research, 38,* 1232–1251.

Ramig, L. O., & Dromey, C. (1996). Aerodynamic mechanisms underlying treatment-related changes in vocal intensity in patients with Parkinson disease. *Journal of Speech and Hearing Research, 39*(4), 798–807.

Ramig, L. O., Pawlas, A. A., & Countryman, S. (1995). *The Lee Silverman Voice Treatment.* Iowa City, IA: National Center for Voice and Speech.

Ramig, L. O., Sapir, S., Countryman, S., Pawlas, A., O'Brien, C., Hoehn, M., & Thompson, L. (2001). Intensive voice treatment (LSVT) for individuals with Parkinson disease: A two-year follow-up. *Journal of Neurology, Neuropsychiatry and Psychiatry, 71*(4), 493–499.

Ramig, L. O., Sapir, S., Fox, C., & Countryman, S. (2001). Changes in vocal intensity following intensive voice treatment (LSVT) in individuals with Parkinson disease: A comparison with untreated patients and normal age-matched controls. *Movement Disorders, 16*(1), 79–83.

Rehman, H. U. (2000). Progressive supranuclear palsy. *Postgraduate Medical Journal, 76,* 333–336.

Rigrodsky, S., & Morrison, E. (1970). Speech changes in parkinsonism during L-dopa therapy: Preliminary findings. *Journal of the American Geriatric Society, 18,* 142–151.

Robbins, J. A., Logemann, J. A., & Kirschner, H. S. (1986). Swallowing and speech production in Parkinson's disease. *Annals of Neurology, 19,* 283–287.

Robertson, S. J., & Thomson, F. (1984). Speech therapy in Parkinson's disease: A study of the efficacy and long term effects of intensive treatment. *British Journal of Disorders of Communication, 19*, 213–224.

Rubow, R., & Swift, E. (1985). A microcomputer-based wearable biofeedback device to improve transfer of treatment in Parkinsonian dysarthria. *Journal of Speech and Hearing Disorders, 50*, 178–185.

Sanabria, J., Ruiz, P. G., Gutierrez, R., Marquez, F., Escobar, P., Gentil, M., & Cenjor, C. (2001). The effect of levodopa on vocal function in Parkinson's disease. *Clinical Neuropharmacology, 24*(2), 99–102.

Santacruz, P., Uttl, B., Litvan, I., & Grafman, J. (1998). Progressive supranuclear palsy: A survey of the disease course. *Neurology, 50*(6), 1637–1647.

Sapir, S., Pawlas, A., Ramig, L. O., O'Brien, C., Hoehn, M., & Thompson, L. A. (2001). Speech and voice abnormalities in Parkinson disease: Relation to severity of motor impairment, duration of disease, medication, depression, gender and age. *Journal of Medical Speech–Language Pathology, 9*(4), 213–226.

Sarno, M. (1968). Speech impairment in Parkinson's disease. *Archives of Physical Medicine and Rehabilitation, 49*, 269–275.

Schrag, A., Ben-Shlomo, Y., & Quinn, N. (2000). Prevalence of progressive supranuclear palsy and multiple system atrophy: A cross-sectional study. *Lancet, 352*(9192), 1771–1775.

Schulz, G. M., & Grant, M. K. (2000). Effects of speech therapy and pharmacologic and surgical treatments on voice and speech in Parkinson's disease: A review of the literature. *Journal of Communication Disorders, 33*, 59–88.

Schulz, G. M., Peterson, T., Sapienza, C. M., Greer, M., & Friedman, W. (1999). Voice and speech characteristics of persons with Parkinson's disease pre- and post-pallidotomy surgery: Preliminary findings. *Journal of Speech, Language, and Hearing Research, 42*(5), 1176–1194.

Scott, S., & Caird, F. I. (1983). Speech therapy for Parkinson's disease. *Journal of Neurology, Neurosurgery and Psychiatry, 46*, 140–144.

Serradura, A., & Hill, P. (1989). *Transitional feeding: The team approach to management of swallowing and tube feeding in adults with acquired neurologic deficits:* Fullarton, Australia: Julia Farr Centre.

Siderowf, A. (2001). Parkinson's disease: Clinical features, epidemiology, and genetics. *Neurologic Clinics, 19*(3), 565–578.

Slaughter, J. R., Slaughter, K. A., Nichols, D., Holmes, S. E., & Martens, M. P. (2001). Prevalence, clinical manifestations, etiology, and treatment of depression in Parkinson's disease. *Journal of Neuropsychiatry and Clinical Neurosciences, 13*, 187–196.

Smith, M., Ramig, L., Dromey, C., Perez, K., & Samandari, R. (1995). Intensive voice treatment in Parkinson disease: Laryngostroboscopic findings. *Journal of Voice, 9*, 453–459.

Solomon, N. P., & Hixon, T. J. (1993). Speech breathing in Parkinson's disease. *Journal of Speech and Hearing Research, 36*, 294–310.

Solomon, N., Lorell, D., Robin, D., Rodnitzky, R., & Luschei, E. (1995). Tongue strength and endurance in mild to moderate Parkinson's disease. *Journal of Medical Speech–Language Pathology, 3*(1), 15–26.

Solomon, N. P., Robin, D. A., & Luschei, E. S. (2000). Strength, endurance, and stability of the tongue and hand in Parkinson disease. *Journal of Speech, Language, and Hearing Research, 43*(1), 256–267.

Stebbins, G. T., & Goetz, C. G. (1998). Factor structure of the Unified Parkinson's Disease Rating Scale: Motor examination section. *Movement Disorders, 13*(4), 633–636.

Stewart, C., Winfield, L., Hunt, A., Bressman, S. B., Fahn, S., Blitzer, A., & Brin, M. F. (1995). Speech dysfunction in early Parkinson's disease. *Movement Disorders, 10*(5), 562–565.

Stocchi, F., & Brusa, L. (2000). Cognition and emotion in different stages and subtypes of Parkinson's disease. *Journal of Neurology, 247*(Suppl. 2), II/114–II/121.

Sullivan, M. D., Brune, P. J., & Beukelman, D. R. (1996). Maintenance of speech changes following group treatment for hypokinetic dysarthria of Parkinson's disease. In D. A. Robin, K. M. Yorkston, & D. R. Beukelman (Eds.), *Disorders of motor speech: Assessment, treatment and clinical characterization* (pp. 287–310). Baltimore: Brookes.

Taha, J., Janszen, M., & Favre, J. (1999). Thalamic deep brain stimulation for the treatment of head, voice, and bilateral limb tremor. *Journal of Neurosurgery, 91*, 68–72.

Tanner, C. M., & Aston, D. A. (2000). Epidemiology of Parkinson's disease and akinetic syndromes. *Current Opinion in Neurology, 13*(4), 427–430.

Tasker, R. R. (1998). Deep brain stimulation is preferable to thalamotomy for tremor suppression. *Surgical Neurology, 49*(2), 145–153.

Theodoros, D. G., Thompson-Ward, E. C., Murdoch, B. E., Lethlean, J., & Silburn, P. (1999). The effects of the Lee Silverman Voice Treatment Program on motor speech function in Parkinson disease following thalamotomy and pallidotomy surgery: A case study. *Journal of Medical Speech–Language Pathology, 7*(2), 157–160.

Ward, C. D., & Gibb, W. R. (1990). Research diagnostic criteria for Parkinson's disease. *Advances in Neurology, 53*, 245–249.

Ward, E. C., Theodoros, D. G., Murdoch, B. E., & Silburn, P. (2000). Changes in maximum capacity tongue function following Lee Silverman Voice Treatment program. *Journal of Medical Speech–Language Pathology, 8*(4), 331–336.

Waxman, M. J., Durfee, D., Moore, M., & Morantz, R. A. (1990). Nutritional aspects and swallowing function of patients with Parkinson's disease. *Nutrition in Clinical Practice, 5*(5), 196–199.

Weiner, W. J., & Singer, C. (1989). Parkinson's disease and nonpharmacologic treatment programs. *Journal of the American Geriatric Society, 37*, 359–363.

Weismer, G., Jeng, J. Y., Laures, J. S., Kent, R. D., & Kent, J. F. (2001). Acoustic and intelligibility characteristics of sentence production in neurogenic speech disorders. *Folia Phoniatrica et Logopaedica, 53*(1), 1–18.

Wenning, G. K., Seppi, K., Scherfler, C., Stefanova, N., & Puschba, Z. (2001). Multiple system atrophy. *Seminars in Neurology, 21*(1), 33–40.

Wintzen, A. R., Badrising, U. A., Roos, R. A., Vielvoye, J., Liauw, L., & Pauwels, E. K. (1994). Dysphagia in ambulant patients with Parkinson's disease: Common, not dangerous. *Canadian Journal of Neurological Sciences, 21*, 53–56.

York, M. K., Levin, H. S., Grossman, R. G., & Hamilton, W. J. (1999). Neuropsychological outcome following unilateral pallidotomy. *Brain, 122*, 2209–2220.

Yorkston, K. M., Spencer, K. A., Beukelman, D. R., Duffy, J., Golper, L. A., Miller, R. M., Strand, E. A., & Sullivan, M. (2002). *Practice guidelines for dysarthria: Evidence for the behavioral management of the respiratory/phonatory system* (Tech. Rep. No. 3). Minneapolis, MN: Academy of Neurologic Communication Disorders and Sciences.

Zetusky, W. J., Jankovic, J., & Pirozzolo, F. J. (1985). The heterogeneity of Parkinson's disease: Clinical and prognostic implications. *Neurology, 35*, 522–526.

137

3

HUNTINGTON DISEASE

Kathryn M. Yorkston, Robert M. Miller, and Estelle R. Klasner

Nature of the Problem

This section provides the background required for knowledgeable management of speech and swallowing disorders in Huntington disease. Topics include etiology, description of symptoms, progression, medical management, and a discussion of how the genetic aspects of the disease influence the management of speech and swallowing disorders. A summary of information is found in the "Huntington Disease" handout in the Appendix at the back of the book.

What Is Huntington Disease?

Huntington disease (originally known as Huntington's chorea) is an inherited autosomal dominant degenerative neurologic disease. Thus, each child of an affected parent has a 50% chance of inheritance. Spontaneous mutations also occur in a small percentage of the population. The gene responsible for Huntington disease (HD) was located in a specific chromosome in 1993. The disease is caused by a trinucleotide repeat. In nonaffected individuals, the number of trinucleotide CAG (cytosine-adenosine-guanosine) repeats on the chromosome ranges from 6 to 35, whereas in individuals with Huntington disease, the repeat length varies from 40 to 121 (Reddy, Williams, & Tagle, 1999). The HD gene produces a protein called Huntington whose function is as yet unclear.

Symptoms of Huntington disease include personality changes, chorea, dystonia, incoordination, dementia, eye movement abnormalities, dysarthria, dysphagia, and weight loss. Symptoms typically appear in the fourth decade of life, often after childbearing years, although they have appeared as early as 2 years of age (Oliver & Dewhurst, 1969) and as late as the seventh decade. The disease does not skip generations and is characterized by slow but relentless progression, with death occurring 15 to 20 years after onset. The disease typically progresses more rapidly in juvenile patients. Huntington disease affects 4 to 7 individuals per 100,000 (Hunt & Walker, 1991). Men and women are affected in equal proportion. Although Huntington disease occurs in all races, it occurs less frequently in those of African or Japanese descent.

What Changes in Neural Tissue and Neural Systems Are Associated with Huntington Disease?

Neuropathologic findings consist of atrophy of the striate bodies, which is associated with loss of small neurons. Cortical neurons may also degenerate. Frontotemporal atrophy has been identified using magnetic resonance imaging (MRI). Biochemically, Huntington disease involves a deficiency of the neurotransmitter gamma-aminobutyric acid (GABA) in the basal ganglia. The lack of GABA inhibition may lead to a relative overactivity of the dopaminergic systems. Hypofunction of the cholinergic neurons has also been suggested.

TABLE 3.1	Clinical Variants of Huntington Disease

Westphal's Variant

- Rigidity is predominant clinical manifestation
- Rarely occurs in adult onset (5%)
- More common in juveniles (50%)

Juvenile Huntington Disease

- Begins before age 20
- Comprises 5% to 10% of Huntington disease population
- Predominant motor sign is rigidity
- Dysarthria and oculomotor alterations are prominent
- Convulsions occur in 30% to 50% of cases
- Heredity is generally paternal
- Evolves more rapidly than adult form

Subchoreatic State

- Begins late in life (between sixth and eighth decades)
- Progression is slower than classic form
- Minimal intellectual decline

Note. Adapted from "Huntington's Disease," by M. S. Haddad and J. L. Cummings, 1997, *Clinics of North America, 20*(4), 791–807.

What Symptoms Are Associated with Huntington Disease?

Symptoms include a triad of motor, emotional, and cognitive disturbances. The movement disorders and cognitive changes result in a number of functional limitations, including abnormal gait, dysarthria, dysphagia, weight loss, and loss of independence in activities of daily living such as feeding and dressing. In addition to the classic form of Huntington disease, three variants also occur. The distinguishing features of these variants are listed in Table 3.1.

MOTOR DISTURBANCES

Motor disturbances are composed of both involuntary movements and abnormal involuntary movements. Chorea is a hallmark feature of Huntington disease. In fact, the disease was originally termed Huntington chorea because of the co-occurrence of rigidity and dystonia with chorea. Chorea is characterized by involuntary, arrhythmic, and irregular movements of the body. Underlying electomyographic activity is variable and may include features such as cocontraction of agonist and antagonist muscles (Berardelli et al., 1999). Hypertonia early in the disease changes to rigidity during progression. A small proportion of individuals with the disease never have significant chorea; rather they experience a rigidity-predominant form known as the Westphal variant. Voluntary movement disorders are associated with deficits in planning, sequencing, executing, and completing tasks (Nance, 1998). Speech and swallowing problems are the result of both involuntary and voluntary movements.

EMOTIONAL DISTURBANCES

Depression and irritability are the most common psychiatric symptoms of Huntington disease; however, anxiety, obsessiveness, and apathy alternating with impulsive or aggressive behavior are also seen. These psychiatric symptoms often are present before the onset of motor or cognitive changes (Hofmann, 1999). Depression occurs in up to 40% of individuals with Huntington disease and may relate to the high suicide rate in this population (Lipe, Schultz, & Bird, 1993; Schoenfeld et al., 1984). A low frustration tolerance is commonly an initial emotional change noted by friends and family (Cummings, 1995). This low tolerance may affect both communication interactions and interactions related to eating and feeding issues. Associations between emotional and cognitive changes may be present. For example, individuals with obsessive or compulsive symptoms showed greater impairment on neuropsychological tests than did individuals without the symptoms (Anderson, Louis, Stern, & Marder, 2001).

COGNITIVE DISTURBANCES

Cognitive changes are another hallmark of Huntington disease. Basal ganglia lesions are associated with cognitive changes as well as disturbances in the control of movements (Middleton & Strick, 2000). Cognitive changes may be noted early in the course of the disease. Mayeux, Stern, Herman, Greenbaum, and Fahn (1986) found that intellectual impairment is a major factor in reducing a person's functional capacity in the early stage of Huntington disease. Early changes have been found in cognitive efficiency, memory, and sensorimotor function (Lundervold & Reinvang, 1991). With progression, a broader range of functions becomes involved. There is a strong relationship between changes in mental status and chorea (Webb & Trzepacz, 1987). Thus, it is likely that a person with Huntington disease will need to cope with dual cognitive and motor impairments.

Dementia in Huntington disease is considered a subcortical type and has characteristics different from the dementias associated with Alzheimer's disease and progressive supranuclear palsy. Pillon, Dubois, Ploska, and Agid (1991) describe disruptions in concentration and acquisition of new information in the Huntington disease population. This is consistent with positron emission tomography (PET) studies revealing decreased glucose metabolism in frontal, parietal, and striatal regions (Goto et al., 1993).

It is critical to understand cognitive changes in individuals with Huntington disease in order to appropriately manage the increasing motor involvement. Cognitive limitations may decrease the ability of people with Huntington disease to compensate for the motor problems that affect speech and swallowing functions. A generalized cognitive slowing compromises the ability to initiate conversation and a marked decrease in verbal communication (Klasner & Yorkston, 2000). Constraints imposed by cognitive limitations dictate both the timing and strategies for training.

Individuals with Huntington disease experience obvious and debilitating cognitive changes. Because language and cognition are highly related, it is not surprising that language skills are also affected. Table 3.2 summarizes some recent investigations in this area. The conclusion of this research is that many aspects of language may be affected by Huntington disease, including spontaneous production, naming, and auditory comprehension. Thus, language needs to be carefully assessed in the development of an intervention plan for dysarthria associated with this disorder. Language assessment is particularly critical when dysarthria is severe enough to require augmentative communication techniques. Many augmentative communication

TABLE 3.2	Language Deficits in Huntington Disease		
Language Task	**Findings**		**Reference(s)**
Connected Speech	• Reduced number of words • Decreased syntactic complexity • Decreased melody line • Decreased phrase length • Decreased articulatory agility • Inceased paraphasic errors • Word finding problems		Illes, 1989 Gordon & Illes, 1989 Speedie et al., 1990
Naming	• More visually based errors than normals • Decreased confrontation naming		Lawrence, Watkins, Sahakian, Hodges, & Robbins, 2000 Wallesch & Fehrenbach, 1988
Auditory Comprehension	• Decreased understanding of subtle prosodic aspects • Reduced Token Test scores • Discourse comprehension		Speedie et al., 1990 Wallesch & Fehrenbach, 1988 Murray & Stout, 1999

devices demand good language skills because they rely on written language production. Furthermore, any novel approach to communication requires the learning of new skills, an ability that may be impaired by the disease.

How Is the Diagnosis of Huntington Disease Made?

Diagnosis of Huntington disease is made on the basis of a number of clinical judgments (Hunt & Walker, 1991).

1. *Positive family history of the disease.* Although family history seems straightforward because the disease is inherited and does not skip generations, confusion can occur in cases in which parental history is unclear or in the event of premature death of the parent before onset of symptoms.

2. *Occurrence of chorea and psychiatric disorders without other apparent cause.* Early cognitive changes may be misdiagnosed as schizophrenia.

3. *A pattern of progressive deterioration.*

4. *Imaging studies such as CT (computerized tomography) scan, MRI, and PET scan.* Imaging studies may all become positive as the disease progresses.

Huntington disease differs from other degenerative disorders described in this text because it is possible to know that one is likely to acquire the disease before the onset of symptoms. Tests are now available that predict the risk of inheriting the disease. The advent of presymptomatic testing has spurred research to study the psychologic consequences of deciding whether to undergo the testing (Meiser & Dunn, 2001; Williams, Schutte, Evers, & Holkup, 2000).

How Is Functional Progression Measured?

Even though the symptoms associated with Huntington disease are well described, the timing of onset and progression of the various motor, emotional, and cognitive symptoms remain uncertain, especially in the early and middle stages of the disease (Kirkwood, Su, Conneally, & Foroud, 2001). Staging of the severity of Huntington disease is a difficult but necessary activity if therapeutic efforts are to be evaluated. A staging system is necessary for planning intervention with any progressive disorder. Although the signs and symptoms of Huntington disease are distinctive, the extent, rate, and natural course of the disability vary considerably from individual to individual. Because so many factors influence the overall level of function, it is inappropriate to use a single factor as a means of staging the disease. For example, measurement of motor function alone does not adequately characterize the natural course of the disorder. Individuals with relatively severe motor involvement and preserved cognitive skills may function well, whereas individuals with relatively minor motor involvement in the presence of serious cognitive and emotional problems may function poorly.

The most common scheme for rating the consequences of Huntington disease is the Unified Huntington's Disease Rating Scale (UHDRS) (Huntington's Study Group, 1996). It assesses the components of motor performance, cognition, behavior, and functional capacity. The motor component consists of 31 questions rated on a 4-point scale. The cognitive component is drawn from five neuropsychologic tests, and the behavioral component consists of 28 items assessing severity and frequency of mood, aggression, and other behavioral abnormalities. The UHDRS has been shown to be effective in tracking the progression of the disease and documenting the effectiveness of intervention (Marder et al., 2000; Reilmann et al., 2001; Siesling, van Vugt, Zwinderman, Kieburtz, & Roos, 1998).

How Does the Inheritance of Huntington Disease Influence Management of Speech and Swallowing Problems?

The hereditary nature of Huntington disease has important implications for planning speech, language, and swallowing interventions. The individual with Huntington disease will frequently have witnessed a family member's experience with the same condition. The individual will have had many years to anticipate his or her own symptoms. In addition, he or she may have the extra burden of possibly passing the disease on to the next generation. This knowledge will undoubtedly have an influence on the individual's perspective on the disease and treatments available (Meiser & Dunn, 2001; Sobel & Cowan, 2000). Every family with Huntington disease handles the knowledge of being part of a family with an identified inherited illness differently. Knowing the family's feelings about Huntington disease, the future, and the at-risk status is essential because it is most likely that the speech clinician will have an ongoing relationship with the family and these issues may be raised during therapy sessions (Hakiman, 2000).

The affected individual and family members are often well aware of the decline of communication and swallowing skills that accompany Huntington disease. Acceptance of services offered will be influenced by this previous exposure. If speech and language services were not effective in the past with other family members, the individual may not be willing to participate in treatment. Family communication patterns have likely been influenced by Huntington disease over a long period of time. The family may have developed effective strategies to communicate with the affected individual. The speech–language pathologist should make every effort to become familiar with the successful strategies designed by the family and, if possible, use those strategies as the foundation for further intervention. The speech–language pathologist may be called upon to facilitate communication situations in a variety of settings that can include doctors' offices, genetic counseling sessions, and legal-related appointments. In addition, the speech–language pathologist may also be asked to treat other family members affected by the disease simultaneously or at a future time.

What Is the Medical Management of Huntington Disease?

At this time there is no cure for Huntington disease, and medical treatment deals only with symptoms. Unfortunately, pharmacologic treatment of one symptom may aggravate others (Quinn & Schrag, 1998; van Vugt & Roose, 1999). For example, tricyclic antidepressants can alleviate depression but aggravate dysphagia (Hunt & Walker, 1991). Typical antipsychotics may decrease the choreiform movements early in the course of the disease but may also produce undesirable side effects such as tardive dyskinesia and worsening cognition (Hurley, Jackson, Fisher, & Taber, 1999). Leroi and Michalon (1998) conducted a systematic review of literature related to the clinical management of the psychiatric aspects of Huntington disease. Their conclusion was that each patient must be treated on a case-by-case basis because of serious limitations in the existing evidence base. In addition to drug treatment of symptoms, early reports of the benefits of neural transplantation are available (Bachoud-Levi, Remy, Nguyen, & Brugieres, 2000). Current information about drug trials for Huntington disease can be found on the Heredity Disease Foundation Web site (http://www.hdfoundation.org/).

Physical and occupational therapies typically focus on determining how chorea has altered the person's performance of activities of daily living (ADLs). Range of motion and strengthening exercises are performed to stabilize proximal joints and maintain stability. Physical and occupational therapists may also use facilitory and inhibitory techniques. Biofeedback and traditional relaxation techniques are applied in early stages of the disease. Family training is particularly critical in Huntington disease because of the cognitive decline and frequent occurrence of functional limitations early in the course of the disease.

Speech Disorders

Involuntary, unpredictable movements may occur in any part of the speech production mechanism. Intervention is directed at whichever systems are most affected and at eliminating maladaptive habits the speaker may have formed.

What Speech Characteristics Are Associated with Huntington Disease?

Motor speech production in Huntington disease reflects the underlying movement disorder. Chorea is associated with involuntary contractions of muscle groups, which cannot be predicted by the speaker. They may occur in any aspect of speech, including respiratory, laryngeal, and oral articulatory movements. An early description of the variable speech pattern characteristic of the hyperkinetic dysarthria of Huntington disease appears in Swift (1929; cited in Darley, Aronson, & Brown, 1975):

> The vocal cords may tighten to raise the pitch and the lung muscles may contract, to heighten intensity; or other muscles may jerk and vitiate the utterance of consonants and vowels. The sentence thus varied may be repeated again perfectly. Usually the same sentence variation never occurs in exactly the same form again. It cannot therefore be considered a sign that uniformly varies each sentence; but must be looked upon as a pitch and intensity change with sound vitiations that occur irregularly. (p. 205)

Darley et al. (1975) characterize movements associated with hyperkinetic dysarthria as excessive, irrelevant, and involuntary. These excessive movements are superimposed on purposeful speech production. They summarized the speech characteristics of individuals with hyperkinetic dysarthria as follows:

> The hyperkinetic dysarthria of chorea is characterized by a highly variable pattern of interference with articulation; episodes of hypernasality, harshness, and breathiness; and unplanned variation in loudness. In the speaker's apparent attempt to avoid the inevitable interruptions and to compensate for them, his rate of speech is variably altered, phonemes and intervals between words are prolonged, stress is equalized, and inappropriate silences appear. (p. 210)

A cluster of speech features is unique to hyperkinetic dysarthria and Huntington disease. Sudden forced inspiration or expiration was noted in 20% of the speakers with chorea studied by Darley et al. (1975). This is the only neurologic group that displays this particular deviation. Other hallmark features of speakers with chorea are irregular articulatory breakdowns, occurring in more than 60% of these speakers; phonatory impairment (harsh voice quality, excess loudness variations, and strained-strangled sound); and a variety of changes in prosody. Prosodic changes include both features that suggest prosodic insufficiency (monopitch, monoloudness, reduced stress, and short phrases) and those that suggest prosodic excess (prolonged intervals, inappropriate silences, prolonged phonemes, and excess and equal stress).

What Management Approaches Are Available for Speech and Cognitive Language Difficulties in Huntington Disease?

Speech symptoms associated with Huntington disease vary considerably in severity. In some individuals, motor disturbances are restricted to the limbs and body and do not interfere with speech production. For others, speech production is so severely impaired that natural speech is no longer a functional means of communication. For most individuals, cognitive language difficulties occur in a mild form early on in the disease and become more severe as the disease progresses. Cognitive difficulties become so severe that the individual generally can no longer live on his or her own by the end stage of the disease.

The following suggestions are organized according to the severity of the dysarthria and cognitive deficit. They represent both clinical suggestions pertinent to individuals with hyperkinetic dysarthria and suggestions for traditional intervention techniques focusing on particular symptoms such as abnormal respiratory behaviors. Because of disease progression and unpredictable occurrence of a variety of symptoms, no single treatment course will be effective throughout the disease. Therapy techniques must be responsive to the changing motor, cognitive, and emotional needs of the individual. To our knowledge, there have been no published reports documenting the efficacy of these procedures in people with Huntington disease. See Table 3.3 for a summary of approaches to speech intervention in Huntington disease.

MILD DYSARTHRIA AND COGNITIVE CHANGES

In mild dysarthria associated with Huntington disease, changes in speech production are obvious to both speaker and listener but do not interfere with speech intelligibility. Individuals are rarely referred for speech services at this point because communication abilities are not compromised. If these speech changes interfere with the ability to participate in activities that require excellent speech production (such as those required in the clergy, teaching, or aspects of the legal profession), a symptomatic approach is generally employed. For example, if phonatory stenosis is present in the laryngeal system, a focus on this aspect of speech production may be appropriate. A number of approaches to intervention for phonatory stenosis are available. Techniques such as chewing, yawning, and instrumental monitoring of hard glottal attack have as their goal the normalization of laryngeal tone during phonation. Relaxation techniques may be useful in speakers who have mild phonatory disturbance associated with Huntington disease. Stress and intonation drills may also be beneficial (Prator & Swift, 1984; Yorkston, Beukelman, Strand, & Bell, 1999).

Potentially maladaptive behaviors should be identified and eliminated. For example, some speakers with Huntington disease may speak at rapid rates in an apparent attempt to hurry through an utterance before a movement disturbance occurs. Making the speaker aware of the rapid rate and emphasizing the importance of maintaining a rate consistent with physiologic capacities can prove helpful in maintaining intelligible speech for longer periods of time.

Mild cognitive changes may begin to occur at this stage on an intermittent basis. Difficulty processing complicated information and completing sequentially complex tasks may occur occasionally. The individual with Huntington disease may want to make others aware of these difficulties and begin to establish a structured routine and to delegate responsibilities in order to reduce tasks to those that continue to be manageable. An effort to avoid situations that stress cognitive and communicative abilities should also be made. A variety of memory and organizational aids may also be useful at this time.

MODERATE DYSARTHRIA AND COGNITIVE CHANGES

People with moderate dysarthria have changes in speech that are severe enough to compromise speech intelligibility. Some simple behavior training may be appropriate, but caution is warranted because carryover of these techniques in natural settings may be limited by the speaker's cognitive impairment and difficulty with learning. Speaking on inhalation rather than exhalation is frequently observed at this stage and interferes with a number of aspects of speech production including rate, prosody, and stress patterning. Elimination of abnormal respiratory behaviors will go a long way toward maintaining an adequate level of speech intelligibility. Standard relaxation techniques and practice of rhythmic breathing patterns may facilitate appropriate respiratory support and breath groups during speech production (Klasner, 1995; Klasner & Yorkston, 2000).

In addition to behavioral techniques to improve speech production, teaching strategies to guide or control communication interactions in the face of increasing dysarthria can be helpful. Individuals with moderate dysarthria complicated by cog-

TABLE 3.3   A Summary of Intervention Approaches for Management of Dysarthria in Huntington Disease

Severity of the Dysarthria	Description	Intervention Approaches
Mild	• Changes in speech are obvious • Choreic movements are superimposed on speech movements • Intelligibility not reduced	• Prosody drills • Techniques to reduce phonatory stenosis • Maintenance of appropriate rate
Moderate	• Choreic movements interfere with speech intelligibility	• Teach strategies to manage difficult communication situations and resolve breakdowns • Behavioral technique to improve speech production
Severe	• Natural speech is no longer functional	• Natural speech with supportive partner • Alphabet boards • Making choices • Calendars and memory aids • Conversational starters • Miniatures • Yes/no system

nitive problems often need assistance with strategies to resolve communication breakdowns. Communication partners need to be willing to assume more responsibility for the success of communicative interactions. We typically do not attempt to teach complex and elaborate partner management behaviors. Rather, our approach is to teach a simple sequence of steps that frequent communication partners can use every time a listener has not understood a message. An example of such a sequence follows:

1. Inform the speaker when you have not understood the message.

2. Watch the speaker for other cues to facilitate understanding.

3. Ask for a repetition of the message once, using the same words.

4. Go to an alternative approach by either asking for a repetition of the main word or verbally spelling a misunderstood word.

As the disease progresses, cognitive difficulties occur more frequently and affect functioning to a greater extent. Many factors (slow response time, inability to retrieve information, and susceptibility to interference with task-related behaviors) compromise the ability to communicate effectively (Murray, Ramage, & Hopper, 2001). Because of reduced speech intelligibility, the intellectual abilities of the individual with Huntington disease are often underestimated. Individuals with Huntington disease are likely to comprehend more than they are able to express. Speech and language intervention should be aimed at capitalizing on the individual's preserved abilities and providing whatever support is needed to maintain communication (Klasner & Yorkston, 2000; Sullivan, Bird, Alpay, & Cha, 2001).

External prompting systems have shown some promise in assisting the individual with Huntington disease in maintaining communication and carrying out structured activities (Klasner & Yorkston, 2001; Turkstra, 2001). Linguistic supplementation strategies (scripting simple standard conversations) and cognitive supplementation strategies (breaking tasks down into manageable steps) allow the individual with Huntington disease to continue to participate in conversational exchanges despite substantial speech and language formulation difficulties.

SEVERE DYSARTHRIA

In severe dysarthria associated with Huntington disease, natural speech is no longer understandable. Severe motor deficits frequently limit the ability to write, type, or directly select words or phrases—skills that are needed to use most augmentative and alternative communication (AAC) devices. In addition, cognitive decline limits the ability to learn and use many complex augmentative communication systems. To our knowledge, there are no reports in the literature of successful application of augmentative communication technology in Huntington disease. Therefore, the following section reviews some general principles of intervention in this population and describes a series of light-tech options that may serve as communication systems for people with advanced Huntington disease.

The principles of communication management of severe dysarthria in Huntington disease are constrained by the nature of the motor and cognitive deficits and the relentless progression of symptoms.

1. Select simple systems that take advantage of previously learned skills and do not demand a great deal of new learning. Some of these techniques and approaches are described later in this chapter.

2. The second principle follows from the first. Initiate training in alternative communication approaches early, perhaps before they are mandatory and communication becomes frustrating. Early practice of simple communication techniques helps to establish them and develop procedural memory. Cueing and prompting techniques should be incorporated in the communication systems.

3. Avoid techniques that are difficult or that require "getting better at them." For example, a keyboard that the individual is marginally able to use today may be completely useless tomorrow if motor disturbances worsen.

4. Rely on well-trained partners. As the course of Huntington disease advances, sheltered, highly structured environments are the norm for the patient. Well-trained partners help to structure communication interactions and are an integral part of many of the simple communication approaches described here.

The following are possible components or elements of a communication system for a person with severe dysarthria and advanced Huntington disease. The elements may be used singly but are frequently combined, depending on the communication task at hand. You will find these techniques to be simple and not dependent on complex technology. However, all require a supportive communication partner who will structure the communication environment.

Natural Speech with Supportive Partners

Natural speech is a component of many communication systems for severely dysarthric speakers. Individuals with Huntington disease are no exception. They have used natural speech all their lives and often will continue to use it even in the face of increasing motor deficits. Management plans need to encourage use of natural speech as long as possible. On one hand, speech is a quick, easy, and solidly ingrained habit. On the other hand, attempting to decode highly distorted speech may be a frustrating experience for a communication partner. Typically, there is a transitional period that bridges the gap between ability to produce understandable natural speech and total dependence on alternative communication. In the Huntington disease population, this transition may involve a "supported communication" phase. Individuals with Huntington disease typically are not able to read signals (Seidman-Carlson & Wells, 1998) or effectively resolve communication breakdowns. Rather than attempting to teach the person with Huntington disease how to manage with highly distorted speech, our focus is on the communication partner. We train the partner to lead the speaker with severe dysarthria through a series of intelligibility enhancement strategies. The handout "Tips for Understanding Severely Dysarthric Speech" in the Appendix at the back of the book gives suggestions that you can individualize for each patient and family.

Alphabet Boards

An alphabet board containing letters, numbers, and selected phrases may be an important element of communication for individuals with Huntington disease. Mild or moderate movements of the arm and hand can be accommodated by enlarging the display size. Large white-on-black letters may be an option to compensate for visual problems.

Alphabet boards can be used in a number of ways. The person can spell out messages letter-by-letter. If the individual continues to have some natural speech, the alphabet board can be used to supplement that speech—for example, by pointing to the first letter of each word spoken. This has the beneficial effect of slowing speaking rate and providing the partner with extra information about the intended word. Use of this technique in the Huntington disease population may be rare, because this population often is constricted in moving both the arms and the head, which limits the ability to indicate letters.

Making Choices

Offering the person a choice among a small number of alternatives is a critical strategy. The use of a choice-making technique has been described with children who have profound developmental delays (Beukelman & Mirenda, 1998) and with adults who have severe aphasia (Garrett & Beukelman, 1992; Garrett & Yorkston, 1997). Individuals with Huntington disease can be offered choices of foods, clothing, music to listen to, rooms to spend time in, and so on. Choices can be offered using real objects, object symbols, or written words. The choice should be offered in a natural setting in "a nonevaluative atmosphere, which is an atmosphere in which 'right' and 'wrong' choices have not been predetermined by the facilitator" (Beukelman & Mirenda, 1998). Table 3.4 contains an example of a script for a choice-making technique presented by Garrett and Beukelman (1992, pp. 265–266).

Calendars and Memory Aids

Because of the frequent occurrence of memory problems in Huntington disease, compensatory techniques should be considered as the disease advances. Because it is not possible to correct the underlying problem, the most appropriate approach is to modify the environment to provide the person with relevant external structure and cues. These memory cues may take the form of calendars, alarm clocks, written schedules, or logbooks. Develop specific strategies individually, depending on the patient's capabilities and needs. Sohlberg and Mateer (1989) suggest the following memory notebook sections for use with patients with traumatic brain injury, and this organization may be relevant for patients with Huntington disease as well:

- *Orientation.* Narrative autobiographical information containing personal data

- *Memory log.* Forms for charting hourly information about what the patient has done; diary of daily information

- *Calendar.* Calendars with dates and times that allow the patient to track appointments and dates

- *Things to do.* Forms for recording errands and intended future actions

- *Transportation.* Floor plans and maps of important environments

- *Feelings log.* Forms to chart the patient's feelings about specific incidents or times

- *Names.* Forms to record names and identifying information about new people

Use of external memory aids with people who have Huntington disease is frequently complicated by severe motor problems. If a patient is unable to manipulate the aid independently, then partner support is necessary. If handwriting is difficult for the patient, partners will need to enter items in the calendar or daily log.

Conversation Starters

The array of communication needs of adults with severely limited speech is broader than simply expressing basic needs. Social closeness is also an important communication

TABLE 3.4

Choice-Making Script

Skill

To choose items to meet grooming needs during daily routines

Patient Subgoals

1. To look at the partner when addressed by name
2. To visually attend to and scan presented objects
3. To take, indicate, or grasp objects.
4. To choose a desired object by gazing, grasping, or pointing after the clinician sets a context, offers a choice of objects in the patient's field of vision, and offers a verbal choice. ("Do you want to wear the red shirt or the Garfield shirt?")

Sample Activities

Choosing a shirt and pants for a daily outfit; choosing a nail polish color

Materials

Two colors of nail polish, or a choice of two appropriate dressing items

Sample Script

Nurse or Clinician:	(calls patient's name) Julia!
Patient:	(doesn't look up)
Nurse or Clinician:	(repeats) Julia!
Patient:	(looks up)
Nurse or Clinician:	Your nail polish is really chipped! (pauses to wait for appropriate gaze to referent)
Patient:	(no response)
Nurse or Clinician:	(picks up patient's hand: examines nails) Look at your nails! You really need some new polish. (pauses—waits for interest or gaze)
Patient:	(looks at own hand)
Nurse or Clinician:	Want to polish them? (pauses—waits for sign of affirmation)
Patient:	(looks back down at nails)
Nurse or Clinician:	(interprets this indicator as affirmation) Oh, you do! I think it's time, too. Let's see what colors you have in your drawer. (slowly gets out nail polish in an attempt to encourage gaze and visual attention to actions)
Nurse or Clinician:	Well, you have a few colors that would go with your outfit (points to patient's shirt). Hmm. Coral, red . .
Patient:	(continues attending)
Nurse or Clinician:	(puts both bottles on lap tray and pauses)
Patient:	(continues attending)
Nurse or Clinician:	The red would look nice (holds bottle up) but so would the coral! (holds bottle up and pauses)
Patient:	(no response)
Nurse or Clinician:	Do you want the red polish? (pauses and holds bottle up) Or the coral? (pauses and holds bottle up)
Patient:	(maintains eye gaze longer on red bottle)
Nurse or Clinician:	Sure, I think the red polish would look great!

Continue with the activity of polishing nails, incorporating affirmation, turn taking, and choicemaking whenever possible.

Note. From "Augmentative Communication Approaches for Persons with Severe Aphasia," by K. L. Garrett and D. R. Beukelman, 1992, in *Augmentative Communication in the Medical Setting* (pp. 265–266), edited by K. M. Yorkston, Austin, TX: PRO-ED. Copyright 1992 by PRO-ED, Inc. Reprinted with permission.

activity. Topic setters are a means of establishing a conversation. New information pockets (Garrett & Beukelman, 1992, p. 295) are means of organizing and accessing mementos, scraps of information, and appointments cards. Items of interest can be placed in a resealable plastic bag, a plastic zipper bag, or a three-ring binder, where they are easily accessible. The person with Huntington disease can be encouraged to share information or news or to start a conversation by displaying an item. The communication partner can then ask a series of appropriate yes/no questions about the item. In some nursing homes, these memento pockets are kept in a display case outside the patient's door. There they function both as conversation starters and as aids to help patients locate their own rooms.

Miniboards

Topic-specific miniboards or minidisplays have been described for use with children who have severe communication problems (Beukelman & Mirenda, 1998; Mirenda, 1985). Each board may contain vocabulary appropriate to a single topic or event, such as playing a card game or celebrating a holiday. Minidisplays are typically mounted in a particular location. For example, vocabulary pertinent to traveling might be posted in the car whereas vocabulary pertinent to the morning dressing routine might be posted bedside. The miniboards concept developed out of the appreciation that vocabulary needs vary considerably from one setting to another, that vocabulary for a particular setting is highly predictable, and that access is more difficult if all vocabulary items are contained in a single large book or on a single board.

Yes/No System

Establishing an easy and reliable means of indicating yes or no is a mandatory element of communication management for adults who use augmentative communication. Although specifics of intervention vary somewhat from one population to another, a number of parameters are similar across populations. See Yorkston (1992) for examples of using yes/no systems with several adult populations.

The following steps are recommended in developing a reliable yes/no system. The reproducible "Establishing a Yes/No System" form in Appendix 3.1 at the end of this chapter gives a protocol for developing a reliable yes/no response that follows these steps.

1. *Identify a reliable motor response.* In individuals with severe chorea, finding a reliable response may be a difficult task because neither hand signals nor head nods may be reliable movements. Some people who are unable to signal by pointing may be able to squeeze their partner's hand, perhaps squeezing the right hand for yes and the left for no. Ideally the motor responses should be (a) two distinctive natural gestures that do not require an external device, (b) highly reproducible by the patient, and (c) universal signals (such as thumbs up for yes) that can be recognized even by untrained partners. Several motor responses are suggested in the protocol form.

2. *Confirm cognitive skills required for yes/no communication.* The "Establishing a Yes/No System" form (see Appendix 3.1) gives a short list of simple cognitive screening items taken from Mitsuda, Baarslag-Benson, Hazel, and Therriault (1992). Because the purpose here is cognitive screening, these tasks should be modified to compensate for motor problems.

3. *Train the patient.* Patient training is typically accomplished in two phases. The first is to practice with a series of questions in which the correct answer is obvious to you. (An example is "Do birds fly?") During the second phase, a familiar partner is asked to verify the accuracy of the patient's responses to questions you would not know the answer to. (An example is "Did you go to college?")

4. *Document the approach.* The purpose of documentation is to ensure that all partners recognize the same signals for yes and no. This is especially critical for patients with cognitive limitations, who may not be able to respond flexibly using different gestures for different communication partners. The location of this documentation will, of course, vary depending on the patient's setting. In a nursing home, for example, the yes/no system might be documented in the patient's room, in the patient's medical record, and in the nurse's card file.

5. *Train the communication partners.* Again, the importance of partner training cannot be overemphasized. Partners not only need to be trained in reading the patient's yes/no signals, but also should be taught to ask appropriate questions. For example, Mitsuda and her colleagues (1992, p. 7) report the case of a cognitively intact patient who told them, "When I was in the ICU unit, I couldn't answer anything except a yes or no question, and the doctors would come in, and they would ask me was my foot up or down? So I would just stare at them."

Unfortunately, this account is probably fairly typical of situations encountered by nonspeaking adults. We try to teach communication partners a few simple rules, including the following:

1. Ask only questions that you would be able to answer with yes or no.

2. Ask one question at a time.

3. Wait for a response before asking the next question.

4. Use an organizational strategy in getting the information. For example, start by identifying the general topic, then ask more specific questions.

Individuals with Huntington disease who are experiencing severe cognitive communication and motor deficits are frequently placed in long-term care facilities and require assistance with all areas of daily living. Although difficult, it is vital to maintain communicative interaction. The communication partner becomes responsible for maintaining communication. Keeping the person informed of daily events and discussing the individual's past interests are good strategies to stay connected. The importance of a reliable yes/no system at this stage cannot be overestimated. Keeping communication exchanges short but frequent will also facilitate success. Partners must practice patience and wait for responses because extra processing time will be necessary for the affected individual (Klasner & Yorkston, 2000).

Recently, a remotivation therapy approach was implemented with a group of individuals with advanced Huntington disease (Sullivan et al., 2001). This approach is aimed at promoting socialization and environmental awareness and involves group therapy with 6 to 8 individuals with severely reduced speech intelligibility and extensive cognitive deficits. Topics for discussion were presented in a supportive setting with a trained group facilitator. Positive feedback, validation, and repetition of content were the principal strategies used in this approach. The results of this program were encouraging. Changes were noted in increased attendance and participation in the group and during other activities. An increase in verbal communication was also noted within the group setting.

Swallowing Disorders

Swallowing problems are common but not universal in Huntington disease. Because of the patient's cognitive involvement, much of the responsibility for implementing dietary modifications and swallowing techniques falls on the patient's caregivers.

What Swallowing Characteristics Are Associated with Huntington Disease?

Management of swallowing difficulties is a challenge for a number of reasons. First, the patient's subjective report of swallowing difficulty is not a reliable indicator of the actual problem because of psychiatric, cognitive, or extrapyramidal impairment. Second, any or all components of the swallowing process may be impaired. If chorea of the respiratory muscles is a major component, then movements of the respiratory system will be involuntary and unpredictable. Thus, they may occur during any phase of swallowing. Third, swallowing problems typically occur during the advanced stages of the disorder, when management is made difficult by dementia, limb chorea, and postural problems.

Kagel and Leopold (1992) reported the results of an extensive battery of clinical and radiologic testing of 35 people with Huntington disease. They all had at least moderately advanced disease, with most of them receiving ratings at stages 3 or 4 of the Shoulson and Fahn scale (1979). This clinical population was divided into a hyperkinetic and a rigid-bradykinetic group. Chorea was the dominant movement disorder in the hyperkinetic group. Individuals in this group exhibited such feeding and swallowing behavior as uncontrolled tachyphagia, darting lingual chorea, uninhibited swallowing initiation, and impaired respiratory inhibition during swallowing. Patients in the rigid-bradykinetic group shared many features of parkinsonism, including mandibular rigidity, inefficient mastication, and slowed oral transit. See Table 3.5 for descriptions and possible mechanisms of some common swallowing disruptions noted in Huntington disease.

How Is Swallowing Function in Huntington Disease Evaluated?

As with the assessment of any individual with a progressive neurologic swallowing disorder, fact finding begins with an interview to obtain a detailed history of the general course of the disorder, current status, and dietary history.

TABLE 3.5

Features of Swallowing Disruptions Particularly of Note in Huntington Disease (HD)

Feature	Description	Frequency of Occurrence	Possible Mechanism
Tachyphagia	Rapid uncontrolled swallowing	Very common	It has been speculated that impaired cognitive and intraoral sensory functions may disable a centrally mediated inhibitory process that normally regulates self-monitoring feeding behavior.
			Buccolingual chorea and dementia appear to interact in the early stages of swallowing, resulting in food being transferred impulsively and prematurely.
Respiratory chorea	Involuntary movements of the respiratory system	Approximately 40% of patients	Choreic movements that interrupt the normal reciprocal respiration–deglutition cycle. When present, this lack of synchrony increases the patient's risk of aspiration, but probably is not the sole cause of aspiration in this population.
Eructation	Excessive belching	Approximately 40% of hyperkinetic patients	Most likely associated with chorea and may be the result of choreic expiratory muscle contractions displacing small amounts of gastric air rather than from air trapped by slowed esophageal motility.
Aerophagia	Swallowing of air	10% of HD patients with hyperkinesia	Lingual chorea and repetitive swallows.
Aspiration	Glottic penetration of food or liquids	Less than 10% in hyperkinetic patients may be a conservative figure due to good position for video study and laryngeal chorea; more frequent and involved larger volumes in the rigid-bradykinetic group	Laryngeal chorea producing a rapid, forceful closure of ventricular and true vocal folds may promote laryngeal penetration but impede glottis aspiration. This may redirect the bolus; subsequent swallows may evacuate residual material.

INTERVIEW

Because of the cognitive problems associated with Huntington disease and because swallowing evaluations are most likely to occur in the more advanced stages of the disease, the initial interview is typically conducted with the patient's family or caregivers. Appendix 3.2 at the end of this chapter contains an outline of an interview form for individuals with Huntington disease. In addition to patient identification information, the form contains questions related to medical, dietary, and swallowing and feeding history.

EXAMINATION

Following the interview, the motility, range, strength, and coordination of oral structures should be examined clinically. Respiratory chorea can be observed at rest and during tasks such as holding one's breath, deep inhalation and exhalation, and intentionally slowed respiratory cycles. Videofluoroscopic techniques are useful in observation of all stages of swallowing in individuals with Huntington disease. Of particular interest are the following aspects of swallowing.

Overall Coordination

Aspects of interest include the coordination and timing of oral mastication, bolus retention orally or in the vallecular and pyriform sinuses, airway protection during swallows, diaphragmatic chorea, esophageal motility, and emptying functions.

Oral Stage

In the oral stage of swallowing for people with hyperkinetic-type symptoms, common findings include hyperextension of the neck and trunk, impaired or absent mastication, premature liquid transfer, delayed or repetitive segmented lingual transfer efforts, and intraoral retention after initial transfer.

Pharyngeal Stage

In the pharyngeal stage, common findings for the hyperkinetic group include incoordination, repetitive swallowing along with swallow delay, prolonged laryngeal elevation, choking or coughing on foods and liquids, wet vocal quality, and phonation during swallowing. Others with hyperkinesia were noted to have belching, aerophagia, vomiting, and early satiety.

The rigid-bradykinetic group also manifested mandibular rigidity, slow lingual chorea, and some of the abnormal features seen in the hyperkinetic group (intraoral retention, delayed lingual transfer, prolonged swallow latency, and coughing and choking). Appendix 3.3 is the "Checklist of Swallowing Abnormalities in Huntington Disease." One can indicate the frequency of occurrence of each symptom in the hyperkinetic and rigid-bradykinetic groups on this form.

What Are Approaches to Management for Swallowing Disorders in Huntington Disease?

Like many aspects of management of individuals with Huntington disease, the caregiver must take considerable responsibility for arranging the setup for eating, supervising the meal, and providing verbal cues during eating. With a properly structured environment, intervention programs have been successful. For example, Leopold and Kagel (1985) reported the results of an intervention program in which all 11 individuals treated improved and 73% (8 of 11) returned to an unrestricted diet. These improvements were reported to have persisted for as long as 3 years.

POSTURAL AND POSITIONAL CHANGES

The goal of this type of intervention is to have the person swallow with the chin in a stable and tucked position. Recall that a common finding of videofluoroscopic swallowing evaluations in Huntington disease is hyperextension of the neck and trunk. Supporting the midthoracic to lumbar spine with a foam rubber wedge is frequently beneficial in reducing hyperextension. Positioning the wheelchair lap tray at waist level may also be helpful.

ASSISTIVE DEVICES

A variety of assistive eating devices may be recommended by the occupational therapist. These include nonskid mats, scoop dishes, built-up utensils with short shafts, small bowls, and double-handled cups. Weighted cups and utensils and wrist weights may improve coordination and slow tachyphagia.

SUPERVISION TO CONTROL EATING RATE AND BITE SIZE

Safety and efficiency of eating may be improved by controlling the rate of eating and size of bites. Serving finger foods, bite-sized items that can be manipulated without the need for utensils, may be beneficial. These behavioral changes are most successfully accomplished when the patient is supervised at mealtime by someone who can provide verbal cues. In some cases, implementing an individualized swallowing sequence, such as chew-swallow-cough-swallow, may be appropriate. Cognitive decline may bring behaviors that interfere with eating. Patients may tend to skip certain meals, refuse particular food items or textures, develop unusual cravings or aversions, or eat only one or two food items. In some cases, patients may sleep excessively and miss meals. Others sit and stare at their food or play with the food on their plate. To minimize the effects of these behaviors, caregivers can emphasize foods that are known to be favorites. Sauces, seasonings, and gravies that are favored can be used on multiple foods. Frequent, high-nutrition snacking can be substituted for a traditional meal schedule.

DIETARY CHANGES

Weight loss is common for patients with HD and efforts should be made to minimize it. In advanced disease, patients lose body fat and then lean muscle mass. There are both physical and psychological factors that contribute to this weight loss. Individuals with nearly constant, involuntary, choreoathetoid movements burn calories at a higher rate. At the cellular level, metabolic dysfunction leads to an inability to efficiently utilize calories. Additionally, the inability to effectively feed oneself, chew, and swallow may result in less than optimal caloric intake. Psychological factors such as emotional changes, depression, obsessive behavior, and a shortened attention span contribute to a loss of appetite and inappropriate selection of foods.

In HD the goal is to achieve a protective weight of 10 to 20 pounds above ideal body weight. This may require dietary changes to supplement caloric intake. For example, dietary changes typically involve restricting the person to softer food consistencies for ease of chewing and swallowing. A careful dietary evaluation is also necessary to ensure that the diet provides sufficient calories. Items that can be added to recipes to increase calories include whole milk, cream, cheese, sour cream, butter, avocado, creamy dressings, extra mayonnaise, sauces, and gravies.

ALTERNATIVE FEEDING

Monitoring changes in the patient's weight, hydration, and occurrences of aspiration pneumonia are the keys to judging the success of dietary modifications. If the patient is at risk for aspiration, malnutrition, or dehydration, then alternative feeding approaches should be considered. See Chapter 1 for a discussion of some of these alternatives.

Name: _____ Date: _____

IDENTIFY A RELIABLE RESPONSE

	+	−
Head nod/shake		
Thumbs up/down		
Look up/down		
Eye blinks		
Finger movements		
Right hand vs left hand		
Hand squeezes		
Points to yes/no		
Other:_____		

DESCRIPTION OF THE APPROACH SELECTED:

CONFIRMATION OF COGNITIVE SKILLS

Attending Behavior

	+	−
Responds to spoken name.		
Responds to "look at me."		

Single-Step Commands

	+	−
Close your eyes.		
Squeeze my hand.		

Orientation

	+	−
Is your name XX?		
Is the current year XX?		
Is XX your hometown?		
Are you married?		

PRACTICE EXERCISES

Questions with Known Answers

	+	−
Do birds fly?		
Are elephants little?		
Is the sun bright?		
Do cats swim?		
Does the earth turn?		
Do we eat cars?		
Does a penny float?		

Questions with Unknown Answers

	+	−
Do you have any pets?		
Do you have any children?		
Do you watch soap operas?		
Do you own a house?		
Have you ever gotten a speeding ticket?		
Do you like coffee?		
Have you ever been in New York?		
Do you like to shop?		
Did you go to college?		
Have you ever used a computer?		

YES/NO RESPONSE DOCUMENTED IN:

_____ Medical chart

_____ Patient's room

_____ Card file

_____ Other:_____

LIST OF PERSONS TRAINED:

_____

_____

_____

_____

APPENDIX 3.2

Swallowing Function Interview for Huntington Disease

Name: _____   ID #: _____

Birth date: _____   Date: _____

Referring physician: _____   Current residence: _____

Status of living will: _____   Informant: _____

Reason for referral: _____

_____

_____

_____

MEDICAL HISTORY

Date of diagnosis: _____   Stage of disease: _____

Current medications: _____

Mobility aids: _____

_____

History of aspiration pneumonia: _____

_____

_____

_____

DIETARY HISTORY

Current height/weight: _____   History of weight loss: _____

Current diet: _____

Estimated liquid intake: _____   Estimated caloric intake: _____

Modifications to diet: _____

_____

_____

_____

(continues)

SWALLOWING AND FEEDING HISTORY

Results of previous swallowing evaluation: _____

_____

_____

Results of previous video study: _____

Episodes of coughing or choking: _____

Abnormal eating behaviors: _____

Symptoms of heartburn or reflux: _____

Typical setup for meal: _____   Enjoyment of food: _____

    Seating aids: _____   Saliva management: _____

    Assistive eating devices: _____

    Patient's estimation of swallowing: _____

    Level of supervision: _____

    Other: _____

_____

Chief swallowing complaints: _____

_____

_____

_____

APPENDIX 3.3

Checklist of Swallowing Abnormalities in Huntington Disease

Name: _____   ID #: _____

ORAL STAGE	Date:					
Rapid lingual chorea (1,3)						
Hyperextension of head and trunk (1, 2, 3, 4)						
Absent or inefficient mastication (1, 2, 3, 4)						
Tachyphagia (1, 2, 3, 4)						
Premature liquid transfer (1, 2, 3, 4)						
Delayed lingual transfer of textured food (1, 2, 3, 4)						
Intraoral bolus retention after initial swallow (1, 2, 3, 4)						
Segmented lingual transfer (1, 2, 3, 4)						
Head and trunk anteroflexion (3)						
Mandibular rigidity (2)						
Other:						

PHARYNGEAL STAGE

Swallow incoordination (1, 3)					
Audible swallows (1)					
Repetitive swallows (1, 3, 4)					
Swallow latency (2, 4)					
Prolonged laryngeal elevation (3)					
Repetitive swallows of liquid					
Inability to stop respiration					
Phonation during swallowing					
Choking on liquids (2)					
Choking on food (4)					

(continues)

PHARYNGEAL STAGE (CONTINUED)

Coughing on food (2)					
Laryngeal chorea (3)					
Vallecular retention (3, 4)					
Pyriform sinus retention (3)					
Other:					

ESOPHAGEAL STAGE

Eructation (belching)					
Aerophagia					
Early satiety					
Diaphragmatic chorea					
Esophageal dysmotility					
Proximal bolus redirection					
Slowed bolus transport and emptying functions					
Gastroesophageal reflux					
Other:					

KEY

1 = Occurred in >50% of hyperkinetic patients during clinical examination.

2 = Occurred in >50% of rigid-bradykinetic patients during clinical examination.

3 = Occurred in >50% of hyperkinetic patients during videofluoroscopy.

4 = Occurred in >50% of rigid-bradykinetic patients during videofluoroscopy.

Adapted from Kagel and Leopold (1992).

References

Anderson, K. E., Louis, E. D., Stern, Y., & Marder, K. S. (2001). Cognitive correlates of obsessive and compulsive symptoms in Huntington's disease. *American Journal of Psychiatry, 158*(5), 799–801.

Bachoud-Levi, A., Remy, P., Nguyen, J., & Brugieres, P. (2000). Motor and cognitive improvements in patients with Huntington's disease after neural transplantation. *Lancet, 356*(9246), 1975–1980.

Berardelli, A., Noth, J., Thompsons, P. D., Bolen, E. L., Curra, A., Deuschl, G., van Dijk, J. G., Topper, R., Schwarz, M., & Roos, R. A. (1999). Pathophysiology of chorea and bradykinesia in Huntington's disease. *Movement Disorders, 14*(3), 398–403.

Beukelman, D. R., & Mirenda, P. (1998). *Augmentative and alternative communication: Management of severe communication disorders in children and adults* (2nd ed.). Baltimore: Brookes.

Cummings, J. L. (1995). Behavioral and psychiatric symptoms associated with Huntington's disease. *Advances in Neurology, 65,* 179–186.

Darley, F. L., Aronson, A. E., & Brown, J. R. (1975). *Motor speech disorders.* Philadelphia: Saunders.

Garrett, K., & Beukelman, D. R. (1992). Augmentative communication in aphasia. In K. M. Yorkston (Ed.), *Augmentative communication in the medical setting* (pp. 245–338). Tucson, AZ: Communication Skill Builders.

Garrett, K. L., & Yorkston, K. M. (1997). Assistive communication technology for elders with cognitive and language disability. In R. Lubinski & J. Higginbotham (Eds.), *Communication technologies for the elderly: Vision, hearing, and speech* (pp. 203–234). San Diego, CA: Singular Press.

Gordon, W. P., & Illes, J. (1987). Neurolinguistic characteristics of language production in Huntington's disease: A preliminary report. *Brain and Language, 31,* 1–10.

Goto, I., Taniwaki, T., Hosokawa, S., Otwsuka, M., Ichiya, T., & Ichimiya, A. (1993). Positron emission tomographic (PET) studies in dementia. *Journal of Neurological Science, 114,* 1–6.

Haddad, M. S., & Cummings, J. L. (1997). Huntington's disease. *Psychiatric Clinics of North America, 20*(4), 791–807.

Hakiman, R. (2000). Disclosure of Huntington's disease to family members: The dilemma of knowing but unknowing parties. *Genetic Testing, 4*(4), 359–364.

Hofmann, N. (1999). Understanding the neuropsychiatric symptoms of Huntington's disease. *Journal of Neuroscience Nursing, 31*(5), 309–313.

Hunt, V., & Walker, F. O. (1991). Learning to live at risk for Huntington's disease. *Journal of Neuroscience Nursing, 23,* 179–182.

Huntington's Study Group. (1996). Unified Huntington's Disease Rating Scale: Reliability and consistency. *Movement Disorders, 11,* 136–142.

Hurley, R. A., Jackson, E. F., Fisher, R. E., & Taber, K. H. (1999). New techniques for understanding Huntington's disease. *Journal of Neuropsychiatry and Clinical Neurosciences, 11,* 173–175.

Illes, J. (1989). Neurolinguistic features of spontaneous language production dissociate three forms of neurodegenerative disease: Alzheimer's, Huntington's, and Parkinson's. *Brain and Language, 37*(4), 628–642.

Kagel, M. C., & Leopold, N. A. (1992). Dysphagia in Huntington's disease: A 16-year retrospective. *Dysphagia, 7,* 106–114.

Kirkwood, S. C., Su, J. L., Conneally, P. M., & Foroud, T. (2001). Progression of symptoms in the early and middle stages of Huntington disease. *Archives of Neurology, 58*(2), 273–278.

Klasner, E. R. (1995). Speech treatment for individuals with Huntington's disease. *Special Interest Divisions: Neurophysiology and Neurogenic Speech and Language Disorders, 5*(3), 12–15.

Klasner, E. R., & Yorkston, K. M. (2000). Augmentative communication for Huntington and Parkinson's disease: Planning for change. In D. R. Beukelman, K. M. Yorkston, & J. Reichle (Eds.), *Augmentative and alternative communication for adults with acquired neurologic disabilities* (pp. 241–279). Baltimore: Brookes.

Klasner, E. R., & Yorkston, K. M. (2001). Linguistic and cognitive supplementation strategies as AAC techniques in Huntington disease: A case report. *Augmentative and Alternative Communication, 17*(3), 154–160.

Lawrence, A. D., Watkins, L. H. A., Sahakian, B. J., Hodges, J. R., & Robbins, T. W. (2000). Visual object and visuospatial cognition in Huntington's disease: Implications for information processing in corticostriatal circuits. *Brain, 123*(7), 1349–1364.

Leopold, N., & Kagel, M. (1985). Dysphagia in Huntington's disease. *Archives of Neurology, 42,* 57–60.

Leroi, I., & Michalon, M. (1998). Treatment of the psychiatric manifestations of Huntington's disease: A review of the literature. *Canadian Journal of Psychiatry, 43*(9), 933–940.

Lipe, H., Schultz, A., & Bird, T. D. (1993). Risk factors for suicide in Huntington's disease: A retrospective case controlled study. *American Journal of Medical Genetics, 48*(4), 231–233.

Lundervold, A. J., & Reinvang, I. (1991). Neuropsychological findings and depressive symptoms in patients with Huntington's disease. *Scandinavian Journal of Psychology, 32,* 275–283.

Marder, K., Zhao, H., Myers, R. H., Cudkowicz, M., Kayson, E., Kieburtz, K., Orme, C., Paulsen, J., Penney, J. B., Siemers, E., Shoulson, I., & the Huntington Study Group. (2000). Rate of functional decline in Huntington's disease. *Neurology, 54,* 452–458.

Mayeux, R., Stern, Y., Herman, A., Greenbaum, L., & Fahn, S. (1986). Correlates of early disability in Huntington's disease. *Annals of Neurology, 20,* 727–731.

Meiser, B., & Dunn, S. (2001). Psychological effect of genetic testing for Huntington's disease: An update of the literature. *Western Journal of Medicine, 174,* 336–340.

Middleton, F. A., & Strick, P. L. (2000). Basal ganglia output and cognition: Evidence from anatomical, behavorial, and clinical studies. *Brain and Cognition, 42*(2), 183–200.

Mirenda, P. (1985). Designing pictorial communication systems for physically able-bodied students with severe handicaps. *Augmentative and Alternative Communication, 1,* 58–64.

Mitsuda, P. M., Baarslag-Benson, R., Hazel, K., & Therriault, T. M. (1992). Augmentative communication in intensive and acute care settings. In K. M. Yorkston (Ed.), *Augmentative communication in the medical setting.* Tucson, AZ: Communication Skill Builders.

Murray, L. L., Ramage, A. E., & Hopper, T. (2001). Memory impairments in adults with neurogenic communication disorders. *Seminars in Speech and Language, 22*(2), 127–137.

Murray, L. L., & Stout, J. C. (1999). Discourse comprehension in Huntington's and Parkinson's disease. *American Journal of Speech–Language Pathology, 8*(2), 137–148.

Nance, M. A. (1998). Huntington disease: Clinical, genetic, and social aspects. *Journal of Geriatric Psychiatry and Neurology, 11,* 61–70.

Oliver, J., & Dewhurst, K. (1969). Childhood and adolescent forms of Huntington's disease. *Journal of Neurology, Neurosurgery and Psychiatry, 32*(5), 455–459.

Pillon, B., Dubois, B., Ploska, A., & Agid, Y. (1991). Severity and specificity of cognitive impairment in Alzheimer's, Huntington's, and Parkinson's disease and progressive supranuclear palsy. *Neurology, 41,* 634–643.

Prator, R. J., & Swift, R. (1984). *Manual of voice therapy.* Boston: Little, Brown.

Quinn, N., & Schrag, A. (1998). Huntington's disease and other choreas. *Journal of Neurology, 245,* 709–716.

Reddy, P. H., Williams, M., & Tagle, D. A. (1999). Recent advances in understanding the pathogenesis of Huntington's disease. *Trends in Neurosciences, 22,* 248–255.

Reilmann, R., Kirsten, F., Quinn, L., Henningsen, H., Marder, K., & Gordon, A. M. (2001). Objective assessment of progression in Huntington's disease: A 3-year follow-up study. *Neurology, 57,* 920–924.

Schoenfeld, M., Myers, R. H., Cupples, L. A., Berkman, D., Sax, D. S., & Clark, E. (1984). Increased rate of suicide among patients with Huntington's disease. *Journal of Neurology, Neuropsychiatry, and Psychiatry, 47,* 1283–1287.

Seidman-Carlson, R., & Wells, D. L. (1998). The ability to comprehend affective communication in individuals with Huntington disease. *Journal of Gerontological Nursing, 12,* 16–23.

Shoulson, I., & Fahn, S. (1979). Huntington's disease: Clinical care and evaluation. *Neurology, 29,* 1–3.

Siesling, S., van Vugt, J. P., Zwinderman, K. A., Kieburtz, K., & Roos, R. A. (1998). Unified Huntington's Disease Rating Scale: A follow up. *Movement Disorders, 13*(6), 915–919.

Sobel, S. K., & Cowan, B. D. (2000). Impact of genetic testing for Huntington disease on the family system. *American Journal of Medical Genetics, 90,* 49–59.

Sohlberg, M. M., & Mateer, C. A. (1989). Training use of compensatory memory books: A three stage behavioral approach. *Journal of Clinical and Experimental Neuropsychology, 11*(6), 871–891.

Speedie, L., O'Donnel, W., Rabins, P., Pearlson, G., Poggi, M., & Gonzalez-Rothi, L. J. (1990). Language performance deficits in elderly depressed patients. *Aphasiology, 4*(2), 197–205.

Sullivan, F. R., Bird, E. D., Alpay, M., & Cha, J. J. (2001). Remotivation therapy and Huntington's disease. *Journal of Neuroscience Nursing, 33*(3), 136–142.

Swift, W. B. (1929). The speech in medicine. *Medical Journal and Record, 130*, 192–195.

Turkstra, L. S. (2001). Treating memory problems in adults with neurogenic communication disorders. *Seminars in Speech and Language, 22*(2), 147–155.

van Vugt, J. P. P., & Roose, R. A. C. (1999). Huntington's disease: Options for controlling symptoms. *CNS-Drugs, 11*(2), 105–123.

Wallesch, C. W., & Fehrenbach, R. A. (1988). On the neurolinguistic nature of language abnormalities in Huntington's disease. *Journal of Neurology, Neuropsychiatry, and Psychiatry, 51*, 367–373.

Webb, M., & Trzepacz, P. T. (1987). Huntington's disease: Correlations of mental status with chorea. *Biological Psychiatry, 22*, 751–761.

Williams, J. K., Schutte, D. L., Evers, C., & Holkup, P. A. (2000). Redefinition: Coping with normal results from predictive gene testing for neurogenerative disorders. *Research in Nursing & Health, 23*(4), 260–269.

Yorkston, K. M. (Ed.). (1992). *Augmentative communication in the medical setting.* Tucson, AZ: Communication Skill Builders.

Yorkston, K. M., Beukelman, D. R., Strand, E. A., & Bell, K. R. (1999). *Management of motor speech disorders in children and adults.* Austin, TX: PRO-ED.

4
MULTIPLE SCLEROSIS

Nature of the Problem

This section describes the neuropathology and epidemiology of multiple sclerosis (MS). Information on medical management of the disease including both drug treatment and rehabilitation is provided. A review of symptoms, including cognitive problems and psychosocial issues, affords a context for the information on speech and swallowing that follows. A summary of information is found in the "Multiple Sclerosis" handout in the Appendix at the back of the book.

What Is Multiple Sclerosis?

Multiple sclerosis is an acquired, inflammatory, demyelinating disease of the central nervous system (CNS). The term *multiple sclerosis* refers to the "many scars" that appear in the white matter of the nervous system during the disease. The disease is most frequently diagnosed in young to middle-aged adults. It is described as a progressive neurologic condition; however, early phases are often characterized by a remitting–relapsing course. The scattered lesions in the central nervous system produce varying combinations of motor, sensory, and cognitive impairments.

What Changes in Neural Tissue or Neural Systems Are Associated with MS?

Inflammatory white matter lesions continuously appear, resolve, and recur, even during periods when the clinical course is quiet. Initially these lesions are edematous. Activated macrophages strip away the myelin and eventually leave the axon bare. Patches of destroyed myelin are later replaced by scar tissue, producing lesions known as plaques. Neurologic dysfunction results primarily from blockage of nerve conduction through the demyelinated area. Additional symptoms caused by demyelination may relate to increased nerve excitability (sustained paresthesia or abnormal sensations of burning or prickling), the inability to sustain high-frequency transmission (muscle weakness and rapid fatigue), or ephaptic cross-activation (paroxysmal symptoms or symptoms that suddenly recur or intensify) (Cobble, Dietz, Grigsby, & Kennedy, 1993). Not all lesions result in neurologic deficits. Some, called silent lesions, are apparent on neural imaging but do not cause clinical signs or symptoms.

Who Is at Risk for MS?

MS is the most common neurologic disorder of young and middle-aged adults. It is the third leading cause of disability in this population after trauma and arthritis. Although the relapsing–remitting pattern typically begins between the ages of 18 and 40, the progressive form of the disease begins somewhat later. There are 250,000 to 350,000 individuals with MS in the United States (Anderson et al., 1992).

Epidemiologic studies suggest that MS is more common in temperate climates and in economically developed countries. The disease is 2 to 3 times more common in the northern half of the United States than in the southern half. Geographic risk is based on childhood residence. This fact has led researchers to propose an environmental exposure in children as a predisposing risk factor. MS appears to be virally induced. MS is 2 to 3 times more common in women than men. Racially, an affected person is more likely to be White than African American and more likely to be African American than Asian American. An individual is roughly 10 times more likely to be diagnosed with MS if parents or siblings have the disease.

There are several theories about the cause of neural changes in MS. The three most common theories involve an autoimmune basis, a viral basis, and a genetic predisposition (Boyden, 2000). Most researchers now believe that the etiology of MS may be a complex interaction among the three theoretic bases that can be summarized as follows, "Best evidence for etiology suggests exposure to a common environmental agent that triggers a dysregulated immune response in genetically susceptible people" (Cobble et al., 1993, p. 862).

How Has Magnetic Resonance Imaging Contributed to the Understanding of MS?

The development of magnetic resonance imaging (MRI) techniques has led to a new understanding of the nature and course of MS and has contributed substantially to the diagnostic process (Lucchinetti, Bruck, & Noseworthy, 2001). MRI involves the application of a powerful magnetic field to the body that causes nuclei to behave like tiny magnets. The signals are picked up by a very sensitive antenna and forwarded to a computer for processing. When first developed, MRI helped to identify subclinical lesions and thus was a major contributor to diagnosis. More recently, MRI has been used to track changes over time and to monitor the impact of drug treatment. Neuroimaging techniques allow researchers to study how lesions evolve and resolve. They also have led to the appreciation that MS is not just a disease of myelin, but that over time the brain atrophies and white cell matter between the lesions of MS may also be abnormal.

A variety of neuroimaging methods are now available, which, taken together, provide a detailed understanding of the neuropathology associated with MS (Joy & Johnston, 2001). Various MRI techniques are capable of revealing many features of MS: recent inflammatory disturbances, total burden of disease, axon loss, abnormalities within normal-appearing white matter, and critical circuitry involved in response to injury, loss of function, and recovery of function (Miller, Grossman, Reingold, & McFarland, 1998).

The correlation between conventional MRI and function status of an individual with MS has been described as modest (Miller et al., 1998). Research studies using MRI often observe areas of new lesions even when the individual is not experiencing any change in function and is still in the relapsing phase of the disease. These findings suggest a previously unsuspected level of activity and pathology throughout the course of the disease. In other words, the disease is active and progressive in a substantial number of individuals even early in the disease. Miller and colleagues suggested several reasons for the lack of strong correlation between conventional MRI findings and level of disability: (a) various problems with measurement (measurement error in quantifying MRI parameters), (b) difficulty in quantifying relapses, (c) the nonlinearity of common measures of disability, and (d) use of scales that measure both impairment and disability. They also suggest that MS is a very complex phenomenon in which specific aspects of the disability may not be simply or directly associated with underlying pathophysiology. Newer nonconventional MRI strategies may provide a closer link between underlying pathology and clinical symptoms in MS (Matthews & Arnold, 2001).

What Are the Symptoms of MS?

Symptoms associated with MS vary extensively, depending on the size, age, activity, and location of the lesions. Table 4.1 lists central nervous system sites and impairments commonly seen in MS. The following sections describe common symptoms associated with MS, including motor, sensory, and cognitive changes; fatigue; depression; pain; and heat sensitivity.

MOTOR SYMPTOMS

Motor symptoms including spasticity, weakness, spasm, ataxia, and tremor are common in MS. Spasticity is generally associated with an increase in muscle tone and occurs in about 70% of the population (Goodin & Northern California MS Study Group, 1999). It occurs when muscle groups fail to work; when one muscle is flexed, its opposing muscle relaxes. Many individuals with MS experience weakness along with spasticity. In progressive stages of the disease, exaggerated extensor or flexor tone can cause forceful activation of muscles (extensor or flexor spasms). Ataxia is characterized by incoordination of muscular activity and in MS is commonly associated with tremor (involuntary, rhythmic, oscillatory movements of a body part) (Alusi, Worthington, Glickman, & Bain, 2001).

SENSORY SYMPTOMS

Sensory changes are also common in MS and may include decrease in touch, pain, or position sense. Symptoms may also include numbness, tingling, burning, shooting

TABLE 4.1	Common Sites of CNS Lesions and Impairment in MS	
CNS Site	**Impairment**
Cerebrum, especially periventricular areas, frontal lobes	Cognitive, affective (mood), and behavioral changes
Spinal cord, especially cervical region	Weakness, spasticity, numbness, bowel and sexual dysfunction
Brain stem	Vertigo, nystagmus, internuclear ophthamoplegia, dysarthria, dysphagia
Cerebellum and basal ganglia	Ataxia and tremor
Optic nerves	Optic neuritis

Note. Adapted from "Rehabilitation of the Patient with Multiple Sclerosis," by N. D. Cobble, M. A. Dietz, J. Grigsby, and P. M. Kennedy, 1993, in *Rehabilitation Medicine: Principle and Practice* (2nd ed.), by J. A. DeLisa (Ed.), Philadelphia: Lippincott.

electrical sensations, and pain. Changes in vision may result from demyelina[...] the optic nerve (Anderson & Cox, 1998; Soderstrom, 2001). Visual changes occu[...] approximately 85% of individuals with MS and are the first symptoms in about 35 [...] (Wikstrom, Poser, & Ritter, 1980). Symptoms of optic neuritis include rapid vision loss, pain associated with eye movement, dimmed vision, abnormal color vision, and altered depth perception (Joy & Johnston, 2001). Uhthoff's symptom, a loss of central vision associated with an increase in body temperature, also occurs in MS (Selhorst & Saul, 1995).

COGNITIVE CHANGES

Appreciation of the nature and extent of cognitive changes in MS has come about only in the last several decades. In the 1970s, MS was considered a "motor" condition and it was estimated that only 5% of individuals experienced cognitive change (Richardson, Robinson, & Robinson, 1997, cited in Joy & Johnston, 2001). By the 1990s, when more extensive neuropsychological studies had been conducted, estimates increased to approximately half of the MS population (Rao, 1995). The underestimation has been attributed at least in part to the fact that cognitive changes are often subtle and difficult to detect in brief office visits (Fischer, 2001).

Like many aspects of MS, cognitive impairment in the disease varies considerably from person to person. This variability is due at least in part to the location, number, and activity of lesions. Excellent reviews of the growing number of studies of neuropsychological function in MS are available (Fischer, 2001; Rao, 1995; Zakzanis, 2000). There is a general consensus that cognitive changes are not global but rather target specific cognitive processes. These deficits have been called "subcortical dementia" (Rao, 1986), characterized by the absence of aphasia, by memory retrieval failure with relatively intact encoding and storage capacity, by impaired conceptual reasoning skills in the context of near-normal intellect, by slowed information processing time, and by personality disturbances, characterized by apathy, depression, or euphoria. Memory changes are also commonly reported in 20% to 40% of individuals with MS (Fischer et al., 1994). Rao (1986) describes memory impairment as affecting retrieval strategies from both short- and long-term memory. Short-term memory capacity and recognition memory are usually not impaired. This pattern of memory deficits is similar to the one seen in individuals with focal lesions affecting fronto-limbic system neural connections.

Because not all individuals with MS experience cognitive decline, it is important to understand the factors that may or may not place individuals at greater risk for cognitive impairment. Some factors such as motor function or disease duration are not good predictors of cognitive function. The degree of cognitive impairment is not strongly correlated with the degree of neurologic disability (Amato et al., 1995; Franklin, Nelson, Filley, & Heaton, 1989). In a study of 100 individuals with MS reported by Rao, Leo, Bernardin, and Unverzagt (1991), 52 were considered cognitively intact and 48 cognitively impaired. No significant differences between the groups were found on measures of physical disability or illness duration.

Other factors such as total lesion burden (the percentage of the brain that shows lesions on MRI scans) have been correlated with cognitive impairment (Rovaris & Filippi, 2000). Franklin and colleagues (1989) suggest that serious loss of cognitive function is likely in individuals with MS who have these characteristics:

1. Chronic, progressive disease

2. Frontal release signs or apraxia or both, prominent in the lower extremities

3. Depression or bipolar disorder refractory to treatment

4. Cognitive difficulties at work or home, particularly in the areas of memory, attention, or complex problem-solving skills

5. Moderate to severe periventricular abnormality on MRI scans, even early in the disease course in the absence of progressive neurologic deficits

Cognitive dysfunction has also been noted during acute disease exacerbation (Foong et al., 1998).

In-depth neuropsychologic testing may be appropriate with individuals who exhibit features associated with cognitive decline. Objective neuropsychologic testing is considered the "gold standard" for determining whether or not cognitive changes are present (Fischer et al., 1999). Results of this testing can be used to help individuals with MS to identify areas of strength as well as weakness. Accurate identification of cognitive status in MS is important for a number of reasons. Cognitive changes may have important effects on many aspects of everyday functioning, including the ability to work. Even mild changes in cognitive function or affect may be particularly distressing to patients and their families. Reischies, Baum, Brau, and Hedde (1988) examined the relationship between presence of cognitive impairment and several aspects of quality of life. They found that people with cognitive impairment engaged in fewer social and avocational activities, were less likely to be working, and exhibited more psychopathology than those with intact cognition.

Cognitive changes may affect language skills. Individuals with MS have reported difficulty with word finding and changes in verbal or written organization (Yorkston, Klasner, & Swanson, 2001). Researchers have also tested high-level language abilities of individuals with MS. For example, Wallace and Holmes (1993) reported differences in performance among 4 individuals with MS and controls on certain subtests of the *Arizona Battery for Communication Disorders* (Bayles & Tomoeda, 1991). These subtests included Object Description, Generative Naming, Concept Definition, Generative Writing, and Picture Description.

Lethlean and Murdoch (1993) administered a battery of language tests to 17 individuals with MS and matched controls. Results indicated subtle, high-level language problems, including problems with naming; comprehension of concepts requiring logicogrammatical operations; repetition of sentences and digits; word fluency; tasks requiring verbal explanation or verbal reasoning; reconstruction of sentences; definitions of words; and interpretation of absurdities, ambiguities, and metaphors. Comprehension, reading ability, and writing ability were preserved in individuals whose sensory and motor abilities allowed them to complete the tasks. Murdoch and Lethlean (2000) suggest the presence of language subgroups in MS. In a study of 60 individuals with MS, they found four subgroups: (a) severe pervasive language impairment (2% of subjects), (b) moderate to severe language impairment (13%), (c) mild to moderate language impairment (32%), and (d) essentially normal language abilities (53%). The implication of these recent studies is that clinicians need to be aware that language deficits are possible in this population. These deficits may be associated with general slowness of information processing, cognitive changes, or fatigue.

FATIGUE

In the Multiple Sclerosis Council for Clinical Practice Guidelines (Miller & Multiple Sclerosis Council for Clinical Practice Guidelines, 1998), fatigue is defined as a subjective lack of physical or mental energy that interferes with daily activities. It is often reported as the most common symptom of MS, experienced by 76% to 92% of the population (Ford, Trigwell, & Johnson, 1998). One third of individuals with MS report fatigue as their worst symptom (Krupp, Alvarez, LaRocca, et al., 1988). The causes of MS fatigue are poorly understood but one theory suggests slowing or alteration of neurotransmitter release and increased nerve conduction times (Joy & Johnston, 2001). Individuals with MS report that the fatigue they experience is "different" and unique to the disease (Yorkston et al., 2001). MS fatigue is multidimensional and interacts with physical and cognitive issues as well as depression (Kinkel, 2000). Individuals with MS describe fatigue in many ways including such terms as weakness, lack of stamina, feeling "spacey," having poor concentration, boredom, or general malaise (Joy & Johnston, 2001). Thus, they suggest both a physical and cognitive association. Recent assessment tools are beginning to distinguish between mental and physical fatigue (Ford et al., 1998). Fatigue is made worse by heat, stress, or physical activity. It limits social, work, and role performance (Deatrick, Brennan, & Cameron, 1998; Schwartz, Coulthard-Morris, & Zeng, 1996). Fatigue is strongly correlated with disability (Goodin & Northern California MS Study Group, 1999), but not well correlated with MRI findings (Bakshi et al., 1999).

AFFECTIVE DISORDERS

Affective disorders—those that relate to emotion or feeling—are common in MS. Disorders include depression, euphoria, apathy, and irritability (Minden & Schiffer, 1990). Depression is a mood disorder that is associated with loss of interest or pleasure. Psychological distress, including depression, occurs frequently in individuals with MS. Estimates of major depression at any point in time range from 27% to 54% (Minden & Schiffer, 1990). Lifetime prevalence is approximately 50% (Mohr & Cox, 2001). These rates are higher than either the general population or other neurologic populations. Depression in MS may either be reactive, a response to the many losses associated with the disorders, or related to the brain lesions. There is also some specu-lation that depression may be a side effect of other medications (Neilly, Goodin, Goodkin, & Hauser, 1996). In a summary of studies of depression, Mohr and Cox (2001) concluded that absolute level of cognitive or physical impairment is not directly related to depression. Rather, they suggest that an individual's perception of uncertainty, the variability of the disease, and the perceived intrusiveness into aspects of daily living are related to depression and adjustment.

HEAT SENSITIVITY

An increase in temperature often causes the appearance of new symptoms or the worsening of old ones. Temperature elevations may be due to ambient air temperature changes, fever from an infection, or exercise. Heat sensitivity in MS is thought to be the result of loss of myelin which serves as a neural insulator.

How Is the Diagnosis of MS Made?

The diagnosis of MS is difficult because clinical signs and course vary greatly. In fact, guidelines have been developed to classify patients into groups such as definite MS versus probable MS, based on clinical and laboratory evidence (Poser et al., 1983). The following characteristics lead to a diagnosis of MS (Cobble et al., 1993):

Age. 10 to 59 years

Attacks (bouts, episodes, exacerbations). Attacks are occurrences of a symptom or symptoms of neurologic dysfunction, with or without objective confirmation, lasting more than 24 hours. Two separate occurrences months apart or progression of neurologic dysfunction lasting longer than 6 months is necessary. Past occurrences are acceptable with documentation by a competent examiner.

Separate lesions. Separate signs or symptoms are present that cannot be explained on the basis of a single lesion.

Features typical of MS. MS is known to involve certain parts of the central nervous system much more frequently than others. Diagnosis is strengthened if sites of lesion are typical.

Other disorders. Diagnosis is also dependent on the absence of a better explanation for the signs and symptoms. A variety of disorders involve multiple central nervous system sites. Because some of these disorders are treatable, accurate diagnosis is critical.

Thus, multiple lesions need to be identified that are discrete both in terms of time (bouts separated by months) and space (different locations in the CNS). Although the diagnosis continues to be a clinical one, MRI findings are often used as support (McDonald et al., 2001; Poser & Brinar, 2001). Although there is little correlation between clinical status and MRI findings, these findings are useful in identifying subclinical levels of lesion activity. The need for early diagnosis has become particularly critical recently, because the course-altering drugs have been shown to be most effective in early stage of the disease.

What Is the Typical Course of Changing Function in MS?

Before describing patterns of progression in MS, a common approach to the measurement of function is reviewed. The severity of MS has been assessed clinically using a variety of scales. See Joy and Johnston (2001) for a review. Measurement of function in MS is particularly important because of the variability inherent in the disease and because functional scales are often used to measure the effectiveness of treatment, including drug trials.

Technically, functional status is a composite measure and refers to the ability to perform activities of daily living. Although many scales are available, the Expanded Disability Status Scale (EDSS; Kurtzke, 1983; Kurtzke & Page, 1997) is most frequently cited. This is a measure of physical and social functioning specific to MS. Although the title of the scale suggests that it focuses on disability or limitation of activities of daily living, it actually rates various aspects of impairment based on clinical signs identified during the neurologic examination. The scale covers eight separate neurologic systems (pyramidal tract, cerebellum, brain stem, sensory, bowel and bladder, visual, mental, and other). Scores are weighted, not simply added, to obtain an overall scale score from 0 to 10. The EDSS is not linear. Rather, it is bimodal with more individuals in the high or low range than the mid-range. Generally, the lower scale scores indicate lower levels of disability. Scores of less than 4 indicate that the individual is fully ambulatory.

TABLE 4.2   Patterns of Disability Over Time in MS

Pattern	Characteristics	Approximate Percentage
Relapsing–remitting	Episodes of acute neurologic dysfunction followed by recovery and a stable course between relapses	70%–85% begin with this course
Primary–progressive	Progressive from onset	10%–15%
Secondary–progressive	A progression of neurologic dysfunction with or without superimposed occasional relapses, minor remissions, and plateaus	50% of relapsing–remitting develop into secondary–progressive within a decade
Progressive–relapsing	Gradual neurologic deterioration from onset with subsequent superimposed relapses	Rare

Like the signs and symptoms of MS, the pattern of progression of the disorder is variable. Table 4.2 lists four patterns of progression. Note that an episode of acute neurologic dysfunction may be called a relapse, attack, or exacerbation, and is associated with symptoms that last longer than 24 hours in the absence of a fever. A relapsing–remitting pattern is the most common, with most individuals initially exhibiting this course. Some individuals in this category are considered benign with little or no disability over 10 to 15 years. About half of the individuals with relapsing–remitting MS will develop a secondary progressive course. This is characterized by a progression of symptoms with the exacerbations. Individuals with primary–progressive MS never experience periods of remission between attacks. Finally progressive–relapsing MS is characterized by both progressive disease from onset and acute attacks.

The prognosis in early MS is more favorable if the age of onset is less than 35 years and if a single symptom rather than multiple symptoms are evident. Symptoms such as optic neuritis and sensory symptoms are considered more favorable than early motor or cerebellar symptoms (Cobble et al., 1993). Although MS is considered a progressive disorder, life expectancy is normal for 85% of individuals with the disease. Death typically is not directly attributable to an MS plaque causing a terminal event such as respiratory failure. Rather, death is typically caused by complications such as pneumonia, renal involvement, decubitus, septicemia, or depression-related factors (Cobble et al., 1993).

How Is MS Managed?

The approaches to the management of MS fall into two categories: drugs that either alter the course of the disease or alleviate symptoms and rehabilitation efforts that focus on improvement of function.

DRUGS FOR MS

Until the last decade, drug management in MS focused on relieving the symptoms of the disease, but not on altering either the frequency of relapse or the rate of progression. In the 1990s the term "disease-modifying therapy" began to emerge with the introduction of a number of drugs known as immunomodulatory agents or the "ABC" drugs (Avonex, Betaseron, and Copaxone). These drugs have been studied in carefully controlled clinical trials and have been shown to alter the clinical course of the disease by reducing the number and severity of attacks in individuals with relapsing–remitting MS (Comi, 2000; Noseworthy, Lucchinetti, Rodriguez, & Weinshenker, 2000; Weinstock-Guttman & Jacobs, 2000). See Polman and Uitde-haag (2000) for a summary of the clinical trials and their outcomes. These drugs have also been shown to alter disease features measured by MRI. When individuals taking the drugs are compared to controls, they have fewer new lesions, less brain atrophy, and reduced total burden of the disease. Studies including measures of neuropsychological function suggest beneficial effects especially in the domains of information processing and learning/memory (Fischer et al., 2000). For an update on recent clinical drug trials, readers are referenced to the National MS Society Web site (www.nationalmssociety.org).

The timing of intervention appears be critical. Studies suggest that course-altering drugs are most effective in the early relapsing–remitting phase of the disease and are much less effective with progressive disease. There is a trend toward starting the drug early in an effort to prevent or reduce the early axonal damage that has been identified in MRI studies (Comi, 2000). The U.S. National MS Society in a consensus statement endorsed treatment as soon as a definite diagnosis of relapsing MS is made (National MS Society, 2001).

Despite these encouraging advances, the drugs are costly and are not viewed as a cure for the disease. Researchers suggest that because of the heterogeneity of the myelin destruction process, no single agent will be sufficient to control the disease (Weinstock-Guttman & Jacobs, 2000). Injections are not pleasant, and side effects include flulike symptoms (Gottber, Gardulf, & Fredrikson, 2000; Walther & Hohlfeld, 1999) and possible depression (Feinstein, 2000).

During acute relapses, steroids may be given in short bursts at high doses to shorten the duration of exacerbation. Other antiviral and immunomodulating treatments such as adrenocorticotropic hormone (ACTH) are also given to shorten the recovery period. Prevention of secondary complications of the disease is also critical. Medical management of acute exacerbations also includes supportive measures such as relative rest, bladder and bowel management, sensorimotor assistance and protections (range of motion, positioning, skin protection, etc.), swallowing precautions, and treatment of vertigo and nausea.

A variety of pharmacologic agents may be employed to target the symptoms of MS. This type of intervention is not directed at a cure of the underlying disease; rather, it is aimed at reducing the level of functional limitation. For example, drugs are available for the management of spasticity, cerebellar incoordination, emotional lability, depression, fatigue, and so on.

What Is the Role of Rehabilitation in the Management of MS?

Despite the fact that drugs may alter the course and relieve the symptoms of MS, individuals are still left with residual neurologic damage (Kraft, 1999). The disability associated with this damage can be addressed through rehabilitation. Rehabilitation by a multidisciplinary intervention has become a standard of practice (Barnes,

Gilhus, & Wender, 2001). This rehabilitation varies, depending on the current clinical situation. For example, intervention during an acute relapse phase is different from that appropriate for static residual disability. In the former case, medical and physical interventions focus on supporting recovery and helping the person adjust to new residual impairments, if any. For static residual disability, the emphasis is on symptomatic treatment and rehabilitation to maximal function, with a home program to maintain gains. Because MS is a progressive condition, individuals are "over-rehabilitated," that is, trained in therapeutic strategies they can use if the condition worsens (Kraft, 1998). For a review of rehabilitation studies, see Thompson (2000).

Rehabilitation interventions address the symptoms of the disease including the following:

- *Weakness.* If weakness is a symptom, a general conditioning exercise program within the limitations of fatigue and heat sensitivity may prevent disuse atrophy for people with mild to moderate impairment. For those with more severe impairment, range of motion should be maintained, and bracing and splinting may be appropriate.
- *Fatigue.* The fatigue experienced by individuals with MS is different from that experienced by healthy adults. It is speculated that the mechanism may be related to the increased energy required for nerves to transmit through and around demyelinated areas. Fatigue is frequently associated with social and vocational limitations. Fatigue has been treated with central nervous system stimulants and with moderate conditioning exercises.
- *Spasticity.* Typical treatment includes medication such as Baclofen and daily stretching exercises. Peripheral phenol motor point nerve blocks may provide temporary localized relief.
- *Incoordination, ataxia, tremor, and dysmetria.* No intervention for these symptoms is always successful. Drugs to diminish the amplitude of tremor may be evaluated. Compensatory strategies such as stabilization for body parts and weighted cuffs may also be used.

A variety of adaptive equipment and assistive devices may be used to compensate for functional limitations in MS. Ambulation aids may include canes, forearm crutches, ankle–foot orthoses, walkers, and wheelchairs. A variety of adaptive equipment and techniques are helpful in activities of daily living such as grooming and dressing. Note that which techniques are appropriate depends on the underlying impairment. For example, wrist weights that compensate for tremor may not be appropriate for individuals for whom weakness is a significant problem. A more complete list of techniques for other activities of daily living can be found in Bhasin, Jensen, Lenling, Robbins, and Shapiro (1991).

Rehabilitation efforts frequently include the management of cognitive changes. This management begins with a careful understanding of the nature of the deficits. Adequate neuropsychological testing is especially critical in the MS population because of the prevalence of frontal lobe involvement. Because individuals with this type of disorder have difficulty with executive function (planning and carrying out an activity) in the presence of good verbal skills, they may appear to be unmotivated because they fail to follow through on plans. Structure, cueing, and breaking a task into small steps may be needed to bring about changes in behaviors. Neuropsychological counseling has been shown to improve social behaviors such as egocentric speech (Benedict et al., 2000). Memory problems are the most common cognitive impairment reported by individuals with MS (Sullivan, Edgley, & Dehoux, 1990). These individuals also report that external aids such as calendars, daily planners, and notepads are useful in compensating for the memory problems. Recent studies of cognitive training strategies have been positive. For example, when training memory strategies, researchers found that individuals with MS learned the strategies more quickly and required less training than individuals with head injury (Allen, 1998). In another example, individuals with MS performed similarly to controls when they were given an adequate amount of time to process information (Demaree, DeLuca, Gaudino, & Diamond, 1999).

How Is Employment Affected by MS?

Employment is a critical issue in MS because the disease typically occurs in young adults in the years of greatest career development. A number of large-scale studies of employment patterns of individuals with MS are available (Edgerton, Tuerck, & Fisher, 1975; Edgley, Sullivan, & Dehoux, 1991; Jackson, Quaal, & Reeves, 1991; Kornblith, LeRocca, & Baum, 1986; LaRocca, Kalb, Scheinberg, & Kendall, 1985; O'Day, 1998). In spite of new course-altering drugs, advances in assistive technology, and the passage of the Americans with Disabilities Act (ADA) in 1990, unemployment rates are high: between 70% and 80% for individuals with MS. Most individuals with MS have held jobs at some point in their lives and reported that symptoms of the disease contributed to their lack of employment. A commonly reported pattern is a move from a higher demand position to a position that places lesser demands on the individuals, followed by a move to retirement or unemployment. Fatigue and muscle weakness were found to have the greatest effect on employment (Jackson et al., 1991). Mobility problems, perceived cognitive problems, age, and lack of education were also implicated as reasons for unemployment (Edgley et al., 1991).

Rehabilitation techniques may assist individuals with MS who wish to maintain employment. Specific accommodations including physical access to the workplace, working part-time, flexible schedules, creating opportunities for intermittent rest, providing assistance with physically taxing duties, adaptive technology, and control over the pace of work may be helpful in maintaining employment (Jongbloed, 1996; Robinson, 2000). A variety of techniques to compensate for tremor, weakness, fatigue, and changes in sensation in the workplace are available (see Table 4.3).

TABLE 4.3

Compensatory Techniques for Individuals with MS in the Workplace

Adaptive Device or Technique	Symptom			
	Tremor	Weakness	Fatigue	Sensation
Make sure surfaces and seating are at proper height		Especially neck, back, trunk	X	X
Sit as much as possible	X	X	X	X
Type or dictate if writing is poor or difficult	X	X		
Use shoulder rest for phone		X	X	X
Eliminate need to hold phone; use speaker phone or headphone	X	X	X	X
Consolidate trips away from work area		X	X	X
Build up pens/pencils with foam rubber or commercial pen grips	X			
Use keyguard for computer keyboard	X			
Use cart or two-wheeler to transport items	X	X	X	X
Use C-clamps, vises, sturdy clips, clipboards, weights to stabilize items	X	Unilateral		
Change location of controls to operate machinery (example: convert foot pedals to hand controls or vice versa)	X	X		X
Extend handles or build up tool/equipment handles	X	X	X	X
Use headstick or mouthstick to substitute for lost function	X	X	X	
Arrange flexible work schedule	X	X	X	
Use wheelchair or three-wheeler at work		X	X	
Obtain "handicapped parking permit" and/or park close to entrance		X	X	

Note. Adapted from "Occupation Therapy," by C. Bhasin, D. Jensen, M Lenling, K. Robbins, and R. T. Shapiro, 1991, in *Multiple Sclerosis: A Rehabilitation Approach to Management*, by R. T. Shapiro (Ed.), New York: Demos. Copyright 1991 by Demos Publications. Adapted with permission.

Speech Disorders

Speech disorders have long been associated with MS. Charcot's original descriptions of MS in 1868 included three hallmark features: nystagmus, intention tremor, and scanning speech. This early desciption has undergone considerable revision. The following section reviews the evidence that (a) the speech disorder involves more than "scanning speech" and (b) although common, dysarthria is not universally associated with MS. Also included in this section is a discussion of special issues related to assessment of dysarthria in MS.

What Are the Typical Speech Characteristics of Individuals with MS?

Scanning speech is described as slow and drawling, with words spoken as if measured or scanned, a pause after every syllable, and syllables pronounced slowly and hesitantly (Darley et al., 1975). In their review of 168 individuals with MS at the Mayo Clinic, however, they found so-called scanning speech is not the most typical pattern associated with MS. Dysarthria in MS is not attributable solely to cerebellar involvement; rather it has components of both ataxic and spastic dysarthria. The speech characteristics of individuals with MS dysarthria are described as follows:

> The most prominent speech deviations in MS are impaired control of loudness, harshness, and defective articulation. Impaired use of vocal variability for emphasis, impaired pitch control, hypernasality, inappropriate pitch level, and breathiness are observed with lesser degrees of frequency. (Darley et al., 1975, p. 242)

Since the Mayo Clinic studies, techniques involving acoustic analysis have been used to describe the articulatory timing and vocal characteristics of dysarthria in MS (Hartelius, Buder, & Strand, 1997; Hartelius, Nord, & Buder, 1995).

How Common Is Dysarthria in MS?

Although dysarthria is not universal in MS, it is an important feature in a substantial proportion of the population. Prevalence figures will vary slightly, depending on how dysarthria is defined and measured. Fifty-nine percent of those studied in the Mayo Clinic group "present an overall speech performance that would be considered essentially normal in terms of its impact upon a listener" (Darley et al., 1975, p. 238). When individual speech features are tallied separately, a slightly different picture emerges. Figure 4.1 illustrates the speech deviations found in the Mayo Clinic study of MS. Note that respiratory and phona-

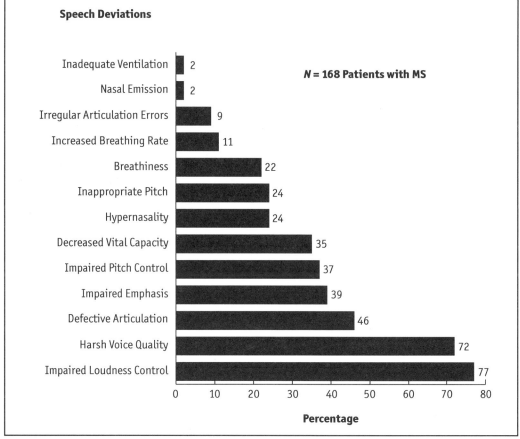

Figure 4.1. Percentage of individuals with MS who exhibit various speech deviations. *Note.* Adapted from *Motor Speech Disorders,* by F. L. Darley, A. E. Aronson, and J. R. Brown, 1975, Philadelphia: Saunders.

tory features occurred most frequently, with 77% of the population exhibiting impaired loudness control and 72% harsh voice quality. Defective articulation occurred in 46% of the group.

Self-report questionnaires about communication difficulties associated with MS indicate that a smaller proportion of the population reports speech difficulty (Beukelman, Kraft, & Freal, 1985; Hartelius & Svensson, 1994). When individuals were grouped by severity of overall disease, the percentage reporting speech problems varied as a function of the stage of the disease. For the group that was characterized as having no problems with ambulation or arm and hand function, 33% reported speech changes. For the group with ambulation problems only, 29% reported speech changes. For the group with ambulation problems and weakness or lack of arm and hand control, 46% reported speech changes. Finally, for the most severe group, those with ambulation problems, weakness, and lack of arm and hand control, 67% reported speech changes. The increasing prevalence of dysarthria as the disease progresses is consistent with the findings of Darley and colleagues (1975). Figure 4.2 illustrates overall speech adequacy as a function of the neural systems involved. Note that speech is least adequate (a higher score) for those with multiple neural system involvement. The most severe dysarthria is associated with cerebral, brain stem, and cerebellar involvement.

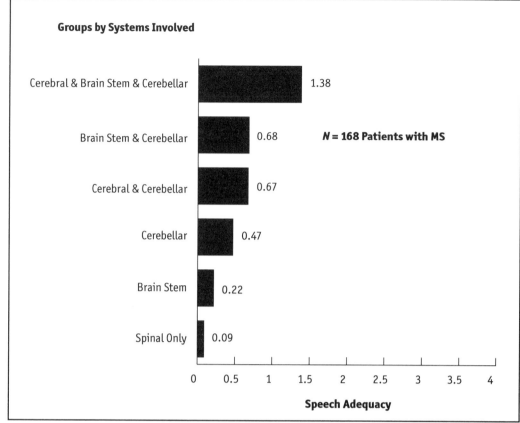

Figure 4.2. Speech adequacy ratings of individuals with MS as a function of the neural system or systems involved; 0 indicates no impairment and 4 indicates most severe impairment. *Note.* Adapted from *Motor Speech Disorders,* by F. L. Darley, A. E. Aronson, and J. R. Brown, 1975, Philadelphia: Saunders.

What Speech Assessment Issues Are Particularly Important in MS?

Like most speech assessments, the evaluation of individuals with MS consists of an interview and clinical examination.

INTERVIEW

Because the course of MS is so variable, a detailed interview is critical. The following topics may be included.

Medical History

A careful medical history should focus on the course of the disease, the history of the nature and timing of exacerbations, and the course of the speech involvement.

Communication Needs

People with MS vary greatly in terms of their communication needs and the environments in which they find themselves. In the early stages of the disease, some are actively pursuing careers in which demands for public contact and superior speech are high. Later, they may find themselves in a much more sheltered environment, where they are not functionally limited by mildly distorted speech. Therefore, a careful discussion of communication needs is necessary.

Associated Problems

Depending on the size, location, and activity of lesions, people with MS may experience a variety of problems that have an impact on communication. For example, fatigue, a common symptom of MS affects the presence and severity of speech symptoms. A history of cognitive impairments should be obtained because these difficulties may exacerbate communication problems and interfere with work or other activities of daily living. Finally, presence or absence of affective disorders such as depression, euphoria, or emotional lability should be established.

Patient's Perception of the Extent of the Problem

The level of functional limitation imposed by a speech disorder varies greatly from individual to individual. Some individuals with barely noticeable dysarthria will complain that they are at a disadvantage because of the disorder. Others will complain of the high level of effort needed to maintain adequate communication. On the other hand, some individuals with more severe dysarthria will experience no functional limitation. We ask questions seeking information about how patients judge the severity of their disorder and how it limits them as they carry out their daily activities. We also attempt to understand how effortful communication is for them.

CLINICAL EXAMINATION

A thorough physical examination is needed because of the variable nature of the disease (see Chapter 1 for a complete description and protocol form). In addition to this examination, we typically obtain the following speech sample.

Sustained Phonation

The sustained phonation measure gives not only an indication of respiratory and phonatory control but also vocal stability, vocal quality, and loudness regulation. The instructions we give are, "Take a breath and give me a long 'ah'; make it long, steady, and clear." If the speaker has vocal stability problems, we will supplement the instructions with some alternate instructions, perhaps suggesting a more appropriate lung volume level. These various attempts give an indication of the speaker's ability to modify phonatory production. Production of short samples of sustained phonation (3–5 seconds) may also be useful in reflecting "best performance." These shorter productions place fewer respiratory control demands on the speaker than do longer productions.

Diadochokinetic Rates

Rapid alternating movement rates are obtained for the single syllables "pa," "ta," and "ka." These tasks give a good indication of the rate and regularity problems common in ataxia. Our instructions are to produce the syllables "as rapidly as you can, but make the syllables precise and distinct from one another." If the speaker does not succeed in making the syllables distinct, we instruct him or her to slow down. In this way, we can estimate the fastest rate at which consonant precision can be maintained. Presence of continuous voicing should also be noted because this is a symptom of poor phonatory control. If the speaker produces a series of voiced rather than voiceless consonants, we give instructions to slow down until the "ba" becomes a "pa."

Reading of a Standard Passage

We ask the speaker to read a standard passage such as the "Grandfather Passage." Connected speech allows you to evaluate prosodic aspects of speech such as respiratory patterning. A variety of questions can be answered with this task: How frequently is the speaker breathing during speech? Do these breaths occur at syntactically appropriate locations? Is the speaker initiating utterances at appropriate lung volume levels? Does loudness decay as a function of inappropriately low lung volume levels? Is stress patterning appropriate?

Randomly Selected Sentences

We ask the speaker to read a series of randomly selected sentences of various lengths (Yorkston, Beukelman, & Tice, 1996). These sentences are recorded and transcribed as a measure of speech intelligibility and rate. We will frequently ask a speaker to repeat sentences that were produced too rapidly or with imprecise articulation. In this way, we can estimate the speaker's ability to repair poorly produced utterances.

How Is Dysarthria in MS Managed?

As is true of the other dysarthrias described in this text, intervention for dysarthria in MS depends on the general characteristics and severity of the problem. Table 4.4 summarizes treatment approaches for individuals with normal speech and mild, moderate, or severe dysarthria.

MILD DYSARTHRIA

Individuals with MS and mild dysarthria typically exhibit changes in vocal quality that do not interfere with normal speaking rate or intelligibility. Vocal instability may

TABLE 4.4 Summary of Speech Intervention in MS

	Normal Speech	Mild Dysarthria	Moderate Dysarthria	Severe Dysarthria
Presenting Features	No observable changes	Vocal tremor Harsh voice Symptoms worsen with fatigue	Decreased speech naturalness Reduced speaking rate Harsh voice	Natural speech no longer functional
Intervention	Confirm normalcy Answer questions	Teach energy conservation techniques Teach loudness regulation techniques	Encourage maintenance of appropriate speaking rate Teach appropriate respiratory patterning Supplement speech with alphabet board	Compensate for severe visual/ motor problems Select appropriate vocabulary

be more obvious on sustained phonation than in connected speech. Voice quality may be harsh. These vocal quality changes rarely limit a speaker's ability to function in speaking situations other than those that require increased loudness such as noisy environments. Individuals with mild dysarthria may complain that symptoms worsen with fatigue.

Teaching energy-conservation techniques and techniques to regulate loudness level are two approaches to intervention for mild dysarthria in MS. These techniques share a common focus on respiratory control. People with ataxia generally do not have weak respiratory muscles; rather, the muscles often are quite strong but uncoordinated. Individuals with weakness will have difficulty achieving the steady subglottal air pressures needed for speech production. Individuals with ataxia, on the other hand, may produce subglottal air pressures far in excess of normal but be unable to produce the steady, relatively low pressure level required for conversational speech. A respiratory pattern stabilization program (Yorkston, Beukelman, Strand, & Bell, 1999) may be appropriate for individuals with ataxia and MS. A list of some abnormal speech breathing behaviors in mild dysarthria follows (Yorkston et al., 1999):

1. The speaker initiates phonation at inappropriate lung volume levels that are either too high or too low.

2. The speaker initiates breath groups either without taking a preparatory inhalation or by taking an excessively large inhalation.

3. The speaker initiates breath groups at inconsistent lung volume levels.

4. The speaker consistently produces utterances that are excessively loud or quiet or vary considerably in loudness levels.

5. The speaker does not terminate a breath group at an appropriate lung volume level, but rather continues to speak until reaching an excessively low lung volume.

Although people with mild involvement typically do not have severe respiratory patterning problems, they will frequently complain of fatigue. The abnormal speech breathing patterns listed previously may contribute to fatigue.

The following steps are included in a respiratory pattern stabilization program:

1. *Establish the appropriate lung volume level.* The first step in stabilizing the respiratory pattern of someone with dysarthria is to identify the range of functional lung volume levels and to establish the most appropriate level at which to initiate speech. For speakers with no impairment, this level is approximately 60% of total lung volume. This may also be a good starting point for individuals with mild dysarthria and MS. Instruments that display respiratory movements are helpful in providing immediate feedback to the speaker.

2. *Examine chest wall shape.* Although there may not be one "best" respiratory shape for speech, some speakers have adopted chest wall shapes that are extremely fatiguing and maladaptive. For example, raising the shoulders in an effort to increase rib cage circumference is more fatiguing than are moderate abdominal and chest wall movements.

3. *Eliminate abnormal respiratory behaviors.* Individuals with dysarthria, especially those with cognitive impairments, may develop unusual respiratory behaviors. For example, they may inhale deeply and then exhale most of the air before they speak, or they may breathe only when they have completely run out of air. Unusual behaviors like these should be identified and eliminated.

Hartelius, Wising, and Nord (1997) described an intervention technique in which the goal is to increase vocal efficiency. Because speakers with MS may have a pattern of ataxia combined with spasticity, the focus of intervention is relaxed and co-ordinated phonation. Exercises include attention to posture, general relaxation, relaxed abdominal breathing with deep inhalation, and controlled exhalations. Most of those treated with this approach benefited in terms of articulatory precision, voice, and naturalness. Cases also have been reported in which the Lee Silverman Voice Treatment (LSVT) improves voice loudness in individuals with progressive MS (Sapir et al., 2001). See Chapter 3 for a more complete description of LSVT.

MODERATE DYSARTHRIA

Individuals with MS and moderate dysarthria typically exhibit the changes in voice quality described for mild dysarthria. In addition, their speech may be characterized by reduced naturalness. A variety of changes in speech prosody are apparent, including slow speaking rates and a stress pattern that has been called excessive and equal.

In addition to the energy-conservation techniques and techniques to normalize respiratory patterns that were described for mild dysarthria, rate-control techniques may be appropriate for individuals with moderate dysarthria. Training in rate control may be particularly important for patients with a sudden increase in ataxia caused by a recent exacerbation. These individuals may not have adapted to the sudden change in their motor control. The following approaches to rate control are reviewed in more detail elsewhere (Yorkston et al., 1999).

Paced Speech

Candidates for paced speech are individuals who are more easily understood if they speak slowly. Candidates must also demonstrate learning ability and must be willing to devote time to practicing and mastering the new motor skills. Feedback about speaking rate can be provided in a variety of ways. Visual feedback can be provided from the intensity by time tracing of programs such as the "Visipitch" (Kay Elemetrics Corp., 2 Bridgewater Lane, Lincoln Park, NJ 07035). Speakers can be taught to increase the overall duration of practice sentences using instructions such as "Fill up the screen." Computerized pacing programs are also available (Beukelman, Yorkston, & Tice, 1997). Passages are presented on the computer screen along with timing information that approximates the rhythmic durational relationships among words in normal speech. Pauses at syntactic boundaries also can be added. When a target rate is entered, the passage appears on the computer screen with a cursor cueing the target rate. Speakers can practice independently once a set of practice materials and the appropriate rates have been established in therapy. Many hours of practice are typically necessary to establish a new optimum speaking rate.

Respiratory Patterning

Respiratory patterning is an approach to rate-control training that focuses on appropriate phrasing and breath patterning. Speakers are taught to chunk utterances into small, meaningful units that are separated with pauses. This chunking into syntactic units and the addition of pauses has the effect of prolonging overall utterance duration and, for many speakers, improving speech intelligibility.

Alphabet Board Supplementation

Alphabet board supplementation is a technique in which speakers point to the first letter of each word as they say it. This approach has the effect of slowing speech and providing the listener with the initial letter of each word. Candidates for the technique are those with sufficient hand function to point to letters on a board. Individuals who use this technique typically are experiencing difficulty making themselves understood and are willing to sacrifice speech naturalness for improved intelligibility.

SEVERE DYSARTHRIA

People with severe dysarthria caused by MS are typically in the late stages of the disorder and are experiencing involvement of multiple neural systems. Natural speech is no longer a functional means of communication in all settings. Providing these individuals with augmentative or alternative means of communication is particularly challenging. Their ability to use their hands for writing or keyboard access is likely to be limited by spasticity, ataxia, or intention tremor. Direct selection access to augmentative communication systems may be limited even with aids such as keyguards. Visual problems may also limit use of augmentative systems that require reading. Cognitive and behavioral problems may reduce the ability to learn to use augmentative systems.

In reviewing the management of communication needs for individuals with end-stage MS and severe dysarthria, Porter (1989) highlighted the benefits of early intervention. Porter described a case in which consultation came late in the course of the disease, at a time when the patient had totally lost the ability to speak and had severe visual and motor problems. The course of intervention was complicated by difficulty with vocabulary selection, limited time to acquire and learn to use technology, and rapidly changing abilities. Honsinger (1989) also described a case in which late intervention was complicated by behavioral problems characterized by outbursts of crying and screaming. The following discussion of intervention will highlight two challenges often faced when serving this population.

Techniques To Compensate for Severe Visual–Motor Problems

Motor deficits in MS are often complicated by severe, progressive visual problems. The first step in developing an intervention plan is careful assessment. The following are questions to ask during the visual examination of individuals with severe dysarthria and late-stage MS (Honsinger, 1989), in order to help you develop communication displays that the patient can read.

1. What is the status of visual acuity?
2. Are there problems with peripheral vision?
3. Are field cuts or field neglect present?
4. What is the patient's response to motion?
5. What are the patient's tracking skills?
6. What are the effects of color and position of visual information?

In developing visual displays, it is appropriate to assume that visual problems will continue to progress. Use of bold print and proper positioning of material in the visual field may be helpful. Honsinger (1989) reported a case in which large print was supplemented with speech output to provide the user with auditory as well as visual feedback. In this case, the display panel might contain the word, "Read." When this item was selected, the speech output would be "Please read to me." Partner-assisted auditory scanning approaches may also be used to compensate for a patient's combined motor and visual deficits. For example, each general category on the communication system may contain a list of selections. The partner reads the list of categories until the patient signals that the desired category has been reached. The partner then reads the list of items in that category, and the patient signals his or her selection.

Vocabulary Selection

Issues of vocabulary selection are critical for people with end-stage MS. Because of the combination of visual and motor deficits just described, rate of communication is often very slow. Therefore, inclusion of whole messages is desirable. These individuals tend to be in sheltered environments and may interact only with familiar people. Porter (1989) stresses the need for individualized messages. In addition to traditional categories such as people, physical feelings or needs, activities, and food or drink, patients who are terminally ill may also wish to have categories containing religious or spiritual terms, emotions, and financial terms.

Swallowing Disorders

Swallowing problems in MS are increasingly likely as the disease progresses. These problems are complicated by difficulty with feeding associated with hand tremor. The following section describes the frequency and characteristics of swallowing disorders in MS along with typical intervention strategies.

How Often Do Swallowing Problems Occur in MS?

The majority of individuals with MS do not experience difficulty swallowing. Reports range from 10% (Garfinkle & Kimmelman, 1982) to over 40% (Abraham, Scheinberg, Smith, & LaRocca, 1997; Hartelius & Svensson, 1994; Thomas & Wiles, 1999). Self-reports of chewing and swallowing problems increase with advancing disease. In early stages 19% reported chewing and swallowing difficulty, whereas in late stages 51% reported difficulty (Hartelius & Svensson, 1994). In a survey of more than 100 individuals with MS, respondents reported that the following types of swallowing difficulties occurred at least "fairly often":

- Choking on food or drink (27%)
- Swallowing solids (16%)
- Swallowing liquids (13%)
- Drink or saliva escaping between lips (13%)
- Chewing difficulty (12%)

In a large study of 525 consecutive outpatients with MS, neither age nor gender was related to the development of dysphagia symptoms. However, subjects who were more disabled, as measured by the EDSS, were more likely to have dysphagia symptoms. Further, those with greater impairments in cerebellar, brain stem, and cognitive functions were more apt to have dysphagia symptoms (Abraham et al., 1997). Thomas and Wiles (1999) report similar findings with regard to the relationship between dysphagia and the level of disability and cerebellar/brain stem function. They add that both impaired vital capacity and depression scale scores correlated with the presence of dysphagia. It is important to note that about half of the patients with objective signs of dysphagia did not complain of a problem (Thomas & Wiles, 1999).

Perhaps more common than swallowing problems is feeding difficulty associated with hand tremor. Transport of food to the mouth may be aided by devices such as weighted cuffs that dampen the intention tremor (Broadhurst & Stammers, 1990; Dahlin Webb, 1986).

What Are the Characteristics of Swallowing Disorders in MS?

Because the cerebellum plays such a small role in the control of swallowing, swallowing disorders may be related to multiple neural lesions, particularly lesions in the brain stem and those involving bilateral corticobulbar tracts. Logemann (1983) suggests that reduced pharyngeal peristalsis and delayed swallowing reflex are the most common features of swallowing disorders in MS. Difficulty initiating a swallow and, less frequently, choking on liquids or sticking of solids is reported (Kirschner, 1989). Not infrequently, individuals with MS will deny swallowing difficulties, even when care providers and family members report problems. Furthermore, studies using pharyngeal and esophageal manometry have demonstrated abnormalities in people who remain asymptomatic for dysphagia (Daley, Code, & Anderson, 1962). To our knowledge, there is no functional scale for assessing severity of swallowing disorders in MS. Therefore, a general scale of swallowing function such as the one that appears in Table 4.5 may be applied in this population.

What Are the Typical Interventions for Swallowing Difficulty in MS?

Intervention varies depending on the severity of the problem or the stage of the disease.

EARLY STAGES OF THE DISEASE

People in early stages of MS will typically complain of occasional difficulty with choking on food or liquid, particularly thin liquids and, most commonly, tap water.

TABLE 4.5	Swallowing Performance Scale

1. Normal
2. Within function limits (WFL): abnormal oral or pharyngeal stage but able to eat regular diet without modifications or swallowing precautions.
3. Mild impairment: mild dysfunction in oral or pharyngeal stage requires a modified diet without need for therapeutic swallowing precautions.
4. Mild–moderate impairment with need for therapeutic precautions: mild dysfunction in oral or pharyngeal stage, requires modified diet and therapeutic precautions to minimize aspiration risk.
5. Moderate impairment: moderate dysfunction in oral or pharyngeal stage, aspiration noted on examination, requires modified diet and swallowing precautions to minimize risk of aspiration.
6. Moderate–severe dysfunction and requires supplemental enteral feeding support: moderate dysfunction in oral or pharyngeal stage, aspiration noted on examination; requires modified diet and swallowing precautions to minimize risk of aspiration; needs supplemental enteral feeding support.
7. Severe impairment: severe dysfunction with significant aspiration or inadequate oropharyngeal transit to esophagus, NPO, requires primary enteral feeding support.

Note. Adapted from "A Database Information Storage and Reporting System for Videofluorographic Oropharyngeal Motility (OPM) Swallowing Evaluations," by M. P. Karnell and E. MacCracken, 1994, American Journal of Speech-Language Pathology, 3(2), 54–56. Copyright 1994 by the American Speech-Language-Hearing Association. Adapted with permission.

Findings on clinical examination will often be within normal limits, and patients will deny a history of aspiration pneumonia or weight loss. When questioned in detail, the person will frequently associate the choking episode with a lapse in attention, a distracting eating environment, or an episode of laughter caused by emotional lability. Fatigue may contribute to difficulties in swallowing, particularly when deterioration of function is brought about by an elevation in body temperature. Patients may need counseling and instruction in the following techniques:

1. Removing distractions from the mealtime environment (avoidance of television and active conversations)

2. Increasing attention to the act of eating and heightening awareness of food taste, temperature, and texture

3. Maintaining optimal body posture during meals (sitting fully upright with the neck slightly flexed)

4. Maintaining adequate hydration

5. Avoiding overly warm environments

6. Using the Heimlich maneuver in the event of an obstructive choking episode

LATE STAGES OF THE DISEASE

Individuals in later stages of MS typically experience multiple neural system involvement. After a complete swallowing evaluation, appropriate techniques can be implemented, depending on the constellation of symptoms observed. These may include behavioral changes such as postural adjustments, changes in diet, or other swallowing precautions such as supervision during mealtimes. In advanced cases, the swallowing musculature may become inadequate to protect the airway and the protective cough reflex may no longer be adequate. Weakness and fatigue may preclude adequate fluid and caloric intake and there may be a lack of enjoyment of meals. If this is the case, a percutaneous endoscopic gastrostomy (PEG) or other alternative route for nutritional support may be considered.

References

Abraham, S., Scheinberg, L. C., Smith, C. R. , & LaRocca, N. G. (1997). Neurologic impairment and disability status in outpatients with multiple sclerosis reporting dysphagia symptomatology. *Journal of Neurologic Rehabilitation*, *11*(1), 7–13.

Allen, D. N. (1998). Teaching memory strategies to persons with multiple sclerosis. *Journal of Rehabilitation Research & Development*, *35*(4), 405–410.

Alusi, S. H., Worthington, J., Glickman, S., & Bain, P. G. (2001). A study of tremor in multiple sclerosis. *Brain*, *124*, 720–730.

Amato, M. P., Ponziani, G., Pracucci, G., Bracco, L., Siracusa, G., & Amaducci, L. (1995). Cognitive impairment in early-onset multiple sclerosis: Pattern, predictors and impact on everyday life in a 4-year follow-up. *Archives of Neurology*, *52*(2), 168–172.

Anderson, D., & Cox, T. (1998). Visual signs and symptoms. In D. W. Paty & G. C. Ebers (Eds.), *Multiple sclerosis* (pp. 229–256). Philadelphia: Davis.

Anderson, D. W., Ellenberg, J. H., Leventhal, C. M., Reingold, S. C., Rodriques, M., & Silberberg, D. H. (1992). Revised estimates of the prevalence of multiple sclerosis in the United States. *Annals of Neurology*, *31*, 333–336.

Bakshi, R., Miletich, R. S., Henschel, K., Shaikh, Z. A., Janardhan, V., Wasay, M., Stengel, L. M., Ekes, R., & Kinkel, P. R. (1999). Fatigue in multiple sclerosis: Cross-sectional correlation with brain MRI findings in 71 patients. *Neurology, 53*(5), 1151–1153.

Barnes, M. P., Gilhus, N. E., & Wender, M. (2001). Task force on minimum standards for health care of people with multiple sclerosis: June 1999. *European Journal of Neurology, 8*, 215–220.

Bayles, K. A., & Tomoeda, C. K. (1991). *Arizona Battery for Communication Disorders.* Tucson, AZ: Canyonlands.

Benedict, R. H., Shapiro, A., Priore, R., Miller, C., Munschauer, F., & Jacobs, L. D. (2000). Neuropsychological counseling improves social behavior in cognitively-impaired multiple sclerosis patients. *Multiple Sclerosis, 6*(6), 391–396.

Beukelman, D. R., Kraft, G. H., & Freal, J. (1985). Expressive communication disorders in persons with multiple sclerosis. *Archives of Physical Medicine and Rehabilitation, 66*(10), 675–677.

Beukelman, D. R., Yorkston, K. M., & Tice, R. (1997). *Pacer/tally rate measurement software.* Lincoln, NE: Tice Technology Services.

Bhasin, C., Jensen, D., Lenling, M., Robbins, K., & Shapiro, R. T. (1991). Occupation therapy. In R. T. Shapiro (Ed.), *Multiple sclerosis: A rehabilitation approach to management.* New York: Demos.

Boyden, K. M. (2000). The pathophysiology of demyelination and the ionic basis of nerve conduction in multiple sclerosis: An overview. *Journal of Neuroscience Nursing, 32*, 49–58.

Broadhurst, M. J., & Stammers, C. W. (1990). Mechanical feeding aids for patients with ataxia: Design considerations. *Journal of Biomedical Engineering, 13*(3), 209–214.

Cobble, N. D., Dietz, M. A., Grigsby, J., & Kennedy, P. M. (1993). Rehabilitation of the patient with multiple sclerosis. In J. A. DeLisa (Ed.), *Rehabilitation medicine: Principles and practice* (2nd ed., pp. 861–885). Philadelphia: Lippincott.

Comi, G. (2000). Why treat early multiple sclerosis patients? *Current Opinion in Neurology, 13*, 235–240.

Dahlin Webb, S. R. (1986). A weighted wrist cuff. *American Journal of Occupational Therapy, 40*(5), 363–364.

Daley, D. D., Code, C. F., & Anderson, H. A. (1962). Disturbances of swallowing and esophageal motility in patients with multiple sclerosis. *Neurology, 59*, 250–256.

Darley, F. L., Aronson, A. E., & Brown, J. R. (1975). *Motor speech disorders.* Philadelphia: Saunders.

Deatrick, J. A., Brennan, D., & Cameron, M. E. (1998). Mothers with multiple sclerosis and their children: Effects of fatigue and exacerbations on maternal support. *Nursing Research, 47*(4), 205–210.

Demaree, H. A., DeLuca, J., Gaudino, E. A., & Diamond, B. J. (1999, November). Speed of information processing as a key deficit in multiple sclerosis: Implications for rehabilitation. *Journal of Neurology, Neuropsychiatry, and Psychiatry, 67*, 661–663.

Edgerton, M. T., Tuerck, D. B., & Fisher, J. C. (1975). Surgical treatment of Moebius sydrome by platysma and temporalis muscle transfers. *Plastic and Reconstructive Surgery, 77*, 305–311.

Edgley, K., Sullivan, M. J., & Dehoux, E. (1991). A survey of multiple sclerosis: II. Determinants of employment status. *Canadian Journal of Rehabilitation, 4*(3), 127–132.

Feinstein, A. (2000). Multiple sclerosis, disease modifying treatments and depression: A critical methodological review. *Multiple Sclerosis, 6*, 343–348.

Fischer, J. S. (2001). Cognitive impairment in multiple sclerosis. In S. D. Cook (Ed.), *Handbook of multiple sclerosis* (pp. 233–252). New York: Marcel Dekker.

Fischer, J. S., Foley, F. W., Aikens, J. E., Ericson, G. D., Rao, S. M., & Shindell, S. (1994). What do we really know about cognitive dysfunction, affective disorders and stress in multiple sclerosis? A practitioner's guide. *Journal of Neurologic Rehabilitation, 8*, 141–164.

Fischer, J. S., LaRocca, N. G., Miller, D. M., Ritvo, P. G., Andrews, H., & Paty, D. (1999). Recent developments in the assessment of quality of life in multiple sclerosis (MS). *Multiple Sclerosis, 5*, 251–259.

Fischer, J. S., Priore, R. L., Jacobs, L. D., Cookfair, D. L., Rudick, R. A., Herndon, R. M., Richert, J. R., Salazar, A. M., Goodkin, D. E., Granger, C. V., Simon, J. H., Grafman, J. H., Lezak, M. D., O'Reilly Hovey, K. M., Perkins, K. K., Barilla-Clark, D., Schacter, M., Shucard, D. W., Davidson, A. L., Wende, K. E., Bourdette, D. N., & Kooijmans-Coutinho, M. F.

(2000). Neuropsychological effects of interferon beta-1a in relapsing multiple sclerosis. Multiple Sclerosis Collaborative Research Group. *Annals of Neurology, 48,* 885–892.

Foong, J., Rozewicz, L., Quaghebeur, G., Thompson, A. J., Miller, D. H., & Ron, M. A. (1998). Neuropsychological deficits in multiple sclerosis after acute relapse. *Journal of Neurology, Neuropsychiatry, and Psychiatry, 64*(4), 529–532.

Ford, H., Trigwell, P., & Johnson, M. (1998). The nature of fatigue in multiple sclerosis. *Journal of Psychosomatic Research, 45*(1), 33–38.

Franklin, G., Nelson, L., Filley, C., & Heaton, R. (1989). Cognitive loss of multiple sclerosis: Case reports and review of literature. *Archives of Neurology, 46,* 162–167.

Garfinkle, T. J., & Kimmelman, C. P. (1982). Neurologic disorders: Amyotrophic lateral sclerosis, myasthenia gravis, multiple sclerosis, and poliomyelitis. *American Journal of Otolaryngology, 3,* 204–212.

Goodin, D. S., & Northern California MS Study Group. (1999). Survey of multiple sclerosis in Northern California. *Multiple Sclerosis, 5,* 78–88.

Gottber, K., Gardulf, A., & Fredrikson, S. (2000). Interferon-beta treatment for patients with multiple sclerosis: The patient's perception of side-effects. *Multiple Sclerosis, 6,* 349–354.

Hartelius, L., Buder, E. H., & Strand, E. A. (1997). Long-term phonatory instability in individuals with multiple sclerosis. *Journal of Speech, Language, and Hearing Research, 40*(5), 1056–1072.

Hartelius, L., Nord, L., & Buder, E. H. (1995). Acoustic analysis of dysarthria associated with multiple sclerosis. *Clinical Linguistics & Phonetics, 9*(2), 95–120.

Hartelius, L., & Svensson, P. (1994). Speech and swallowing symptoms associated with Parkinson's disease and multiple sclerosis: A survey. *Folia Phoniatrica et Logopaedica, 46,* 9–17.

Hartelius, L., Wising, C., & Nord, L. (1997). Speech modification in dysarthria associated with multiple sclerosis: An intervention based on vocal efficiency, contrastive stress, and verbal repair strategies. *Journal of Medical Speech–Language Pathology, 5*(2), 113–140.

Honsinger, M. J. (1989). Midcourse intervention in multiple sclerosis: An inpatient model. *Augmentative and Alternative Communication, 5*(1), 103–110.

Jackson, M. F., Quaal, C., & Reeves, M. A. (1991). Effects of multiple sclerosis on occupational and career patterns. *Axone, 13*(1), 16–17, 20–22.

Jongbloed, L. (1996). Factors influencing employment status of women with multiple sclerosis. *Canadian Journal of Rehabilitation, 9*(4), 213–222.

Joy, J. E., & Johnston, R. B. (Eds.). (2001). *Multiple sclerosis: Current status and strategies for the future.* Washington, DC: National Academy Press.

Karnell, M. P., & MacCracken, E. (1994). A database information storage and reporting system for videofluorographic oropharyngeal motility (OPM) swallowing evaluations. *Journal of Speech–Language Pathology, 3*(2), 54–60.

Kinkel, R. P. (2000, October). Fatigue in multiple sclerosis. *International Journal of MS Care* (Suppl.), pp. 1–16.

Kirschner, H. S. (1989). Causes of neurogenic dysphagia. *Dysphagia, 3*(4), 184–188.

Kornblith, A. B., LaRocca, N. G., & Baum, H. M. (1986). Employment in individuals with multiple sclerosis. *International Journal of Rehabilitation Research, 9*(2), 155–165.

Kraft, G. H. (1998). Rehabilitation principles for patients with multiple sclerosis. *Journal of Spinal Cord Medicine, 21*(2), 117–120.

Kraft, G. H. (1999). Rehabilitation still the only way to improve function in multiple sclerosis. *Lancet, 354*(9195), 2016–2017.

Krupp, L. B., Alvarez, L. A., LaRocca, N. G., et al. (1988). Fatigue in multiple sclerosis. *Archives of Neurology, 45,* 435–437.

Kurtzke, J. F. (1983). Rating neurologic impairment in multiple sclerosis: An expanded disability status scale (EDSS). *Neurology, 33,* 1444–1452.

Kurtzke, J. F., & Page, W. F. (1997). Epidemiology of multiple sclerosis in US veterans: VII Risk factors for MS. *Neurology, 1*(489), 204–213.

LaRocca, N., Kalb, R., Scheinberg, L., & Kendall, P. (1985). Factors associated with unemployment of patients with multiple sclerosis. *Journal of Chronic Diseases, 38*(2), 203–210.

Lethlean, J. B., & Murdoch, B. E. (1993). Language problems in multiple sclerosis. *Journal of Medical Speech/Language Pathology, 1*(1), 47–59.

Logemann, J. (1983). *Evaluation and treatment of swallowing disorders.* Boston: College-Hill Press.

Lucchinetti, C., Bruck, W., & Noseworthy, J. H. (2001). Multiple sclerosis: Recent development in neuropathology, pathogenesis, magnetic resonance imaging studies and treatment. *Current Opinion in Neurology, 14,* 259–269.

Matthews, P. M., & Arnold, D. L. (2001). Magnetic resonance imaging of multiple sclerosis: New insights linking pathology to clinical evolution. *Current Opinion in Neurology, 14,* 279–287.

McDonald, W. I., Compston, A., Edan, G., Goodkin, D., Hartung, H. P., Lublin, F. D., McFarland, H. F., Paty, D. W., Polman, C. H., Reingold, S. C., Sandberg-Wolheim, M., Sibley, W. A., Thompson, A., van den Noort, S., Weinshenker, B. Y., & Wolinsky, J. S. (2001). Recommended criteria for multiple sclerosis: Guidelines from the international panel on the diagnosis of multiple sclerosis. *Annals of Neurology, 50*(1), 121–127.

Miller, D., & Multiple Sclerosis Council for Clinical Practice Guidelines. (1998). *Fatigue and multiple sclerosis: Evidence based management strategies for fatigue in multiple sclerosis.* Washington, DC: Paralyzed Veterans of America.

Miller, D. H., Grossman, R. I., Reingold, S. C., & McFarland, H. F. (1998). The role of magnetic resonance techniques in understanding and managing multiple sclerosis. *Brain, 121,* 3–24.

Minden, S. L., & Schiffer, R. B. (1990). Affective disorders in multiple sclerosis: Review and recommendations for clinical research. *Archives of Neurology, 47,* 98–104.

Mohr, D. C., & Cox, D. (2001). Multiple sclerosis: Empirical literature for the clinical health psychologist. *Journal of Clinical Psychology, 57*(4), 479–499.

Murdoch, B. E., & Lethlean, J. B. (2000). High-level language, naming and discourse abilities in multiple sclerosis. In B. Murdoch & D. G. Theodoros (Eds.), *Speech and language disorders in multiple sclerosis* (pp. 131–155). London: Whurr.

National MS Society. (2001). *National MS Society Disease Management Consensus Statement.* Retrieved October 18, 2001, from www.nationalmssociety.org

Neilly, L. K., Goodin, D. S., Goodkin, D. E., & Hauser, S. L. (1996). Side effect profile of interferon beta-1b in MS: Results of an open label trial. *Neurology, 46,* 552–554.

Noseworthy, J. H., Lucchinetti, C., Rodriguez, M., & Weinshenker, B. G. (2000). Multiple sclerosis. *New England Journal of Medicine, 343*(13), 938–952.

O'Day, B. (1998). Barriers for people with multiple sclerosis who want to work: A qualitative study. *Journal of Neurologic Rehabilitation, 12*(3), 139–146.

Polman, C., & Uitdehaag, B. M. J. (2000). Drug treatment of multiple sclerosis. *British Medical Journal, 321,* 490–494.

Porter, P. B. (1989). Intervention in end stage of multiple sclerosis: A case study. *Augmentative and Alternative Communication, 5*(2), 125–127.

Poser, C., Paty, D., Scheinberg, M., McDonald, W., Davis, F., Ebers, G., Johnson, K., Sibley, W., Silberg, D., & Tourtellotte, W. (1983). New diagnostic criteria for multiple sclerosis: Guidelines for research protocols. *Annals of Neurology, 13,* 227–231.

Poser, C. M., & Brinar, V. V. (2001). Diagnostic criteria for multiple sclerosis. *Clinical Neurology and Neurosurgery, 103*(1), 1–11.

Rao, S. M. (1986). Neuropsychology of multiple sclerosis: A critical review. *Journal of Clinical and Experimental Neuropsychology, 8,* 503–542.

Rao, S. M. (1995). Neuropsychology of multiple sclerosis. *Current Opinion in Neurology, 8,* 216–220.

Rao, S. M., Leo, G. J., Bernardin, L., & Unverzagt, F. (1991). Cognitive dysfunction in multiple sclerosis: I. Frequency, patterns and predictions. *Neurology, 41,* 658–691.

Reischies, F. M., Baum, K., Brau, H., & Hedde, J. P. (1988). Cerebral magnetic resonance imaging findings in multiple sclerosis: Relation to disturbance of affect, drive, and cognition. *Archives of Neurology, 45*(10), 1114–1116.

Richardson, J. T., Robinson, A., & Robinson, I. (1997). Cognition and multiple sclerosis: A historical analysis of medical perceptions. *Journal of the History of the Neurosciences, 6,* 302–319.

Robinson, J. E. (2000). Access to employment for people with disabilities: Findings of a consumer-led project. *Disability and Rehabilitation, 22*(5), 246–253.

Rovaris, M., & Filippi, M. (2000). MRI correlates of cognitive dysfunction in multiple sclerosis patients. *Journal of Neurovirology, 6*(Suppl. 2), S172–175.

Sapir, S., Pawlas, A., Ramig, L. O., Seeley, E., Fox, C., & Corboy, J. (2001). Effects of intensive phonatory–respiratory treatment (LSVT) on voice in two individuals with multiple sclerosis. *Journal of Medical Speech–Language Pathology, 9*(2), 141–151.

Schwartz, C. E., Coulthard-Morris, L., & Zeng, Q. (1996). Psychosocial correlates of fatigue in multiple sclerosis. *Archives of Physical Medicine and Rehabilitation, 77*, 165–170.

Selhorst, J. B., & Saul, R. F. (1995). Uhthoff and his symptom. *Journal of Neuroophthalmology, 15*(2), 63–69.

Soderstrom, M. (2001). Optic neuritis and multiple sclerosis. *Acta Ophthalmologica Scandinavica, 79*(3), 223–227.

Sullivan, M. J., Edgley, K., & Dehoux, E. (1990). A survey of multiple sclerosis. Part I: Perceived cognitive problems and compensatory strategies use. *Canadian Journal of Rehabilitation, 4*(2), 99–105.

Thomas, F. J., & Wiles, C. M. (1999). Dysphagia and nutritional status in multiple sclerosis. *Journal of Neurology, 246*, 677–682.

Thompson, A. J. (2000). The effectiveness of neurological rehabilitation in multiple sclerosis. *Journal of Rehabilitation Research & Development, 37*(4), 455–461.

Wallace, G. L., & Holmes, S. (1993). Cognitive–linguistic assessment of individuals with multiple sclerosis. *Archives of Physical Medicine and Rehabilitation, 74*, 637–643.

Walther, E. U., & Hohlfeld, R. (1999). Multiple sclerosis: Side effects of inteferon beta therapy and their management. *Neurology, 53*, 1622.

Weinstock-Guttman, B., & Jacobs, L. D. (2000). What is new in the treatment of multiple sclerosis? *Drugs, 59*(3), 401–410.

Wikstrom, J., Poser, S., & Ritter, G. (1980). Optic neuritis as an initial symptom in multiple sclerosis. *Acta Neurologica Scandinavica, 61*, 178–185.

Yorkston, K. M., Beukelman, D. R., Strand, E. A., & Bell, K. R. (1999). *Management of motor speech disorders in children and adults.* Austin, TX: PRO-ED.

Yorkston, K. M., Beukelman, D. R., & Tice, R. (1996). *Sentence Intelligibility Test.* Lincoln, NE: Tice Technology Services.

Yorkston, K. M., Klasner, E. R., & Swanson, K. M. (2001). Communication in context: A qualitative study of the experiences of individuals with multiple sclerosis. *American Journal of Speech–Language Pathology, 10*(2), 126–137.

Zakzanis, K. K. (2000). Distinct neurocognitive profiles in multiple sclerosis subtype. *Archives of Clinical Neuropsychology, 15*(2), 115–136.

Appendix

HANDOUTS FOR PATIENTS AND FAMILIES

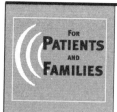

Normal Speech Production

► Normal speech is produced with a complex series of movements that combine breathing (respiration), producing a voice (phonation), forming speech sounds by constricting the airstream with the lips and tongue (articulation), producing a nasal or nonnasal sound (resonance), and adding stress and rhythm (prosody). Figure A.1 shows the structures that are used for speech. The muscles we use for breathing provide the energy source for speech. When speaking, you must be able to take in enough air and control how you release it through the vocal folds. The vocal folds (voice box) give sound to the air coming from the lungs. Air flowing between the moving vocal folds produces sound. Changes in the amount of air flowing through the vocal folds and in the position of the vocal folds produce pitch and loudness changes. The tongue, lips, jaw, and soft palate must then move rapidly and work together to make different speech sounds. Finally, so we don't sound monotonous, we add stress and rhythm to our speech. Doing all of this requires precise, rapid, and coordinated movements of the muscles in all the body parts used for speech.

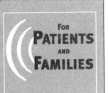

Normal Speech Production *(continued)*

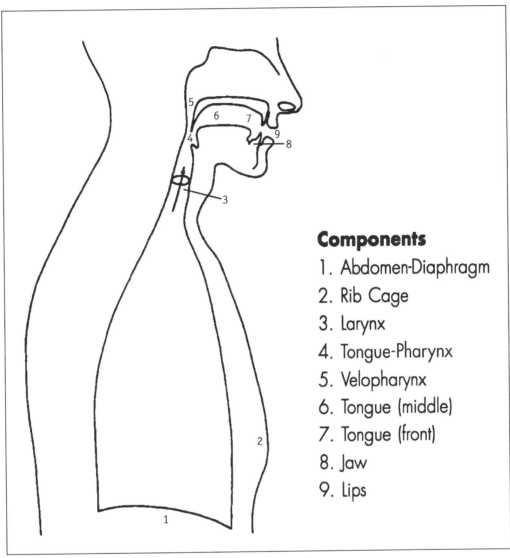

Components
1. Abdomen-Diaphragm
2. Rib Cage
3. Larynx
4. Tongue-Pharynx
5. Velopharynx
6. Tongue (middle)
7. Tongue (front)
8. Jaw
9. Lips

FIGURE A.1. Parts of the body used in speech.

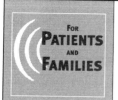

Dysarthria

▶ When we make the complex series of movements for speech, many muscles are active. These muscles must move in the right direction, with the right speed and force, and at the right time in order for speech to be clear and precise. When there is a problem with the brain that causes the muscles to be weak, to move slowly, or to not move together, speech will not sound normal and may be difficult to understand. This speech disorder is called *dysarthria*. There are different types of dysarthria, depending on what part or parts of the brain are affected. People who have a stroke, Parkinson disease, amyotrophic lateral sclerosis (ALS or Lou Gehrig's disease), multiple sclerosis, or Huntington disease may have dysarthria.

▶ Sometimes people who have dysarthria speak very slowly because their muscles are weak and do not move easily or quickly. This is often true for people who have ALS. Other people may seem to mumble and speak very fast because the lips, tongue, and jaw do not move very far. This sometimes happens with Parkinson disease. Other times, speech may sound slurred or uncoordinated. This is because the muscles cannot vary how hard they work or because they cannot move to exactly the right place at the right time.

▶ A person's voice often changes as well in dysarthria. People with Parkinson disease may have very quiet voices. In other diseases, such as Huntington disease, the loudness of the voice may change without warning. The person's voice can also sound breathy or hoarse if the vocal folds cannot come together all the way or with enough force. In some types of dysarthria, the voice may sound harsh or even "strangled." The voice can also

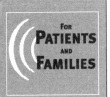
be changed when speakers are unable to produce a constant flow of air from the lungs through the larynx to make the vocal folds vibrate steadily.

▶ If the dysarthria becomes severe, you will be hard to understand. This means that sometimes other people will not be able to understand what you say. There are many things people with dysarthria can do if they are hard to understand. A speech–language pathologist may be able to help you speak more clearly through speech therapy. There are also ways to help your listeners understand you better. Finally, you can learn ways to change your surroundings to make understanding you easier—for example, by cutting out noise. Finally, alternative communication systems can be implemented.

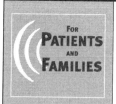

Normal Swallowing

▶ Normal swallowing occurs in four stages: the oral preparatory (chewing) stage, the oral (mouth) stage, the pharyngeal (throat) stage, and the esophageal (food tube) stage. In the oral preparatory stage, food is placed in the mouth and chewed. In the oral stage, the muscles of the tongue, cheeks, and upper part of the throat move the food to the back of the mouth. During the pharyngeal stage, the larynx (voice box) is drawn up toward the base of the tongue, and the tongue moves back to meet the larynx. The vocal folds then close to keep food from going into your windpipe. The soft palate (the back part of the roof of your mouth) lifts to close off the passage to the nose. A muscle at the top of the esophagus relaxes to allow food to enter the esophagus. During the esophageal stage, food is passed down the esophagus to the stomach through a wavelike action of the muscles.

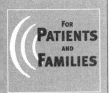

Disorders of Swallowing

▶ If you develop difficulty with swallowing (called *dysphagia*), problems may happen at any of the four stages of swallowing. Here are some symptoms you might have.

▶ Oral Preparatory and Oral Stage Difficulties

- Drooling or leaking of food and drink from the mouth
- Too much saliva
- Difficulty chewing
- Difficulty moving food to the back of the mouth

▶ Pharyngeal Stage Difficulties

- Difficulty starting the swallow reflex—you feel as if you try to swallow several times before you actually feel the food go down
- Nasal regurgitation—when the palate does not move fast or far enough, food may be pushed up into the nose
- A feeling of food "sticking in the throat" when the cricopharyngeus muscle doesn't relax to allow the food to pass into the esophagus
- Choking and coughing if the larynx and tongue don't move at the same time or don't move far enough to block off the windpipe
- *Aspiration pneumonia* happens when food or liquid has actually entered the lungs, perhaps causing an infection

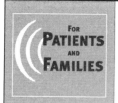

► ## Esophageal Stage Difficulties

Problems at the level of the esophagus are usually caused by blockage, food moving back up into the esophagus from the stomach (reflux), or pain, and are not usually related directly to the problem in the brain.

► ## Slowed Eating

A more common complaint is that, with weakened muscles, it takes a lot longer to eat a meal. Because of the length of time it takes, many people do not eat enough, so they lose weight and don't get the proper nutrition.

► ## Warning Signs of a Swallowing Problem

Here is a list of some warning signs that you might be at risk for or have a swallowing problem. If you notice any of these problems, your swallowing should be checked carefully by a speech–language pathologist or other professional.

- You choke or cough when you eat or drink.
- You lose weight.
- You notice drooling.
- Mealtimes take much longer than they used to.
- You no longer enjoy eating.
- You have difficulty chewing food.
- You have to try several times to start a swallow—food seems to "stick in your throat."
- You have a history of pneumonia.

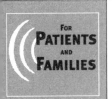
► There probably won't be a cure for your swallowing problem, but there are many things you can do to cope with and lessen the problem. A speech–language pathologist will be able to give you ideas that are likely to help you.

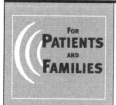

Amyotrophic Lateral Sclerosis (ALS)

▶ Amyotrophic lateral sclerosis is a progressive disease that damages or destroys motor neurons. *Motor neurons* are the nerve cells in the brain that control movement. *Upper motor neurons* start in the higher centers of the brain (cerebral cortex) and carry information to the *lower motor neurons*, which are in the brain stem and spinal cord. The lower motor neurons carry messages to your muscles. You need upper motor neurons for voluntary control of your muscles. If the upper motor neurons are damaged, your muscles become *spastic* (too tight), and your reflexes become too strong. When a lower motor neuron is damaged, then messages cannot be sent out to the muscle it controls, and the muscle becomes *flaccid* (floppy and weak). You may see *atrophy* (wasting away of muscle tissue). The name "motor neuron disease" has been given to several diseases in adults, including ALS, progressive bulbar palsy, spinal muscular atrophy, and primary lateral sclerosis.

The first symptoms of ALS vary, depending on whether upper or lower motor neurons are damaged, and, if lower motor neurons are damaged, on whether these nerve cells are in the brain stem or the spinal cord. The motor neurons that go to the spinal cord control the muscles of your arms and legs. Motor neurons that go to the brain stem control the muscles of your face, tongue, and throat. When the nerve cells in the spinal cord are damaged, you will have less strength and range of movement in your arms and legs. When the nerve cells in the brain stem are damaged, you will have difficulty chewing, swallowing, coughing, and speaking. So two people who have ALS may have very different signs and symptoms. Usually symptoms begin in one arm or leg, later spreading to other limbs or to the muscles of the face and tongue. Sometimes the symptoms start in the face,

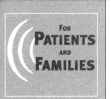
and later move to the arms and legs. Your senses of touch, sight, and hearing are not affected, however. Intelligence and awareness usually remain intact as well. Personality changes are not usually seen.

The cause of ALS is unknown. About 5% to 10% of the time ALS runs in the family, but most of the time it does not. ALS affects adults, usually between the ages of 30 and 60 years. It happens slightly more often in men than women. ALS may progress rapidly or it may plateau for varying lengths of time. There is no known medical or surgical treatment or cure. Therapy is given to help you keep as much strength as possible; to provide you with wheelchairs, communication aids, and other aids; and to teach you how to compensate for your illness.

▶ How ALS Affects Speech

In ALS the muscles can be spastic (too much muscle tone) or flaccid (too little muscle tone). In either case, movement of the muscles is weaker. This causes your movements to be slower and reduced in range. If you have movement problems in the muscles that produce speech, you will have changes in speech that may make your speech hard to understand.

The changes in speech that we hear depend on which speech muscles are affected. If the muscles for breathing are affected, you may have less breath support for speech. If this is the case, you may have difficulty shouting, speaking in a noisy place, or speaking long sentences on a single breath. You may also feel tired after talking for a long time.

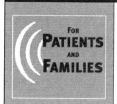

Amyotrophic Lateral Sclerosis (ALS) *(continued)*

If your vocal folds (voice box) are spastic (too tight) and not able to come together smoothly, your voice may sound harsh or strained and strangled. If your vocal folds do not have the strength to come together properly, your voice may sound breathy or harsh. The pitch of your voice may also be too low or too high. When the vocal folds do not move apart as they should, you may hear a "voice" when you breathe in.

Weakness in the muscles of the lips, tongue, jaw, and soft palate (back of the roof of your mouth) may make it difficult to say consonants and vowels clearly, making your speech sound slurred and at times hard to understand. Your voice may also sound very nasal, and air may actually come out of your nose when you speak. ALS speech is frequently slow, labored, and reduced in stress.

▶ How Speech Changes as ALS Gets Worse

You may or may not have had speech problems when you were diagnosed with ALS. But many people will, at some point in their illness, begin to notice changes in voice or start to have problems making speech sounds. Speech changes do not occur in the same way or at the same rate for everyone with ALS because the pattern of nerve cell damage is different for each person. Voice symptoms will usually start with hoarseness, or with your voice sounding more monotonous. Hoarseness may worsen into a "strained-strangled" quality if the muscles are too tight (spastic). On the other hand, your voice may become breathier if the muscles are floppy (flaccid). Often, as your illness progresses,

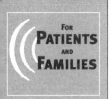
the muscles that open the vocal folds become more involved, making it hard to open the vocal folds all the way. This can cause noise when you breathe in or out deeply.

Speech symptoms will usually start with weakness of the tongue, and then the lips. Sounds like *p*, *t*, and *k* that stop the air all the way become more difficult to make. Because the soft palate gets weak, it won't move as easily to block the flow of air into the nose, so your speech may sound nasal. If the speech symptoms get severe, then tongue movement will be so poor that it will be difficult to make vowel sounds, and your speech will become very difficult to understand.

▶ What Can Be Done About These Speech Problems

A variety of options are available for coping with speech problems. Which one is most appropriate depends on what aspects of speech production are contributing to the speech problems. The best option will also depend on how severe the speech problems are. In order to develop the best plan for managing your speech problems, a thorough evaluation should be completed by a certified speech–language pathologist.

Usually, the speech–language pathologist will help you compensate for your speech problems so your speech is as easy to understand as possible. For example, if the movement of your tongue and soft palate is lessened, opening your jaw farther can sometimes help make your voice sound less nasal and make your vowel sounds clearer. Finding the posture that is easiest to speak in, using shorter phrases, and being aware of when to take breaths are all examples of ways to compensate for poor breath support. It is

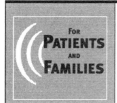
important that a certified speech–language pathologist teach you these strategies and supervise you as you learn them, to make sure you get the best possible treatment.

Some augmentative communication aids may also help you if the dysarthria (speech problem) becomes very severe. *Augmentative communication* means anything that supplements or replaces speech—such as a picture board or gestures or a talking computer. If you can still use your arms and fingers, you might use an alphabet board to point to the first letter of each word you say, giving your listener some context to guess the word you said. If your speech becomes so bad that you cannot be understood at all, no matter how hard you try, you might use a portable typing system to prepare printed messages. Or you might use a computerized system that produces artificial speech. Computers that produce "speech" make it possible (but sometimes difficult) to talk on the telephone.

▶ How ALS Affects Swallowing

With ALS the muscles used for swallowing are weakened. As a result, you may experience swallowing difficulties (dysphagia). Your symptoms will depend on where the weakness is. If you have weakness and lessened range of motion in the tongue, you will have difficulty with the oral phase of swallowing. It may be difficult to move the food around in the mouth for chewing and then to move it to the back of the mouth and into the throat. If the muscles of the throat (pharyngeal wall) are weak, there may be difficulty with the muscle action that pushes the food down, causing food to feel like it's "sticking" in your throat. Thin liquids (like water) can be difficult to manage if your tongue and

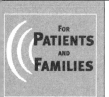
lips are weak. Liquid may escape between the lips, causing drooling. Because the muscles will have difficulty directing the liquid to the right place, it may "go down the wrong pipe" and cause choking. The vocal folds not only produce your voice, they also close when you swallow to keep food or drink from getting into your windpipe and lungs. If the vocal folds are weak, your cough may be weak and may not do a good job of protecting your windpipe. Just as with your speech, no one can cure your swallowing problems. But there are many things you can learn to do to compensate for your swallowing problems.

As your illness gets worse, you may reach a point when you cannot swallow food and liquid anymore. This may happen because the danger becomes too great that food or liquid will get into your lungs, which can cause pneumonia. Or it may become so difficult to eat that you simply cannot eat enough to meet your nutritional needs. At this point, many people with ALS begin to dread mealtimes. If you reach this point, you may wish to consider taking your food by a tube rather than by mouth. A tube can be inserted from your nose to your stomach (nasogastric) or from your mouth to your stomach (orogastric) without surgery. Most people find it more comfortable in the long run to have surgery to insert a tube directly into your stomach (gastrostomy). The most common type of tube currently used is the PEG (percutaneous endoscopic gastrostomy). This tube is inserted permanently, directly into your stomach. A small portion of the tube is taped down on your abdomen so that you can easily access it to take your liquid meal. It can't be seen under your clothes. You will still be able to eat normally, if you like, and use the tube to make sure you get enough liquid and calories each day. Some people like the PEG because it "takes the pressure

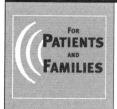

Amyotrophic Lateral Sclerosis (ALS) *(continued)*

off" getting enough food orally. If you are considering tube feeding, your doctor will tell you about the advantages and disadvantages of each type of tube and help you select the best treatment.

Keep in mind that having a feeding tube does not prevent you from eating by mouth. Many people with ALS will eat for enjoyment and supplement eating with tube feedings. Others will use the tube to meet their fluid needs. Other people will use the tube only when they are in a hurry and would prefer not to take the time to eat a full meal. Although the decision to use tube feeding is almost always a difficult one, most people with ALS are pleased with the result. Many indicate that it takes some of the burden of eating off their shoulders.

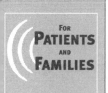

Parkinson Disease

▶ Parkinson disease is a progressive neurologic disease caused by problems in the basal ganglia of the brain. There is a shortage of a neurotransmitter called *dopamine* in part of the basal ganglia called the *substantia nigra*. The lack of dopamine causes certain symptoms. The three most common ones are tremor (shaking), bradykinesia (slow movement), and rigidity (stiffness). The tremor or shaking seen in Parkinson disease is called *resting tremor*. It usually appears first as small shaking movements or "pill-rolling" movements in the hands. Later, the tremor may show up in the arms, the neck, and the legs. The tremor may get worse when you are tired or under stress, and it often lessens or stops during sleep or when you move.

Bradykinesia means slowness of movement and difficulty beginning a movement. For example, someone with Parkinson disease may have difficulty lifting one leg to begin a step. Many automatic movements are reduced, such as swinging your arms when walking or making facial expressions. Sometimes people with Parkinson disease are described as having a "masklike" expression because they look as if they are feeling no emotion. However, this lack of facial expression is really just caused by the bradykinesia.

Rigidity is the term used for increased muscle tone, or stiffness of the muscles. This makes it harder to move a limb quickly through its range of motion. For example, if you try to move the arm of an individual with Parkinson disease quickly up and down around the elbow, it will "catch" every so often, much the way a cogwheel behaves.

Some people with Parkinson disease have the biggest problems with bradykinesia and may also suffer some difficulty with

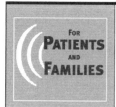
thinking skills (termed *cognitive impairment*). Other people with Parkinson disease have mostly tremor and much less impairment in their cognitive skills. Parkinson disease is progressive, but the rate of progression may be slow and varies greatly from person to person. Although there is no cure for Parkinson disease, there are medications that reduce some of the symptoms of the disease.

▶ How Parkinson Disease Affects Speech

Parkinson disease may affect any or all of the movements of speech production. The three movement problems discussed before—tremor, bradykinesia, and rigidity—affect the muscles you use for speech just as they do the rest of the body. The result is slurred and unclear speech called *dysarthria*. Dysarthria happens when the speech muscles can't move far enough or with enough speed or strength to make the very fine adjustments needed for speech. About 70% of people with Parkinson disease report that their speech and voice are affected by the disease. Although everyone's speech and voice are affected somewhat differently, some characteristics are common in this disease. If the voice is affected, it is usually softer and somewhat breathy or hoarse. Many people notice slurring of the consonant sounds in speech. Also, some people with Parkinson disease sound as if they are speaking very fast because the muscles are moving with greatly reduced range of motion.

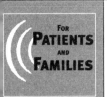

Parkinson Disease *(continued)*

▶ How Speech Changes as Parkinson Disease Gets Worse

Not everyone with Parkinson disease notices speech changes. Speech changes are rarely among the first symptoms of the disease, but may show up many years after diagnosis has been made. The first speech-related symptom typically appears in the voice. The voice gets softer, may sound hoarse or breathy, and may lack expression. As the dysarthria gets worse, speech sounds may become slurred. Movements of the tongue, lips, and soft palate may be limited, and speaking rate may become very rapid. If these symptoms are severe, speech may become difficult to understand. In severe cases, people have difficulty beginning to speak.

▶ What Can Be Done About These Speech Problems

There are several options for people with parkinsonian dysarthria. The best option for you depends on the nature and severity of your particular speech problems. In order to develop the best plan for managing speech problems, a complete evaluation should be completed by a certified speech–language pathologist. Although the problems causing your speech difficulty cannot be cured, a speech–language pathologist can help you learn to adjust for these difficulties and speak more clearly. For example, you might be taught how to speak with a louder voice and with more emphasis. Changing speech habits and bringing your speech under voluntary control requires that you put time and effort into a practice routine. These practice routines should be developed and supervised by a certified speech–language

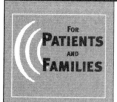
pathologist. A number of devices such as portable speech amplifiers or delayed auditory feedback devices (used to slow speaking rate) are helpful to some people.

People whose speech problems are very severe may use an augmentative communication system. *Augmentative communication* means anything that supplements or replaces speech—such as a picture board or gestures or a talking computer. If you can still use your arms and fingers, you might use an alphabet board to point to the first letter of each word you say, giving your listener some context to guess the word you said. If your speech becomes so bad that you cannot be understood at all, no matter how hard you try, you might use a portable typing system to prepare printed messages. Or you might use a computerized system that produces artificial speech. Computers that produce "speech" make it possible (but sometimes difficult) to talk on the telephone.

▶ How Parkinson Disease Affects Swallowing

In Parkinson disease, any stage of swallowing may be affected. The muscles of the tongue may be rigid, making it difficult to move the food around in the mouth to chew it. Chewing may take longer than normal, and it may be difficult to start a swallow. Swallowing saliva is normally automatic, but you can begin to swallow less often in Parkinson disease. This may cause drooling. The parts of the swallow in which food is moved into the throat and down to the esophagus may be delayed.

A swallowing disorder is of concern because many people with Parkinson disease are unaware of the difficulty, thus placing themselves at risk for sucking food or liquid into the lungs

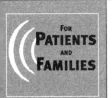

Parkinson Disease *(continued)*

(known as *aspiration*). Aspiration is dangerous because it can cause pneumonia and serious infections. Sometimes people with Parkinson disease deny having problems, even when family members notice them and point them out. People with swallowing problems also find it difficult to maintain their weight and to drink enough liquid every day. Over time, they can develop dehydration and serious malnutrition. A speech–language pathologist or occupational therapist can help you change the way you eat by changing your diet to those foods that are easiest and safest to manage.

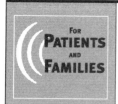

Huntington Disease

► Huntington disease is a progressive, hereditary, neurologic disorder. The disease usually appears in midlife and occurs in 4 to 7 people out of every 100,000. One symptom of the disease is *chorea*, which is excessive, random, and irregular movements. This symptom is caused by an imbalance of chemicals in the basal ganglia of the brain. There is too little of a transmitter called GABA, which causes overactive movement.

The symptoms of Huntington disease include changes in cognitive (thinking) skills and increasingly more debilitating movement disorders. Initially, there may be personality changes and unintentional movements. In later stages, the cognitive changes may progress to dementia (confusion) and memory loss. In addition to the chorea, rigidity (stiffness of muscles) may be present. You may also hear the term *dystonia*, which means abnormal writhing-like movements caused by frequent, maintained contraction of muscles.

► How Huntington Disease Affects Speech

The chorea that people with Huntington disease experience causes unpredicted, uncontrolled, and involuntary contractions of muscle groups. This causes your body to move even when you don't want it to. When these movements happen in the structures you use for speech (like your lips and tongue), the result is dysarthria. *Dysarthria* is a speech problem that happens when the muscles of speech are weak or cannot move with the right speed, direction, force, or coordination needed to make the correct sounds. People with Huntington disease may have difficulty controlling the movements of the breathing muscles, vocal folds (voice box), lips, tongue, and jaw.

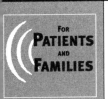

Huntington Disease *(continued)*

The symptoms of the speech problem in people who have Huntington disease are quite variable. People usually will have episodes of hypernasality (too much air going through the nose) and harshness of the voice. There will be unplanned and unexpected increases in loudness and pitch. Some consonants and vowels will sound distorted. As they try to compensate for these unintended movements, their rate of speech will change. They may stretch out sounds and syllables and will tend to use equal stress. There may be sudden forced taking in or letting out of air.

► How Speech Changes as Huntington Disease Gets Worse

Although Huntington disease is a progressive neurologic disease, symptoms don't appear in a particular order. How much speech is affected varies considerably from person to person. Some individuals have chorea only in the limbs, and their speech is not affected. For other people, speech may be severely impaired to the point where alternative systems of communication need to be used. Most people with Huntington disease fall somewhere in the middle. As a rule, however, if the abnormal movements that occur with this disease are getting worse in the muscles of the face and throat, then speaking will likely become more difficult. Nothing can be done to get rid of the changes in the speech muscles. However, therapists called speech–language pathologists can teach you techniques that can help you deal with these problems.

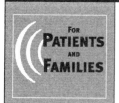

Huntington Disease *(continued)*

▶ What Can Be Done About These Speech Problems

Some individuals with Huntington disease have only mild changes in their speech, and people can still easily understand them. If you have mild dysarthria like this, therapists may work on muscle relaxation and teach you ways to control your stress and intonation. If your speech is more severely affected, therapists will teach you ways to improve your speech and, at the same time, teach you ways to modify your surroundings to make speaking easier for you. The therapist may also teach the people who often talk with you some tricks that will help them understand your speech better. If your speech becomes very bad, augmentative communication may be helpful. *Augmentative communication* means any system such as pictures, a word board, a computer, or gestures that you can use in addition to or instead of speech. It is important to remember, however, that difficulties in thinking or in language skills will affect how you talk and may make it difficult to learn a new system of communication.

▶ How Huntington Disease Affects Swallowing

Swallowing is a problem for many but not all people who have Huntington disease. Swallowing problems vary, depending on how severe the unpredictable movements are and where they occur. For example, if extra movement occurs in the breathing system, the swallow may be out of time with your breathing. Extra movement of the tongue, lips, and jaw will affect how you chew and how easily you can get the food to the back of your mouth to swallow it. Changes in judgment and perception may cause you to take bites that are too large or to eat foods that are not safe.

220

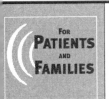
It is also sometimes difficult for individuals with Huntington disease to stay in a position in which it is easy to swallow. An upright position with the head bent slightly toward your chin is the best position. But it may be hard to stay in that position if you have constant movement. Sometimes you may have difficulty getting food from the plate to your mouth because of all the extra movement. You will also need to get lots of calories due to all the extra movement. It is sometimes difficult to eat enough calories because of the extra time it takes to eat. Management of swallowing problems may be difficult in this disease. There are, however, some ways to compensate for or deal with these problems. A certified speech–language pathologist or occupational therapist can help you eat well and safely.

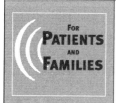

Multiple Sclerosis (MS)

▶ In multiple sclerosis, the myelin or "white matter" in the nervous system begins to break down. Myelin is a sheath or cover over your nerve fibers that helps information get from nerve cell to nerve cell properly. When lesions, or holes, appear in the white matter, this causes a breakdown in nerve impulses, that is, the messages going from nerve to nerve. The result is sensory and motor problems. These disruptions or breakdowns can change how the nervous system works in many ways. For example, if your nerves are too easily excited, you may feel a burning or prickling sensation. If your nerves do not stay active long enough, the result may be muscle weakness.

It is most common for MS to be diagnosed in early to middle adulthood. The disease may be diagnosed after sudden onset of a few mild symptoms, followed by a reduction in these symptoms. Bouts of more severe symptoms are called *exacerbations*. Periods when the symptoms become milder are called *remissions*. Some people have no recurrence of the symptoms and no permanent limitations in their activities. More often, the disease gets slowly worse with periods of exacerbation and remission. A smaller number of people with MS have chronic, or ongoing, illness leading to significant disability within 2 to 10 years.

A variety of symptoms may occur with MS, depending on the size, location, and activity of the nerve fiber lesions at a particular time. If the spinal cord is involved, you may have weakness, spasticity (muscle tightness), some numbness, and bladder and bowel difficulties. If the brain stem (lowest part of the brain) is affected, you may have difficulty swallowing and speaking. If the parts of the brain known as the cerebellum and basal ganglia are involved, ataxia (incoordination) and tremor may occur. Some

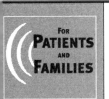
people see changes in their behavior and thinking skills (cognition) if there is damage in the cortex of the brain. Every person with MS will have different patterns of difficulty and a different progression of symptoms.

At the present time there is no cure for MS, although some drugs may reduce the number and severity of exacerbations. Medical management during a flare-up includes supportive measures such as rest, bladder and bowel management, swallowing precautions, and treatment of dizziness and nausea. Many medications can be used to treat the symptoms and allow you to carry out your daily activities.

▶ How MS Affects Speech

Many people who are diagnosed with multiple sclerosis may at some point have difficulty with their speech because of the movement problems they experience. This speech disorder, called *dysarthria*, happens when muscles are weak and do not move as far, as fast, or with the coordination that is needed for precise speech. Dysarthria typically involves many parts of the system used to produce speech, including the tongue, lips, jaw, and soft palate (back part of the roof of the mouth). Because many parts of the brain may be affected in multiple sclerosis, the pattern of speech difficulties is likely to differ from person to person—or may change over time for any one person. Several speech symptoms are commonly seen in multiple sclerosis. It may be difficult to control the loudness of your voice, and your volume may change at inappropriate times without your control. Similar problems may happen to the pitch of your voice. Your consonants may not sound "quite right" because of weakness or

223

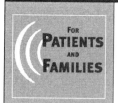

incoordination of the muscles used to move the lips, tongue, or soft palate. Your speech may sound slurred or uncoordinated. Hypernasality (too much air going through the nose) is also possible. Your voice may also sound hoarse or harsh. Some people have what is called "scanning speech," in which they speak very slowly and seem to pause after every syllable.

▶ How Speech Changes as MS Worsens

Because the disease may get worse and then get better for awhile and because so many different parts of the brain may be involved, it is difficult to describe how speech changes as multiple sclerosis progresses. If the disease worsens, however, some changes in speech are typical. For example, as muscles become weaker or movement becomes less coordinated, speech sounds will be harder to make. They will sound more and more distorted. Voice changes are also common as the disease gets worse. The voice may sound increasingly hoarse or harsh, and the pitch may be too high or too low. The voice may also sound "shaky." That is, it may sound wavering due to tremor. Sometimes, these speech changes make it harder for others to understand you. There are some things that can be done to help you be more easily understood or to provide other ways for you to communicate.

▶ What Can Be Done About These Speech Problems

Speech therapy can often be helpful for people who have dysarthria. The type of therapy that is best depends on whether the speech problem is mild, moderate, or severe. If your speech is only mildly affected, therapy might help you conserve your

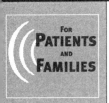
energy and control your pitch and loudness to make your speech sound more natural.

Many people with moderate dysarthria due to multiple sclerosis will have difficulty coordinating respiration (breathing) with voice and articulation (making consonant and vowel sounds). There are many ways therapists can help you control your use of the outgoing airstream for speech. Work on controlling rate is also often helpful. Helping you adjust your phrasing and breath patterns can often help to improve intelligibility. For people with severe dysarthria, augmentative communication is often recommended. *Augmentative communication* means any system such as a picture or word board, a computer, or gestures that you can use with speech or instead of speech.

▶ How MS Affects Swallowing

Because of all the different types of nerve damage in MS, swallowing symptoms are quite variable. Both spasticity (too much stiffness in the muscles) and ataxia (incoordination) may contribute to swallowing problems. There may be slowness of movement or incoordination of movement during the oral stage of swallowing (chewing the food and moving it back to the throat). It may be difficult to swallow food easily, causing the feeling of food "sticking" in your throat.

Other problems that may go along with MS, such as urinary tract infections and fever, may cause *decomposition*, that is, a big reduction of abilities in other areas. Sometimes this happens with swallowing. If a person who has been swallowing fine catches a severe infection, it may result in temporary difficulties

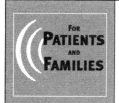

Multiple Sclerosis (MS) *(continued)*

in swallowing. Some people who experience cognitive (thinking) changes may have difficulty swallowing because of changes in judgment. They may take bites that are too big or choose foods that are difficult to chew and swallow. Sensory problems, such as lack of feeling or pain, may interfere with swallowing.

When MS is severe, lessened ability to take air into the lungs and weakness of the vocal folds (voice box) may cause a weak and inefficient cough. This makes it hard to cough out food or drink that goes down "the wrong pipe." It is important to be aware that this may be a problem because food or drink getting into the lungs can cause pneumonia.

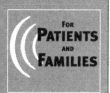

Tips for Understanding Severely Dysarthric Speech

▶ **Controlling the Communication Environment**

1. Make sure the area is as free of distractions as possible. For example, the room should be quiet.

2. Watch the speaker.

3. Attend to communication and don't try to accomplish other tasks at the same time.

▶ **Setting the Stage for Interaction**

1. Be honest and acknowledge the difficulty you are having understanding.

2. Express a sincere interest in understanding the message.

3. Ask permission to jump in by asking questions and giving prompts when necessary.

4. Ask for the topic of the message so you can use context cues to help you.

▶ **Prompting the Speaker**

1. Signal when you have not understood.

2. Repeat the part of the message that you have understood. That way, the speaker doesn't have to say that part again.

3. Ask the speaker to repeat the message in exactly the same way.

4. If you still can't understand, give some prompts, such as "Say it slower next time" or "Please try to say it louder."

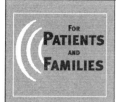
Try making this suggestion: _____

_____

_____

5. If this fails, prompt the speaker to use an alternative system for the part of the message that you cannot understand. Examples include spelling the words out loud or pointing to an alphabet board.

Try using this alternative system: _____

_____

_____

6. Ask targeted yes/no questions to try to complete the message.

7. Acknowledge the failure and say that you will try again later.

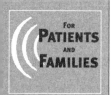

Ways You Can Compensate for Dysarthria

▶ The following suggestions may help if your speech is sometimes difficult to understand. Some suggestions help you talk more clearly; others give your listeners extra clues to help them figure out your message. The checked items are likely to be the best ones for you.

_____ 1. *Speak loudly and slowly.* Concentrate on speaking loudly and clearly. Using extra effort when you speak allows others to hear you better, and also slows your speaking rate. Using loud, slow speech prevents slurring of speech sounds and allows you to add expression to your speech. You may feel as if you are shouting, but others will feel that your speech is more normal if you speak loudly.

_____ 2. *Make your surroundings as "friendly" as possible.* Some communication environments are more difficult than others. Avoid carrying out important conversations in noisy places or in places where your listener cannot watch you as you speak—for example, in dimly lit rooms or in places where your listener is a long distance from you.

_____ 3. *Enlist the help of your listener.* Conversation is a partnership. Be sure to get as much help as you can from your communication partners. For example, ask others to let you know when they can't understand you. In that way you will know when you need to speak more loudly and clearly. With people you talk to often, you might come up with a hand signal they can use instead of interrupting to say, "I don't understand."

229

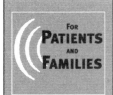
Ways You Can Compensate
for Dysarthria *(continued)*

_____ 4. *Provide context or background for what you are saying.* Knowing the topic of conversation makes it much easier for your listener to "fill in the gaps" when speech is slightly distorted.

_____ 5. *Consider how well people around you hear.* A hearing loss may make your speech very difficult to understand. Make sure that people you talk with often have had their hearing tested if you suspect a hearing problem. Properly fitted hearing aids may make your speech more understandable to them.

_____ 6. *Alphabet board supplementation.* Using a board of alphabet letters, you can point to the first letter of each word as you say it. This makes you talk more slowly, allowing weak muscles more time to form the precise movements of the speech sounds. It also gives your listener information to figure out which word you are saying. If your listener still doesn't understand when you give the first letter, you can resort to spelling out the entire word.

_____ 7. *When to seek more help.* If you cannot change your speech without help and you are having difficulty making yourself understood, it may be time to seek more help. A certified speech–language pathologist can evaluate your speech problems and recommend techniques or devices to make communication easier for you.

_____ 8. *Time important conversations with medication cycles.* Some people with Parkinson disease experience movement problems that get better or worse depending on how

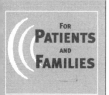

long it has been since they last took their medications. Try to carry out important conversations at the "peak" point in your drug cycle.

_____ 9. *Separate words and phrases with little pauses.* If you pause between words or phrases, your listener will have more clues about when a new word is starting. Some people with Parkinson disease speak too rapidly. Adding some silent time between words also helps to keep you from talking too quickly.

_____ 10. *Exaggerate speech sounds.* Exaggerating the movements of your mouth and tongue gives the weakened muscles time to make the proper movements for different speech sounds. Pay particular attention to emphasizing final sounds in words.

_____ 11. *Compensating for poor breath support.* You may find that your voice gets quieter because it's harder to take a full breath, especially if you have ALS. You may find that people often ask you to "speak up." If this is the case, shorten the number of words you speak on one breath. It is generally a good idea to take a breath before you absolutely need to. If you try to talk as long as you can on one breath, the last several words are usually "squeezed out" only with a lot of effort. This extra effort can be very tiring, and the final words are often hard to understand. If your muscles continue to get weaker, these compensations may no longer be enough. At this time, a speech–language pathologist may recommend amplification. You simply speak into a microphone, which can be hand held, worn around the neck,

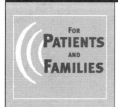
or attached to eyeglasses or a headband, and your voice is made louder by way of a small pocket amplifier.

_____ 12. *Palatal lift prosthesis.* A common complaint in ALS and some other illnesses is extremely nasal speech or fatigue in speaking because of loss of air through the nose. The nasal speech and air leakage are caused by weakened muscles in the palate (roof of the mouth) and upper throat. The soft palate does not rise far enough to close off the passage between the nose and mouth. A speech–language pathologist might fit you with a palatal lift in order to compensate for this problem. The palatal lift consists of a dental retainer secured to the teeth. A shelf attached to the retainer lifts the soft palate, reducing the nasality and nasal air escape. Note that this device is rarely helpful to people with ALS, because they also have difficulty with tongue and lip movement that makes their speech difficult to understand.

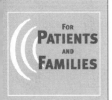

Augmentative Communication

► When speech is no longer meeting important communication needs or when speaking is effortful and tiring, communication is more efficient using alternative means. If you have little or no arm or hand weakness, handwriting is a good way to clarify misunderstandings. Handwriting is the most natural, accessible, and portable means of alternative communication. Handwriting is also more rapid and obviously less expensive than any mechanical or electronic communication device.

If your arm and hand muscles are so weak that handwriting is very difficult or impossible, or hard to read, the speech–language pathologist may introduce an augmentative communication approach. Augmentative communication may include boards or books containing pictures and words, electronic devices, or other strategies. Because of ever-changing computer-based technology, the number and flexibility of augmentative communication devices continue to increase. Generally, however, there are three types of systems: direct selection, scanning, and encoding. *Direct selection* systems require that you have enough control of your movements to make a variety of choices by pointing to or touching specific items. An example of a direct selection system is a typewriter or computer keyboard. *Scanning* systems require less physical control. In this case, the computer (or your communication partner) would move through all the options one at a time. You would indicate when the correct item is reached by activating a switch, nodding to your partner, or signaling in some other manner. *Encoding* systems require very little movement on your part. Each pattern of responses is a code that indicates a specific message, word, or letter. An example of an encoding system is the Morse code system.

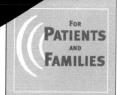
Augmentative Communication (*continued*)

► The type of augmentative communication approach you and your therapist select will depend in part on your physical capabilities. Equally as important in the decision, however, are your specific communication needs: whether you need to communicate at work, with your family, with friends in social situations, and so on. You can imagine that a communication device that allows you to communicate basic needs and self-care requests to relatives and friends who know you well would be quite different from a communication device that allows you to express lengthy, complex messages to strangers in a work setting.

In identifying specific communication needs, you and your therapist will consider (a) what messages you need to communicate, (b) what your listeners need in order to understand, and (c) the environments in which you need to communicate. Here is an example of a checklist to decide on your communication needs:

_____ Do I need to call attention?

_____ Do I need to signal an emergency?

_____ Do I need to ask for basic needs?

_____ Do I need to prepare new messages all the time?

_____ Do I need to prepare lengthy, complex messages?

_____ Do I need to communicate with strangers?

_____ Do I need to communicate in groups?

_____ Do I need to communicate over the phone?

_____ Do I need to communicate with people who are hard of hearing?

_____ Do I need to communicate with people who have difficulty seeing?

____ Do I need to communicate in a wheelchair?

____ Do I need to communicate in bed?

____ Do I need to communicate outdoors?

____ Do I need to communicate in a work setting?

The time may never come when your speech is no longer useful or requires too much effort to use as your only means of communication. However, knowing your physical capabilities and communication needs, the speech–language pathologist will be able to select an appropriate augmentative communication device should you need one.

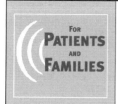

Ways You Can Compensate for Swallowing Difficulties

▶ Because neurologic disorders affect each person differently, all of the following suggestions may not be helpful to you. Also, in degenerative diseases, what may be appropriate at the present may very well change as the disease progresses. You should stay in regular contact with a physician, speech–language pathologist, and dietitian to keep track of your swallowing program. These suggestions might make eating easier for you and lower your risk of choking and aspiration (getting food or liquid in your lungs). The checked items may be the best ones for you.

____ *Sit upright.* Sitting upright in your chair while eating is generally the best position for safe swallowing.

____ *Take small bites.* Place only small amounts of food or liquid in your mouth. Use a teaspoon or small plastic spoon rather than a soup spoon (even for soup). If you are drinking through a straw, take one sip at a time, hold it in your mouth, then swallow.

____ *Think "swallow."* Hold the food or drink in your mouth and think about swallowing, then swallow!

____ *One bite at a time.* Be sure you swallow all the food or drink in your mouth before putting more in. Bits of food can collect in your mouth and cause choking later.

____ *Concentrate.* Always eat slowly and carefully, concentrate only on eating, and don't watch TV or engage in conversation at the same time.

____ *Keep your chin down.* Keeping your chin down as you swallow may make the swallow easier and will lower the chance of food trickling into the windpipe. See the pictures of correct and incorrect swallowing positions (Figure A.2).

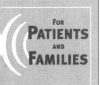
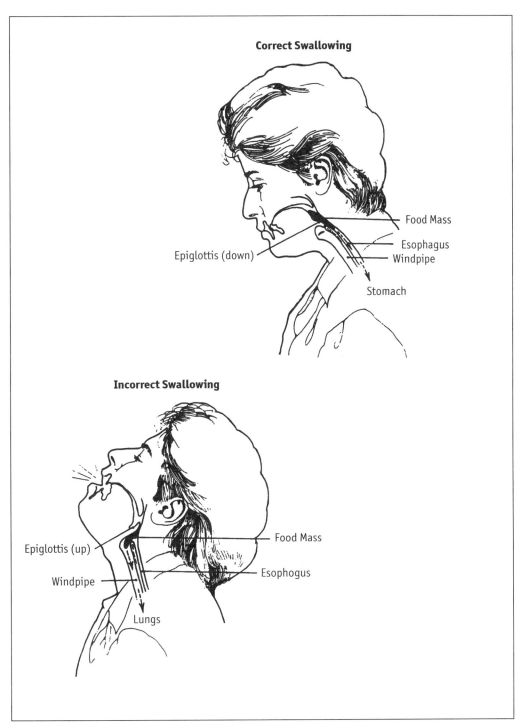

FIGURE A.2. Correct and incorrect swallowing postures.

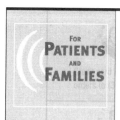
_____ *Place food in the back of your mouth.* If moving food to the back of your mouth is difficult, put the food as far back on your tongue as possible. If the muscles on one side of your face are weak, place the food on the stronger side of your tongue. If your lip muscles are weak, letting food leak out of your mouth, try pinching your lips together with your fingers.

_____ *Eat often.* Eating six small meals rather than three large meals keeps you from tiring your already weakened muscles. Make the most of the time you spend eating by eating nutritious items, not empty calories. It is more efficient to spend the same amount of time and energy drinking a milk shake or eggnog than drinking coffee or tea.

_____ *Remain upright.* It is a good idea to sit upright for a few minutes after eating. That way, if food remains in the mouth or the back of the throat, it will slide down to your esophagus, rather than falling into your windpipe later.

_____ *Drink lots of fluids.* Dehydration causes thick saliva that may be more difficult to swallow than thin saliva. Drinking 2 quarts of liquid per day is recommended.

_____ *Time medications:* If you have Parkinson disease, time when you take your medications to make sure they will have their greatest effect at mealtimes.

_____ *Bring swallowing under voluntary control.* Individuals with Parkinson disease may find that movements that used to be automatic don't happen as often. Because swallowing may not be as automatic as it used to be, concentration is critical. Using special techniques such as a double swallow followed by a voluntary cough may help protect your airway.

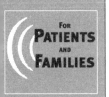

_____ *Choose your foods carefully.* Eating foods that are the easiest texture for you to swallow will help prevent choking problems and keep you from getting too tired.

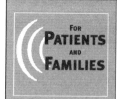
Dietary Changes To Compensate for Swallowing Difficulties

► When the muscles used for chewing and swallowing are weak, the following changes in your diet may be helpful in reducing fatigue and lowering your risk of choking. This is by no means a complete list of food items. Rather, it gives examples of food textures and types that are easy to swallow.

____ *Texture.* Stick to the food textures recommended. For the most part, you should eat easy-to-swallow foods that hold together in the mouth and are easy to control with your tongue and swallowing muscles. Such foods as casseroles, puddings, and custards hold together and are easy to swallow. Dry, flaky foods and foods that are hard to control in your mouth (like peas, corn, and lettuce) are usually not recommended. Examples of other foods that hold together and are easy to swallow are the following:

- Egg dishes such as soufflés or quiches
- Soft cheese
- Egg salad
- Canned fruit
- Ground meat with gravy
- Gelatin
- Creamed vegetables
- Hot cereals
- Au gratin potatoes

____ *Avoid thin liquids.* Be careful with thin liquids (water, coffee, tea, milk) as they may slip into your windpipe before you are ready to swallow. If this is a problem, try thick liquids such as milk shakes, malts, eggnog, nectars, and yogurt.

240

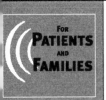
Thin liquids can also be thickened using a commercially available product called "Thick-it."

_____ *Taste*. Flavorful foods can be easier to swallow than bland foods. Try adding brown sugar, honey, herbs, and seasonings to foods. Also drink liquids with lots of flavor, such as citrus juices.

_____ *Temperature*. Foods that are very warm or very cold are generally easier to swallow than are lukewarm foods. Ice-cold liquid is easier to swallow than tap water.

_____ *Avoid these foods*. Avoid foods that are hard or have tough skins, such as raw apples. These are difficult to chew and swallow. Also avoid foods that fall apart in your mouth, such as applesauce, seeds, and nuts. Finally, dry, sticky foods such as plain mashed potatoes, white bread, and peanut butter should be avoided.

_____ *Thick saliva*. If thick saliva in your mouth is a problem, avoid uncooked milk and chocolate products because they cause thicker secretions in some people.

_____ *Don't sacrifice nutrition*. Talk with a dietitian who can help you learn about a diet that will meet your nutritional needs. If eating takes a lot of your time and energy, avoid empty calories.

▶ Maintaining Your Liquid Intake

People with neurologic disorders often complain of choking on liquids as well as solid foods. It is very important to provide your body with plenty of liquids (about 2 quarts a day is a good target). Thick liquids, such as pear or apricot nectars, tomato juice,

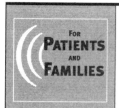
eggnog, milk shakes, instant breakfast products, "Ensure," and creamed soups are easy to swallow. Thin liquids, such as water, apple or orange juice, coffee, and tea are more difficult. Thin liquids are difficult to control because they have no texture and spread out in the mouth. The following suggestions may help you take in enough liquids:

_____ *Avoid liquids that are at body temperature.* Cold liquids tend to stimulate the swallow. We do not usually recommend very hot liquids, because most people prefer to cool them to body temperature before swallowing them.

_____ *Carbonated beverages.* Some individuals find that carbonation adds texture to liquids and makes them easier to swallow.

_____ *Avoid caffeine.* Avoid caffeinic beverages (coffee, tea, and many colas) because caffeine causes water loss.

▶ Controlling Excess Saliva

When excessive saliva is a problem, try any or all of the following suggestions:

_____ *Frequent swallows.* Swallow frequently and clear your mouth. Wipe your mouth often with a tissue or soft cloth.

_____ *Sleeping position.* If you have trouble with choking on saliva while lying down, raise your head so your neck is flexed during sleep, or lie on your side to allow saliva to drain out of your mouth.

_____ *Avoid phlegm-producing foods.* People with difficulty swallowing often report that uncooked milk and milk products,

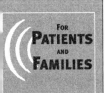
such as ice cream or chocolate, increase phlegm. Boiling milk and substituting sherbet for ice cream are possible solutions.

_____ *Papase.* Some people have noticed that papaya or pineapple juice tends to decrease mucus. Dissolving a papase tablet (an enzyme made from papaya) slowly in your mouth or swabbing meat tenderizer in your mouth can help thin the mucus.

_____ *Medications.* If excess saliva continues to be a problem, talk with a physician about medication to decrease saliva.

_____ *Mints.* Some people say that strongly flavored mints such as Altoids are helpful.

_____ *Maintain liquid intake.* Thick saliva is more difficult to manage than thin saliva. Drinking enough liquid is one of the most important ways to make sure that saliva is thin.

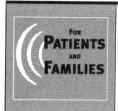

Gastroesophageal Reflux Disease (GERD)

Gastroesophageal reflux disease or GERD is a disorder that affects the muscle connecting the esophagus (food tube) with the stomach. Normally when we eat, this circular band of muscles, called the lower esophageal sphincter (LES), opens to allow the food to pass into the stomach and then closes to prevent food and acidic stomach juices from flowing back into the esophagus. Because this muscle does not work normally, the acidic contents of the stomach back up into the esophagus. Long-term reflux may damage the lining of the esophagus, cause changes to your voice and swallowing, and cause respiratory problems (asthma, chronic bronchitis, and so on).

▶ Symptoms

Heartburn (also called acid indigestion) is a common symptom of GERD. Almost everyone experiences symptoms of gastroesophageal reflux at one time or another. It may feel like a burning in the chest. Symptoms are worst after eating. Many people with heartburn have an acidic or bitter taste in their mouth, especially when they awake in the morning. There is also a "silent" form of GERD in which the person does not experience heartburn but may have an unexplained cough, sore throat, swallowing problems, or hoarseness.

▶ Relationship to Speech and Swallowing

Many individuals with GERD report having trouble swallowing. In severe cases, they may experience the feeling of food being stuck in the throat or even choke. GERD may also cause a chronic sore throat. If stomach acid reaches the larynx (voice

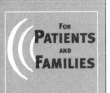
box), it may cause laryngitis and produce hoarseness, a dry cough, the sensation of having a lump in the throat, or the need to repeatedly clear the throat. GERD can also affect breathing by causing asthma-like symptoms or making existing breathing problems worse.

▶ Dietary and Lifestyle Modifications

There are a variety of things that you can do to avoid or reduce reflux.

1. *Dietary changes.* Certain foods and beverages cause the LES to relax and allow stomach contents to regurgitate into the esophagus. Foods to avoid include chocolate, peppermint, fried or fatty food, coffee (both caffeinic and decaffeinated), carbonated drinks, and alcoholic beverages. Other foods can irritate a damaged esophageal lining. These foods include citrus fruits and juices, tomato products, spicy foods, and pepper.

2. *Meal size.* Decrease the size of portions at mealtimes. It is best to eat small, frequent meals.

3. *Body position.* The position of your body will affect GERD. Lying down or bending over can make symptoms worse. Many people feel better if they stand upright or take a walk. Avoid lying down 2 to 3 hours after eating.

4. *Elevate head while sleeping.* Elevate the head of the bed on 6-inch blocks to sleep on an incline. Avoid simply using extra pillows because these only raise your head and may increase the risk of reflux.

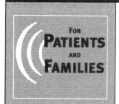
5. *Lose weight.* Lose weight if this is appropriate for you. Obesity increases the pressure on the LES.

6. *Clothing.* Avoid tight clothing, particularly around the abdomen.

7. *Avoid certain drugs.* Avoid the class of drugs called non-steroidal anti-inflammatory drugs. This class includes aspirin, ibuprofen (Motrin, Advil), and naproxen (Aleve). Tylenol (acetaminophen) is a good alternative.

8. *Stop smoking.* Smoking relaxes the LES and promotes reflux. This is another good reason to stop.

9. *Antacids.* Antacids can neutralize acid and provide temporary relief. However, extensive long-term use may cause side effects.

If symptoms persist, your doctor may wish to prescribe medications. A small number of people with GERD may need surgery because of severe reflux that isn't helped by diet and lifestyle changes or medication.

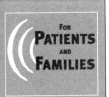

Emergency Plan: First Aid for Choking

► Anyone with swallowing difficulties should have an emergency plan in case of an airway obstruction (total blockage of your windpipe resulting in your being unable to breathe). You, your family or attendant, a physician, and a rescue unit should all work together to make up this plan. The plan should be printed and posted for easy reference. Your risk of choking depends on your diet. Your risk can be lessened by choosing a soft, moist, chopped diet and cutting out items such as steak and roast, leafy or chunked vegetables, and raw fruits. If your airway does become blocked, the following is an emergency plan you might follow:

Try to relax. First, try to relax. Cough forcefully and continue trying to breathe around the blockage. If you are able to breathe, your airway is not blocked.

Have signals. Have a system of signals to direct your family or attendant. For example, an open hand turned out can indicate "Stop, I don't need help" and an open hand placed on the throat can indicate "Please help me."

Do the Heimlich maneuver. If the blockage does not move, try the Heimlich maneuver (abdominal thrust). The goal of the Heimlich maneuver is to push air out of the lungs in a forceful cough.

To perform the Heimlich maneuver on someone else:

- Stand behind the choking person and wrap your arms around his or her waist. Bend the person slightly forward.

- Make a fist with one hand and place it slightly above the person's navel.

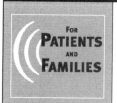
- Grasp your fist with the other hand and press hard into the abdomen with a quick, upward thrust. Repeat this procedure until the object is expelled from the airway.

To perform the Heimlich maneuver on yourself:

- Position your own fist slightly above your navel.

- Grasp your fist with your other hand and thrust upward into your abdomen until the object is expelled. You may also lean forward over the back of a chair to produce this effect.

Call 911. If you are still unsuccessful, a caregiver should call your local emergency phone number for assistance.

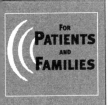

Useful Addresses and Web Sites

General Information

Academy of Neurologic Communication Disorders and Sciences (ANCDS)
P.O. Box 26532
Minneapolis, MN 55426
Phone: 952/920-0484
Fax: 952/920-6098
E-mail: ancds@incnet.com
Web site: http://www.ancds.duq.edu/index.html

American Speech-Language-Hearing Association
10801 Rockville Pike
Rockville, MD 20852
Phone: 301/897-5700
Web site: http://www.asha.org

International Society for Augmentative and Alternative Communication (ISAAC)
49 The Donway West
Suite 308
Toronto, Ontario M3C 3M9
Canada
Phone: 416/385-0351
Web site: http://www.isaac-online.org

National Institute of Neurological Disorders and Stroke
P.O. Box 5801
Bethesda, MD 20824
Phone: 800/352-9424
Web site: http://www.ninds.nih.gov/

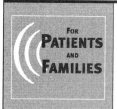
Useful Addresses and Web Sites (continued)

National Organization for Rare Disorders (NORD)
55 Kenosia Avenue
P.O. Box 1968
Danbury, CT 06813-1968
Phone: 203/744-0100, 800/999-NORD (6673)
Fax: 203/798-2291
E-mail: orphan@rarediseases.org
Web site: http://www.rarediseases.org

Amyotrophic Lateral Sclerosis

ALS Association of America (ALSA)
27001 Agoura Road
Suite 150
Calabasas Hills, CA 91301-5104
Phone: 818/880-9007, 800/782-4747
Fax: 818/880-9006
Web site: http://www.alsa.org/

Muscular Dystrophy Association
3300 East Sunrise Drive
Tucson, AZ 85718-3208
Phone: 520/529-2000, 800/572-1717
Fax: 520/529-5300
E-mail: mda@mdausa.org
Web site: http://www.mdausa.org/

Parkinson Disease

American Parkinson Disease Association
1250 Hylan Blvd.
Suite 4B
Staten Island, NY 10305-1946
Phone: 718/981-8001, 800/223-2732, Calif: 800/908-2732
Fax: 718/981-4399
Web site: http://www.apdaparkinson.org

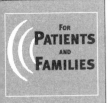
National Parkinson Foundation
1501 N.W. 9th Avenue
Bob Hope Research Center
Miami, FL 33136-1494
Phone: 305/547-6666, 800/327-4545, Fla: 800/433-7022
Fax: 305/243-4403
E-mail: mailbox@parkinson.org
Web site: http://www.parkinson.org/

Parkinson Alliance
211 College Road East
3rd Floor
Princeton, NJ 08520
Phone: 609/688-0870, 800/579-8440
Fax: 609/688-0875
E-mail: admin@parkinsonalliance.net
Web site: http://www.parkinsonalliance.net

Parkinson's Disease Foundation (PDF)
710 West 168th Street
New York, NY 10032-9982
Phone: 212/923-4700, 800/457-6676
Fax: 212/923-4778
E-mail: info@pdf.org
Web site: http://www.parkinsons-foundation.org

Huntington Disease

Hereditary Disease Foundation
3960 Broadway
6th Floor
New York, NY 10032
Phone: 212/928-2121
Fax: 212/928-2172
E-mail: cures@hdfoundation.org
Web site: http://www.hdfoundation.org

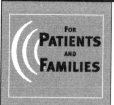

Huntington's Disease Society of America
158 West 29th Street
7th Floor
New York, NY 10001-5300
Phone: 212/242-1968, 800/345-HDSA (4372)
Fax: 212/239-3430
E-mail: hdsainfo@hdsa.org
Web site: http://www.hdsa.org

Multiple Sclerosis

Multiple Sclerosis Association of America
706 Haddonfield Road
Cherry Hill, NJ 08002
Phone: 856/488-4500, 800/532-7667
Fax: 856/661-9797
E-mail: msaa@msaa.com
Web site: http://www.msaa.com

Multiple Sclerosis Foundation
6350 North Andrews Avenue
Ft. Lauderdale, FL 33309-2130
Phone: 954/776-6805, 800/225-6495
Fax: 954/938-8708
E-mail: admin@msfocus.org
Web site: http://www.msfocus.org

National Multiple Sclerosis Society
733 Third Avenue
6th Floor
New York, NY 10017-3288
Phone: 212/986-3240, 800/344-4867 (FIGHTMS)
Fax: 212/986-7981
E-mail: nat@nmss.org
Web site: http://www.nationalmssociety.org

Glossary: Operational Definitions

A

Alimentation.   The process of nourishing the body; alimentation includes mastication, swallowing, digestion, absorption, and assimilation.

Alphabet supplementation.   The provision of a printed alphabet so that the speaker can point to the first letter of each word as it is said. This provides more context for the listener and slows the speaker's rate of speech.

Amplifier.   Any electronic device that makes the speech of someone with very low speaking volume louder.

Amyotrophic lateral sclerosis (ALS).   A progressive degenerative disease of the motor neurons; ALS affects both upper and lower motor neurons, causing weakness and eventually paralysis.

Ankle–foot orthosis (AFO).   A plastic brace worn to stabilize the ankle.

Articulation.   Action of the structures used in production of speech sounds (movement of the tongue, jaw, soft palate, and other structures).

Aspiration.   When food or liquid (bolus) penetrates the airway below the vocal folds; aspiration can occur before, during, or after the pharyngeal response.

Aspirator.   An apparatus for suctioning fluid out of cavities. It is frequently used by individuals with dysphagia to suction saliva from the mouth.

Ataxia.   Discoordination of movement, usually resulting from damage in the cerebellum.

Atrophy.   Wasting away of muscle mass due to lower motor neuron degeneration.

Augmentative communication system.   Any method of nonspeech communication, including books of pictures, communication boards, gestures, or electronic devices.

B

Basal ganglia.   A group of nuclei located in the middle of the brain that is involved with the initiation and regulation of the proper amount of movement.

Bolus.   The food, liquid, or other material placed in the mouth for swallowing.

Bradykinesia.   Slowness of movement, usually due to problems with the basal ganglia.

Breathiness.   A term used to describe voice quality disorders in which incomplete closure of the vocal folds as they vibrate is perceived as excess air wastage.

C

Cachexia.   A state of profound poor health and malnutrition.

Central nervous system.   The brain and spinal cord.

Chorea.   A disorder characterized by excessive irregular, nonrepetitive, randomly distributed involuntary movements.

Cogwheel rigidity.   A continuous state of muscle contraction that causes the extremity to alternately resist and release during movement.

Contractures.   A state of too much muscle tone (too much continuous contraction of muscle tissue) that causes the limbs to fix around the joints; contractures result from fibrosis and shortening of muscle fibers.

Cuirass.   A chest shell ventilator consisting of a firm shell that covers the anterior chest and abdomen and a negative-pressure ventilator, which creates subatmospheric pressure under the shell.

D

Delayed auditory feedback (DAF).   A device that records a person's speech and plays it back with a delay of some number of milliseconds. DAF allows an individual to listen to his or her own speech. The technique has been successful in assisting some people with Parkinson disease to slow their speaking rate.

Dementia.   A deterioration in mental state with absence or reduction of intellectual faculties caused by organic disease.

Diadochokinetic rates.   In speech, diadochokinetic rates refer to measurements of the speed of rapid alternating movements of the articulators (lips, tongue, velum). Clinicians will often measure how many alternating movements (e.g., /pataka, pataka/) a speaker can produce in 5 seconds.

Direct selection.   The means of access to an augmentative communication system in which the user can immediately choose a desired message or letter. (Examples are a typewriter, a computer keyboard, or pointing to a letter on an alphabet board.) Direct selection requires better motor control than a scanning system.

Dopamine.   A neurotransmitter important in basal ganglia functioning. In Parkinson disease, a depletion of this neurotransmitter causes bradykinesia and rigidity.

Durable power of attorney for health care.   The appointment of a person to make one's decisions regarding medical treatment in the event of mental incompetence or reduced decision-making capacity.

Dysarthria.   A general term used for the speech disorders that result when the muscles cannot move with the correct range of movement, speed, force, or coordination. It is caused by damage to the central or peripheral nervous systems. Speech may sound slurred, imprecise, or discoordinated.

Dyskinesia.   A general term denoting a deficit in voluntary movement, dyskinesia sometimes denotes unwanted involuntary movement (such as tardive dyskinesia, which refers to slow, rhythmical, involuntary movements that sometimes occur after use of some psychotropic drugs).

Dysphagia.   Refers to difficulties in any stage of swallowing (chewing, oral transport, pharyngeal contractions, airway protection, and esophageal passage).

E

Emotional lability.   A reduced threshold for emotional responses such as laughter and crying; usually occurs after damage to the brain.

Extrapyramidal system.   A group of subcortical structures, primarily the basal ganglia, that are involved in motor control.

F

Fasciculations.   Spontaneous contractions of a number of muscle fibers supplied by a single motor nerve filament. In ALS, fasciculations may be related to collateral sprouting of nerves. There is no clear relationship between fasciculations and muscle weakness, and fasciculations may appear benignly.

Feeding. Arm and hand coordination and motor planning required to bring food from the plate to the mouth.

Festination. Abnormal and involuntary increases in the speed of walking in an attempt to catch up with a displaced center of gravity; festination is seen in certain neurological diseases such as Parkinson disease.

Fibrillations. Spontaneous contraction of individual muscle fibers no longer under control of a motor nerve.

Flaccid dysarthria. A speech disorder characterized by weak movement of the articulators (especially tongue, lips, and soft palate) due to lack of muscle tone; speech will sound slurred and hypernasal.

Flaccidity. Reduced or absent muscle tone.

G

Gag reflex. A brain stem reflex elicited by contact of a foreign object with the back of the tongue, soft palate, or pharynx, resulting in contraction of the pharynx to push the object up and out of the pharynx or to prevent entrance into the pharynx. This neuromuscular action is the opposite of the neuromuscular coordination used in swallowing. The gag reflex cannot be used to predict the presence or adequacy of a swallow. The gag is protective for refluxed material from the esophagus and stomach. A gag will not be elicited by food being swallowed unless the individual exhibits a strong dislike for the food, which then becomes a foreign stimulus.

Gastrostomy. Surgical creation of a gastric fistula (opening) through the abdominal wall for the purpose of introducing food into the stomach; a gastrostomy is necessary in some degenerative neurologic diseases when chewing and swallowing become too difficult to manage.

H

Harshness. A term used to describe a voice quality suggesting a variety of noisy voices. Particularly important in ALS are strained-strangled harshness and "wet" or "gurgly" harshness.

Hoarseness. A term used to describe an abnormal voice quality that sounds as if one has a mild case of laryngitis.

Huntington disease. An inherited autosomal dominant degenerative neurologic disease, Huntington disease is characterized by cognitive deterioration and increasingly debilitating movement disorders, which often result in dysphagia, dysarthria, and functional disabilities.

Hyperkinetic dysarthria. A speech disorder characterized by "too much movement." The patient will exhibit variable, unpredictable increases in loudness and imprecise consonant production. This type of dysarthria often accompanies Huntington disease.

Hypernasality. A condition in which too much air resonates in the nasal cavity during speech, changing voice quality; hypernasality may occur as a result of a weak soft palate (velum) that doesn't rise up against the pharyngeal wall to completely close off the airstream from the nose.

Hypokinetic dysarthria. A speech disorder characterized by large reductions in range of motion of the articulators during speech, giving the impression of very rapid rate, syllable reduction or omission, and consonant imprecision; occurs as a result of Parkinson disease.

Hypotonia. A decrease in muscle tone.

I

Incidence.   The number of new cases beginning per unit of time and population; incidence is usually expressed as cases per 100,000 population per year.

L

Laryngeal penetration.   Entrance of food or liquid into the portion of the airway above the vocal folds (supraglottic area). Laryngeal penetration can occur in unimpaired individuals and can also occur before, during, or after the pharyngeal swallow.

Levodopa.   A drug used in the treatment of Parkinson disease.

Living will.   A legal document expressing to the health-care team one's desire for using or foregoing life-sustaining procedures in the event of terminal illness with no chance of recovery.

Lower extremity function.   The functional ability of the legs, including strength, ambulation, and coordination.

Lower motor neurons.   The nerve cell from which fibers extend to innervate a peripheral muscle. The lower motor neurons for the face are located in the brain stem; for the limbs, they are in the anterior portion of the spinal cord.

M

Multiple sclerosis (MS).   A progressive neurologic disease caused by degeneration of the myelin, or protective sheath, around neuron fibers; MS is characterized by periods of exacerbation and remission; sensory, motor, and cognitive processes may be affected.

N

Nasal emission.   Air that escapes through the nose, usually audibly, during speech; nasal emission sometimes accompanies hypernasality caused by weak movement of the soft palate.

Nasogastric tube.   A tube that is passed through the nasal cavity, down the pharynx, and into the stomach as an alternative means of feeding.

NPO.   "Nothing by mouth"; patients designated as NPO must receive nutrition and hydration by alternative means such as an IV, a nasogastric tube, or a gastrostomy.

O

Oculogyric crisis.   An attack of involuntary deviation and fixation of the eyeballs, usually upward, that may last for several minutes or hours; sometimes seen with Parkinson disease.

On–off effect.   A functional deterioration that occurs at the end of drug dosage periods; may be characterized by severe and rapid fluctuations in mobility and dyskinesia.

P

Palatal lift prosthesis.   An acrylic prosthetic device worn in the posterior mouth to elevate the soft palate against the pharyngeal wall so air will not leak into the nasal cavities during speech.

Palilalia.   Repetitious use of words and phrases that occurs in some neurologic diseases.

Paralysis agitans.   A term sometimes used for Parkinson disease. The term suggests progressive weakness and delay of voluntary motion, characterized by rigid tremulousness, festinating gait, and slow movement without actual paralysis.

Parkinson disease.   A progressive neurologic disease caused by a shortage of dopamine in the basal ganglia of the brain; Parkinson disease is characterized by resting tremor, bradykinesia, and rigidity.

Percutaneous endoscopic gastrostomy (PEG). A small tube placed into the stomach (under local anesthetic) through the abdominal wall for feeding.

Peripheral nervous system. The sensory and motor nerve cells and fibers outside the brain and spinal cord.

Phonation. Voicing produced by periodic vibration of the vocal folds.

Phonatory instability. A tremulous quality perceived in the voice. Instability is categorized as "flutter" (>10 Hz), "tremor" (3–10 Hz), and "wow" (<2 Hz); the instability may be in intensity or frequency or both.

Prevalence. The number of all cases present in the community at one time per unit of population.

Procedural memory. The ability to learn rule-based automatic behavioral sequences, such as motor skills, conditioned responses, certain kinds of rule-based puzzles, perceptual-motor tasks, and sequences for running or operating things. Procedural learning may occur even though the individual does not remember having done the activity and cannot talk about it.

Progressive supranuclear palsy. A progressive degenerative neurologic disease characterized by symptoms similar to Parkinson disease (rigidity and bradykinesia). Vertical-occular gaze paresis is the most salient feature. Other symptoms may also occur, including cognitive changes, dysarthria, and dysphagia.

Pulmonary Function Test. Evaluation of respiratory functions (such as vital capacity and flow rates).

R

Respiration. The act of breathing.

Respirometer. A device used to measure vital capacity, or the number of liters of air that the lungs are capable of holding and expiring.

Resting tremor. Regular small "shaking" movements, usually of the hand, that occur when the limb is at rest; commonly seen in Parkinson disease.

Rigidity. An increase in muscle tone that is present more or less constantly throughout a movement, as opposed to spasticity, which is present at the start of the movement and is most evident during rapid movements.

S

Sinemet. The brand name for a drug commonly used in treatment of Parkinson disease.

Spasticity. A state of having too much muscle tone; muscles are stiff and movements are slow and difficult.

Spastic dysarthria. A speech disorder characterized by imprecise consonants, distorted vowels, and harsh or strained-strangled voice; caused by hypertonicity and slowing in the muscles used for speech.

Speech intelligibility. How understandable a person's speech is; intelligibility is usually measured as a percentage of words understood by a naive judge who listens to a list of words or sentences that has been read by the speaker.

Spirantization. When extra air can be heard with the production of consonants that aren't usually accompanied by air escape.

Stages of swallowing. Four stages of phases of swallow have been delineated in classic research: oral preparation, oral, pharyngeal, and esophageal. Recent studies indicate that these stages are most clearly distinguished during small bolus swallows. These stages may overlap during large bolus swallows.

Strained-strangled voice. A term used to denote the vocal quality one hears when there is hypertonicity (too much muscle tone or stiffness) in the vocal folds.

T

Tracheostomy. An opening into the trachea through the neck for insertion of a tube to overcome airway obstruction.

Tremor. Regular small "shaking" movements; tremor occurring when a limb is at rest is called "resting tremor" and is commonly seen in Parkinson disease; shaking that occurs when one attempts a specific movement is called "intention tremor" and is usually seen with cerebellar disorders.

U

Upper extremity function. A measure of activities of daily living completed with the arms and hands.

Upper motor neurons. Brain cells in the cortex that initiate voluntary movement; upper motor neuron syndrome is characterized by spasticity and hyperreflexia and occurs when there is damage to the cell itself or at any point along the descending motor fibers (axons).

V

Velopharyngeal mechanism. Refers to the soft palate and its normal action of moving up against the pharyngeal wall (upper throat) to close off the nasal cavities during speech.

Ventilator. A device for artificially providing respiration.

Vital capacity. The amount of air (measured in liters) that can be expelled by the lungs after the person takes as deep a breath as possible.

W

Weakness. Lack of muscle strength for movement caused by too much or too little muscle tone.

About the Authors

Kathryn M. Yorkston, PhD, CCC-SLP, BC-NCD, is head of the Division of Speech Pathology and professor in the Department of Rehabilitation Medicine at the University of Washington, Seattle. She also holds an adjunct appointment in the Department of Speech and Hearing Sciences. Dr. Yorkston has a long history of clinical research and publication in acquired neurologic communication disorders in adults. She serves as the speech–language pathologist in the Neuromuscular Speech and Swallowing Disorders Clinic, an outpatient clinic that focuses on management of individuals with amyotrophic lateral sclerosis and other degenerative disorders. Dr. Yorkston has co-authored the book *Management of Motor Speech Disorders in Children and Adults.* She is a past president of the Academy of Neurologic Communication Disorders and Sciences and currently serves that organization as Chair of the Writing Committee for Practice Guidelines in Dysarthria.

Robert M. Miller, PhD, CCC-SLP, BC-NCD, is a senior lecturer in the Department of Speech and Hearing Sciences at the University of Washington. He is formerly chief of Audiology and Speech Pathology at the Veterans' Administration Medical Center in Seattle, Washington. He holds the position of clinical associate professor in the Departments of Rehabilitation Medicine and Otolaryngology, Head, and Neck Surgery at the University of Washington, Seattle. A nationally recognized expert on management of swallowing disorders, he serves as consulting speech–language pathologist in the Neuromuscular Speech and Swallowing Disorders Clinic at the University of Washington Medical Center. Dr. Miller has authored numerous chapters and articles on the topic of swallowing disorders. He is co-author of the book *Medical Speech Pathology.* He is board certified by the Academy of Neurologic Communication Disorders and Sciences.

Edythe A. Strand, PhD, CCC-SLP, BC-NCD, is a consultant in the Division of Speech Pathology, Department of Neurology at the Mayo Clinic, and an associate professor in the Mayo Medical School. Dr. Strand's research has focused on developmental and acquired apraxia of speech, issues related to intelligibility and comprehensibility in degenerative dysarthria, and the application of data from apraxic and dysarthric patients to current models of speech production and theories of speech motor control. She is an experienced clinician who has worked in the public schools, private practice, and hospital and clinic settings. Her primary clinical interests include assessment and treatment of children and adults with neurologic speech, language, and voice disorders. She has presented numerous talks and workshops on the assessment and treatment of motor speech disorders in children and adults. She is the co-author of the book *Clinical Management of Motor Speech Disorders in Children and Adults* and the co-editor of the book *Clinical Management of Motor Speech Disorders in Children.*